MEDICAL TESTS
AND
DIAGNOSTIC PROCEDURES

———

A Patient's Guide to
Just What the Doctor Ordered

MEDICAL TESTS AND DIAGNOSTIC PROCEDURES

A Patient's Guide to
Just What the Doctor Ordered

Philip Shtasel, D.O., F.A.O.C.R.

 HarperPerennial
A Division of HarperCollins*Publishers*

For Thelma
My 40-year pal, and still counting

———————————

First HarperPerennial edition published 1991

Designed by The Book Company

The Library of Congress has cataloged the hardcover
edition of this book as follows:

———————————

Shtasel, Philip, 1925-
    Medical tests and diagnostic procedures: a patient's
guide to just what the doctor ordered / Philip Shtasel.—
1st. ed.
        p.   cm.
    ISBN 0-06-016245-7
    1. Function tests (Medicine)—Popular works.
2. Diagnosis—Popular works.   3. Patient education.
I. Title.
RC82.S554   1990
616.07′5—dc20   89-45716
ISBN 0-06-272001-5 (paperback edition)
91 92 93 94 95 FG 10 9 8 7 6 5 4 3 2 1

CONTENTS

Part II: Imaging and Laboratory Tests

ACKNOWLEDGMENTS

There are some things that come off better when said than when written. "Thank you" falls into that category. It is far more difficult even when not being limited to a hundred words or less, and even when neatness, originality, and clarity of thought are not being judged, to communicate one's true depth of appreciation and gratitude on the printed page than in person. Enhancers such as "so very much," "I really, really," "from the bottom of my heart," and the like certainly help but can't touch the communication of the voice tone and body language when one looks straight into the eyes of the recipient and lets go. So, to all of you who will be identified below, make believe you are hearing it and not reading it, because to the *thank you so very, very much* let me also add another, better said than read—*without you this couldn't have happened.*

First, the Group One Gang—those who read the first rambling draft of the introduction and whose opinions were sought as to whether or not they felt the project could and/or should fly: Sana Shtasel, Larry Shtasel, Dr. Dov Gorshein, Ann Mooney, Dee Watson, and Ruth Levine. You guys stroked when stroking was really important.

Next, a Gang unto Herself—she who read the same ramble but rather than stroke, kicked, clawed, and went for the jugular: Barbara Lowenstein, my literary agent. To you I owe far more than a client's fee. I owe you the student's recognition of that so very special teacher who taught me how to get it together.

The following list is of those who gave their time and expertise so that all the areas of diagnostic testing that compose this work could be included.

Because of the number I will cite the medical specialties and the person or persons in each who deserve applause. (In keeping with standard protocol, because of the large number I shall withhold individual recognition and applaud you all collectively at the end. *Allergy:* Dr. Sheryl Talbot; *cardiology:* Dr. Gerald Sharff, Dr. Marvin Rosner, and Dr. Stanley Schiff; *dermatology:* Dr. Herbert Goldschmidt; *endocrinology:* Dr. Leslie Rose; *gastroenterology:* Dr. Charles Hurwitz, Dr. Robert S. Fisher, and Ms. Marie Tsolikis; *gynecology:* Dr. Edward Slotnick; *nephrology:* Dr. Julie Rothman; *neurology:* Dr. Laurence Janoff, Dr. Murray Klein, Dr. Rochell Gur, and Ms. Sue Marck; *obstetrics:* Dr. George Davis; *oncology:* Dr. Richard Gordon; *ophthalmology:* Dr. Alexander Brucker and Ms. Ellen Sandberg; *orthopedic surgery:* Dr. Victor Gennaro; *otorhinolaryngology:* Dr. Lynn Summerson and Ms. Louise Feldherr; *psychiatry:* Dr. Derri Shtasel and Dr. Gary Gottlieb; *pulmonology:* Dr. Edward Hamaty; *rheumatology:* Dr. Barry Getzoff; *urologic surgery:* Dr. Robert Swain; *laboratory:* Dr. Robert Biondi; *MRI:* Dr. David Mayer; *ultrasound:* Dr. Neil Berger, Dr. Harvey Nissenbaum, and Dr. Peter Arger; *X-ray:* Dr. Robert Rosenbaum, Dr. Lewis Halin, and Dr. Bruce Bonier.

Susan Randol, associate editor at Harper & Row, my New York Moses, who quietly, gently, and patiently slogged through my quagmire of words and pages and led me to the Promised Land.

And last, but really first, the Whole First Team that has always been my undeniable support system (listed by chronology of coming on board): Sana Shtasel, Derri Shtasel, Larry Shtasel, Gary Gottlieb, Jim Kretz, Corey, and Zoe.

What Your Doctor Didn't Say

Scene 1: *A consultation room. A person in a white coat with a stethoscope dangling from a pocket is sitting in a large desk chair behind an imposing desk. On the desk is a framed picture of a woman, two small children, and a shaggy dog; a small silver trophy with a golfer on its top; an appointment book; and a folder in which the person is making notes. Also present is a second person sitting in a less imposing chair in front of the desk.*

The person in the white coat is your doctor.

The second person is a patient, and it is you.

(*curtain up*)

YOU: It's those headaches again. They used to hit me once or twice a week and I could handle them with aspirins. Now they are almost daily. The throbbing is off the wall. Aspirins don't begin to touch these headaches. Yesterday was the worst. Not only was it an "Excedrin 50," but also I began to see double, felt dizzy, and even thought I was going to throw up.

DOCTOR: Hmm! Headaches are tough. A lot of the time they are stress-related. Given that your schedule qualifies you for the "Ox of the Month" award, that might well be the explanation. But, you say the headaches are getting worse, and there was that episode with the vision, nausea and dizziness. Hmm! It certainly could be your sinuses or even your eyes. But then again, *it could be serious.*

We'll have to get some tests. Let's start with a skull X-ray and a nuclear brain scan. While you're there, we might as well add some sinus films. They probably won't offer much, but we have to go that route first. I'm pretty sure we will have to get a CAT and maybe even an MRI, or both, before this is over. And, I want you to have a carotid Doppler, go for a complete neurologic, get your eyegrounds and visual fields checked out, and have an SMA 12 picked up. I hope a spinal tap and EEG won't be necessary. If all of these prove negative we may have to add a PET, and maybe even get you to a shrink.

O.K.? See my secretary out front. She will make all the arrangements. All you have to do is show up. The whole package will probably take a couple of weeks to get put together. I guess it sounds like a big deal to you, but as I said, it could be serious! But don't worry. Get back to me when everything is done.

(curtain down)

Scene 2: The time is one minute later. The place is the waiting room of the same doctor's office. You enter from the consultation room. Ms. Secretary is talking on the phone.

(curtain up)

Ms. SECRETARY (into the phone): Hold on, I'll be back in a sec. (To you) Well, now. Doctor told me what goodies are in store. Here's the list. Call me tomorrow and I'll give you the times and places. And *have a nice day!*

You: Thanks. I'll call.

(curtain down)

———————————

One- to two-minute dramas such as this are played out tens of thousands of times each day. They are mystery playlets—not so much "whodunits" as "whatdunits"—all with a similar plot. You are the victim. Your doctor is the detective. You identify the events that have aroused concern. These are the clues. Dr. Sherlock must find the culprit—make a diagnosis—since all remedial measures must wait until the villain is identified. But, too often, and most unfortunately, your clues may not be sufficiently specific to permit an instantaneous "make." In those cases additional information is essential and your doctor will see that this is obtained by having you *get some tests* and/or sending you to *see a medical specialist.*

The above plot, as written, seems concise, logical, and suspenseful. The sleuth will track down the "what" using as the magnifying glass the X-rays and other tests that you will have done. A diagnosis will be made and appropriate treatment will be started. You will be pleased and grateful. Right? Wrong! Too often that is not the way it goes. Everything is the same, except that instead of being pleased and grateful, you will be pleased that a diagnosis has been made and angry at how it came about. Your anger—or worse—is a consequence of failed communications. The plot, as presented, is flawed. Some things are missing that result in your ultimate displeasure. What, then, is the script's failure?

Let us examine what hapened in that consultation room. What was it that *your doctor said* after "Hmm" and "it could be serious"? Your doctor said, "Get some tests!" and told you that you need

A skull X-ray

A nuclear brain scan

Sinus films

A CAT

An MRI

A carotid Doppler

A complete neurologic

An eyeground and visual field check

An SMA-12

A spinal tap

An EEG

A PET

A shrink

The fatal flaw in the scenario is what your doctor failed to say! What he omitted was

A skull X-ray, a brain scan, sinus films, a CAT, and an MRI are . . .

A carotid Doppler is . . .

A complete neurologic is . . .

Eyegrounds and visual fields are . . .

SMA-12 is . . .

A spinal tap is . . .

An EEG is . . .

A PET is . . .

A shrink is . . .

These procedures are performed in the following way . . .

Some will cause discomfort . . .

Some are hazardous . . .

Some require special preparation . . .

Some require hospitalization . . .

Why were these basic facts left unanswered or delegated to a clerical person? In some cases it is the doctor's inability to devote the time necessary for these discussions. However, in most cases, the physician, even if well intentioned, is unable to answer all of the above questions. It is now virtually impossible for any doctor to be completely familiar with, and knowledgeable of, the details of each examination that can and should be ordered. In the above minidrama—one that is not remarkably complex—fourteen separate procedures were "ordered" that demanded the involvement and attention of at least seven different medical areas and their specialists:

Radiology and a radiologist for the skull and sinus X-rays, the CAT scan, and the MRI

Neurology and a neurologist for the "complete neurologic" and the possible EEG and spinal tap

Ultrasonography and an ultrasonographer for the carotid Doppler

Ophthalmology and an ophthalmologist for the "eyegrounds and visual fields"

Clinical pathology and a clinical pathologist for the SMA-12

Nuclear medicine and a nuclear medicine physician for the brain scan and PET

Psychiatry and a psychiatrist (a.k.a. shrink)

So the script's flaw is failure to explain. And it is this failure that is responsible for your annoyance, your anxiety, your anger, and even your rage.

What is ringing in your ears as you leave the office is not the exit line, "Have a nice day," but what your doctor said in the consultation room: *"It could be serious."* (Did he really say, "Don't worry"?) As the realization dawns: "My God, does he think I could have a *brain tumor?*" you see clutched in your hand the shopping list of procedures that have been ordered and you hear yourself screaming silently: "What in hell is an MRI and the rest of that stuff? I can forgive him for not knowing exactly what's wrong, but he really could have spent a precious minute explaining this to me! Darn him! He could have at least explained the other stuff."

The "other stuff" is procedure. Procedural things are all the examinations you submit to in the course of your doctor's establishing a diagnosis. They are tests. They are studies. They are specialized examinations. They are additional consultations. They are investigations that may be performed by another physician than the original doctor you consulted. They are searches that may be carried out by a nonphysician—a technologist trained to administer the requested study. They may require going somewhere—to a hospital, to a facility that is uniquely equipped, or to the office of a specialist. They are any and all events that help to answer your first and overarching question to any physician: "What is wrong with me? What do I have?" They are any and all of the activities set into motion by your implicit command: "Make me better! Cure me!"

We are thus left with the following conundrum: If diagnostic procedures are essential to the intelligent practice of medicine, and information and details concerning the nature of these procedures and their impact on the recipient are appropriate, how can this information be obtained if your physician, who initiates these procedures, cannot provide the data? The answer is by using a source—a primer that takes you on an escorted tour through adult diagnostic procedures and provides you with a detailed explanation of all commonly requested "tests," examinations, and consultations—whatever is necessary to reach a diagnosis. This guidebook must prepare you for the total experience. It must tell it like it is! You must know!

This escorted tour must familiarize you with what is both predictable and common to all of the ordinary adult procedures (pediatric studies are not dealt with), and it must also describe each particular procedure or experience in sufficient detail so that you will be prepared for the event.

General Events Common to
All Adult Diagnostic Procedures

Registration Whether the examination takes place in a hospital or in a private office, there will be an up-front moment of reckoning called payment. In a hospital, it will be in the outpatient billing department. In an office it will probably be handled by a billing clerk or the receptionist. What each will want is your method of payment. *Bring all insurance material necessary*, be it a card or appropriate forms. Also, *allow time!* It is impossible to guesstimate how long this will take at any given site, but it will take some. Therefore, allow at least 15 minutes before the examination appointment time to satisfy this dragon.

History Somewhere and somehow before the day is over you will be asked about the reason for the examination. This data is remarkably helpful to the consultant in the evaluation of your problem. The latest craze in obtaining this material is to have you fill out a questionnaire. Cutesy responses such as "You're the doctor—don't you know?" or "Just ask my doctor" do not serve you well. The other end of the spectrum—a long and rambling reconstruction —is also counterproductive. A short and concise explanation will do it.

It is always important for the new consultant to know if you are allergic to anything. If it was some medication in the past or something that was given to you at some other examination, dig out the name of what it was. The more specific you can be, the better.

Medications What you are taking now or have taken in the immediate past is of tremendous import. You will probably be asked. It is often difficult to provide this data unless you are forewarned. So, either bring along everything you are taking or make a list.

Questions will also be asked about your present or past use of alcohol and/ or drugs. Truth is essential. Your questioner is neither a policeman nor a cleric. You will not be judged. So, for your own sake, tell it like it is.

Pregnancy If you know you are pregnant, or even suspect that you may be, *tell,* even if not asked! To paraphrase that old saying, "the life you save might be your baby's." Certain procedures, particularly X-ray examinations, and pregnancy don't go well together.

Records Lots of times you have records of medical procedures you have had done in the past. These might be old reports from different specialists. They might be X-ray films. They might be bills specifying procedures. Anything that might provide data could be helpful and beats "Yeah, I think I did, but it was so long ago . . ." If you don't need a U-Haul to do so, take your records along.

Disrobing Certain examinations require you to disrobe. Appropriate rooms are available for this purpose. What is not always available is appropriate gowns. Often these garments are of the "one size fits all" variety and will not quite fit many. What is comfortable coverage for some may not be for others. What about shoes when everything else is off? Bringing whatever will make you comfortable to all of these exams is appropriate. Nothing else is as reassuring as your own robe and slippers. So, if "hangin' out in the back" makes you moody or as a devout pacifist you want to "avoid the draft," bring your own stuff along.

Disjeweling I made up this word. It means removing all jewelry. This is not always necessary, but it is requested often enough for you to take note. Certain procedures require that only your body be in attendance. To that end, you are requested to remove anything that can move. This would include your eyeglasses or contact lenses, your false teeth if they are of the in-a-glass-of-water-at-night type, and certainly your gems. Often, this request invokes concern over potential loss and/or theft—and rightly so. So, leave whatever can be left at home. (Bring your teeth and glasses, but leave the rings and chains in the box.)

Waiting and Delay Sadly, the problem of waiting and delay is not unique. It exists almost without exception in all areas of medical activity. Don't ask why. I could identify at least a thousand recurrent events that destroy the timetable of appointments. Most are inadvertent—the scheduled 30-minute study that preceded yours became one hour because that patient became unexpectedly ill, or that same 30-minute study extended to one and a half hours because the physician saw something suspicious and had to keep taking extra tests, or a piece of equipment broke down, and so on. Unfortunately, some delays are avoidable and a consequence of insensitivity—the receptionist was busy on a personal call; the technologist had to finish his cigarette; the doctor's stockbroker was on the line with a "hot" one. Whatever. But a patient's response is the same regardless of the cause. Depending on the length of the wait, the reaction is mere irritation to downright rage. Thus this section.

It—the wait and the delay—will occur. Obviously it is not to be condoned. Neither should it go unrecognized. But now is not the time for anger. You have prepared and made the necessary arrangements to be here. It's essential that you do not let your annoyance interfere with the performance of the procedure. Afterward, either to the offender or to your own doctor who sent you for the procedure, let it all hang out! Accept the reality that a delay probably will happen and plan for it. For your own sake and the sake of the best examination that can be done, try this mind-set: "I just won't let it get to me; I'll go through it because I have to—and then good-bye!" Don't have a procedure done on a day that you are on such a tight schedule that the delays start you churning. Do take along something interesting to divert you —a book, a magazine, knitting, a friend. An imprecise rule of thumb is to double the actual examination time that is listed in the tables (found throughout this book in the sections describing particular examinations) to allow for processing, disrobing and the like, and then double that again for the unaccountable delays. A last tip: Call where you are going before leaving home to get an idea of "how the doctor is running." Sometimes this will help. But after all is said and done, remember to be prepared, and *"stay cool."*

Short Procedure Hospitalization

When the procedure that you are to have requires that you stay in a hospital, there is again a series of events that are common to this group of tests and examinations. A word of clarification is appropriate before enumerating them.

The term "hospitalization" once meant a stay within the institution of at least one night. This has been modified recently to include confinement to a bed and all of the specialized management provided by trained personnel for a period that may be only a few hours in total duration. This arrangement is known as a short procedure hospitalization. Almost without exception the tests and/or examinations that necessitate this form of hospitalization require the use of a general anesthetic. However, once you recover consciousness, and are found to be fully stable, you may leave. So, the short procedure experience consists of many common events regardless of the particular test that takes you to the hospital.

Registration The only variation in this event (compared to what was detailed earlier) is that it may take place several days before you actually enter the hospital for your short procedure. At that time you will be told the exact date and time for your "main event."

Preadmission Testing Since you will undoubtedly be receiving a general anesthetic, certain screening tests are required to ascertain that you have no hidden problems that might make the anesthetic unduly hazardous. These usually include a routine laboratory blood profile (description found in Chapter 17), an electrocardiogram (a heart tracing described in Chapter 2), and sometimes an X-ray of the body part that will be examined (see Chapter 18 for descriptions of X-ray studies). These tests will be done following registration.

Meeting the Anesthesiologist An anesthesiologist (a medical specialist skilled in the administration of anesthetic agents) will see you on the day that you register. That person will discuss the choices available to you that will make the procedure tolerable. Usually it will be suggested that you be "put to sleep." If that is not your desire then let your feelings be known to the anesthesiologist, and come to a mutually satisfactory agreement. Also, if you have had any previous anesthetic experience that was difficult, for any reason, discuss that, too.

The Big Day You will arrive at the hospital on the day and at the time that has been previously scheduled, having had nothing by mouth since the night before. You will go directly to the Short Procedures Unit of the hospital where they are expecting you. You will be asked to disrobe and will be given a bed.

Preprocedure Prep Prep is the "in" word for preparation; it is the word that describes what someone, usually a nurse, will do to you before the examination, to get you ready for it. It may be nothing more than giving you some medication, usually by injection into your upper arm muscle—a mild ouch—which will make you both more relaxed and mildly sleepy. Or it may be shaving off some hair in the area to be examined, or perhaps cleansing the part in a special way. At the moment of truth a uniformed person will arrive with the chariot (a wheeled stretcher), will ask you to hop on, and will ceremoniously deliver you to the ball (the operating suite).

BAP: Bring a Pal A pal is anyone who will come to the hospital with you on the day of your short procedure and help you get home. Although you will be fully recovered from both the procedure and the anesthesia you won't be feeling tiptop. You will have been through an ordeal, and a helping hand will be much appreciated.

History, Medications, Pregnancy, Records, Disrobing, Disjeweling, and Waiting and Delays All of these categories are identical to the non-hospital experience and have been described earlier.

Specific Procedures

All of the following chapters are devoted to the description of what you will experience along the highways and byways that you have been directed to travel in search of the pot of gold at the end of the rainbow—a diagnosis!

For logical organization this escorted tour is divided into two parts appropriate to the instructions you receive:

Part I: "Go See . . ."—which is always a person.
Part II: "Go Get . . ."—which is always a procedure.

"Go See . . ." begins as a consultation with a medical specialist whom you will meet, talk to, and be examined by. He or she will undoubtedly advise you that additional procedures will be necessary. When everything needed to be done is finished, the specialist will either inform you of your diagnosis or refer you back to your personal physician for this information.

"Go Get . . ." directs you to a particular examination which is but one of a general group of similar studies—"Go Get an X-ray [general] of your stomach [particular]." These experiences may or may not include your meeting a physician, although all procedures are supervised in their performance, and interpreted as to their meaning, by a medical specialist in that discipline. Although you may not see *her* or *him*, that person is there. She or he is like the director of a movie—never seen, but responsible for the whole thing. Because we have been acculturated to "going to get an X-ray or a blood test," not to "going to see a radiologist or clinical pathologist," I have decided to present the material relating to these (and a few other) specialties in this form. The opinions derived from these procedures are reported to your personal physician, who will incorporate this data with the rest of the information that has developed since you began the pilgrimage. And then—and then —*a diagnosis!*

And finally, some clarification is warranted to explain the meaning of the symbols found in all the tables and elsewhere and to explain why some words are printed in CAPITAL letters throughout all the pages of our tour. The symbol Y stands for yes, N for no. The symbols (−) and (+) stand for degrees of intensity, ranging from (−) to (+ + + +). A (−) is therefore the least intense (the least hazardous, for example), while (+ + + +) is the most intense (for example, the most uncomfortable). Thus the symbols (+) and (−) serve as a rating system for three categories found in the tables: (1) degrees of discomfort; (2) the hazard each procedure entails; and (3) the final score—the bottom line—of the impact of the total experience. How these ratings are derived and how you can relate to their value is described in the Appendix, Table Details.

Capitalized words: Almost without exception any word where all the letters are CAPITALIZED is a medical term that might not be familiar to you. Their definitions can be found in the Glossary at the end of the book.

I

MEDICAL SPECIALISTS

CHAPTER

1

Go See an Allergist

An allergist is a physician who specializes in diseases that result from hypersensitivity of the body to certain substances or physical conditions. Some of these specialists are also trained in the recognition and treatment of diseases of the IMMUNE SYSTEM. To be permitted to assume the title allergist, this person, after graduating from both college and medical school, spends three additional years studying internal medicine or pediatrics and then at least two more years devoted only to those problems that embrace the diagnosis and treatment of allergic manifestations.

Allergy is a problem or a group of problems that may result from some unusual response to a stimulus. When everyone reacts similarly to a stimulus, that is considered normal. Everyone who is stung by a bee experiences sudden pain and then develops a slightly raised and red swelling at the site of the bite. That is expected. Some individuals, however, may experience a variety of severe reactions, including loss of consciousness and, in some cases, even death. These reactions are manifestations of hypersensitivity and are often referred to as allergic responses.

The nature and number of the different stimuli that can induce or provoke abnormal responses must be identified so that appropriate measures can be taken to protect the sufferer. The nature and number can be found by appropriate testing.

For a detailed discussion of each examination, start with the accompanying table. It identifies the procedures that are the usual province of this specialist. Suppose your doctor said, "I think your cat is to blame for what is

Allergy

Procedure	Discomfort* (-) to (+ + + +)	Hazard* (-) to (+ + +)	Hospital (Incl. Short Procedure)	Special Prep.	Extras*	Informed Consent*	Exam Time* (Hrs.)	Bottom Line* (-) to (+ + + +)	Exam Description (Page)
Physical exam	(+)	(-)	N	N	N	N	½	(½+)	5
Laboratory tests	(+)	(-)	N	N	Y	N	¼	(+)	6
Skin tests									
Prick	(½+) to (+ + +)	(-)	N	Y	Y	N	1	(+ +)	6
Scratch	(½+) to (+ + +)	(-)	N	Y	Y	N	1	(+ +)	6
Intradermal	(½+) to (+ + +)	(+)	N	Y	Y	N	1	(+ +)	7
Patch	(½+)	(-)	N	N	N	N	72	(+)	7
Spirometry	(+ +)	(-)	N	N	N	N	½	(+ +)	8
Challenge Tests—*too variable to rate*									8

* See Appendix, Table Details.

happening. I want to do a scratch test to prove it." Find this test and read across its entire line. A quick synopsis of the pertinent data characterizing this study will be listed. (These data are elaborated upon in the Appendix.) The last item on the line is the page number where the study is described in detail.

And finally, after you have read about the examination you are preparing for, reread pages xiv through xvi, General Events Common to All Adult Diagnostic Procedures.

Allergy and Allergy Testing

We are continuously subjected to things from the outside world that our bodies must react to: the air we breathe, the objects we touch, the food we eat. Our bodies cope with these invaders constantly. When this defense system spots a UFO it must immediately decide whether it is friend or foe. If friend, fine. If foe, action is initiated in the form of a warning signal to us that our territorial turf (our bodies) has been violated. This warning may be in the form of sneezing, watery eyes, stuffy nose, headaches, sinus infections, lumps and bumps on our skin, coughing, wheezing, or diarrhea. Sometimes the warning provokes such alarm that our defenses are overwhelmed, and this is sufficient to cause us to collapse, lose consciousness, and even die. This is known as an anaphylactic reaction.

Our bodies have made a treaty with most things and we accept them as friends. Some of us, for reasons that are too complex to discuss here, have a defense system that is faulty, and mistakenly considers as foes many things that the rest of us accept as friends—and treats them accordingly. It therefore becomes necessary to find out what's being misidentified so that an appropriate coping mechanism can be arranged, and also to undo the bodily changes that have been unleashed in the name of defense.

The error in identification and the responses it provokes is called AL-LERGY. The search for the foe we call allergy testing.

The diagnostic procedures for allergy testing consist of a physical examination, laboratory tests, skin tests, spirometry, and challenge tests.

Physical Examination The examination performed will be an amalgam of that which is done by a cardiologist, a dermatologist, and an otorhinolaryngologist. The detailed descriptions of each can be found in chapters 2, 3, and 13.

Laboratory Tests Most of the laboratory tests performed will be blood tests. They go by fancy names such as RAST (radioallergosorbent), FAST (fluorogenic allergosorbent), and even MAST (multiple allergosorbent). But they are, from your standpoint, all the same—they are blood tests and affect you only by their method of collection. See Blood in Chapter 17.

Skin Tests There are several ways that these allergy tests may be done; they are called prick, scratch, intradermal, and patch.

Prick Prepreparation is necessary in the form of discontinuing certain medications, such as antihistamines and antidepressants, for one to two days. The doctor or technologist will probably choose the front of your arm, or perhaps your back, to use for the tests. The part chosen will be bared and cleansed with alcohol. Then trays containing small bottles with dropper tops will be brought out. Each bottle contains a solution with something in it that might be the source of your allergy. A drop of solution from each of the bottles will be placed on your skin. As many as 30 to 35 different drops can be tested at one time. Once the drops are placed in their rows and charted by the doctor, he or she will take a small thin metal needle-like object with a fine fork-tipped end and gently "prick" the center of each drop. If there is discomfort, it is no greater than $(\frac{1}{2}+)$. That is the extent of the test, with the exception of the 15-minute wait to see what will happen. If you are sensitive to a particular agent, you will experience a slight swelling and a slight itching. It's like a mosquito bite. Like that bite, it represents only a minor annoyance—$(\frac{1}{2}+)$, but if there are many such areas of sensitivity, you can be quite uncomfortable—$(++)$ or even $(+++)$. However, left alone, the whole thing will disappear in 15 to 30 minutes. If the reactions are severe you will be given medication that will control them. It is possible that the remedy could make you sleepy, so try to bring a pal along to help you get home. There are no hazards. The whole experience will take about one hour. There will be no real aftereffects by the time you are ready to go home. Keep in mind, however, that since there is a finite number of things that you can be tested for at any one time and because there are so many things that you might have to be tested for ultimately, you may need to have the whole thing repeated over many visits.

Bottom Line: $(++)$ Really more tedious than aversive.

Scratch The procedure differs from the prick test only in that a small scratch is made on the skin of your arm with a very fine needle before the drop of solution is placed on it. This is instead of the prick. It is only slightly more uncomfortable than the prick, so it is rated the same as the other. Everything else is identical.

Intradermal *Intra* means "within"; *dermal* refers to the skin. This procedure differs from the others in that the testing solutions are injected under your skin rather than being placed on it. This technique is employed when your doctor suspects that sensitivity is present despite a negative prick or scratch test. The concentration of the offending agent is higher in this method and therefore may evoke a positive response where none was detected by the other procedures. However, the higher concentration can result in two problems. The first is a larger number of false positive results; that is, results that indicate a sensitivity which is really not present. The second, and more significant, problem is the hazard of a more significant and serious reaction than the "mosquito-bite" variety.

The injections are made, as a rule, in the upper and outer part of your arm. The skin is first cleansed. The injection is made with an extremely fine needle so that you perceive it only as a mild prick ($\frac{1}{2}+$). The rest is the same as for the other skin tests, to see if there is a response. The discomfort is similar—($\frac{1}{2}+$) to ($+++$)—depending on the number and severity of responses. There is a ($+$) hazard in this method. The time is the same—about one hour. You won't experience lingering effects unless you required medication, and then you will be sleepy for a few hours. Don't forget your pal.

Bottom Line: ($++$) Like the other skin tests, more tedious than aversive.

Patch This type of skin test is performed when you have a particular type of rash, one that is thought to be due to something that touches or is in contact with your skin. A common offender is the metal nickel, which is used in certain types of jewelry. When it is worn against the skin it may induce the particular reaction known as contact dermatitis.

Samples of all possible offenders are placed onto individual patches of material that are then affixed to a longer strip of material that can be taped onto your back. This is done after your back has been cleansed. The tape takes only a minute to position and it produces neither discomfort nor hazard. You can then go home, but you must return in two days for a "reading." The strip is removed and you then wait about half an hour. The allergist will examine your back for evidence of a reaction—which, if present, will be red, scaly, and itchy. This could last for several days, and if particularly annoying, can be treated with creams that you will be given.

Bottom Line: ($+$) The worst part is having to skip taking a shower.

Spirometry   Spirometry is one of a group of tests to measure pulmonary (lung) function. (All of these procedures are described in detail in Chapter 14.) This particular test measures the amount of air that you can both take into your lungs—inhalation—and breathe out of your lungs—exhalation. It is done when there is concern that a certain lung condition (asthma) may exist and may be a result of allergy.

When the test is performed, the doctor first clamps your nostrils shut with a clothespin kind of gadget. He or she then asks you to breathe into a piece of tubing equipped with a mouthpiece that is connected to a special machine. At first you will be asked to breathe normally. Then you will be instructed to take in as deep a breath as you can. Then you will be told to get rid of as much air as you can. This will be repeated several times. Occasionally, the doctor may ask you to inhale a special medication from a nebulizer (a small, hand-held instrument that creates a fine mist of any liquid placed into it) and repeat the deep breath in and out, 15 or so minutes later, to see if the medicine affects your performance.

The entire procedure takes only a few minutes to perform, but it may be difficult for some to do. It requires a lot of effort to "blow it all out," and may cause you to experience muscle aching along the side of your chest. In some people it may induce coughing or even wheezing. If you are asked to do the test after taking medication you may experience increased nervousness or awareness of an increase in your heart rate. These symptoms will pass in a few minutes. Therefore, the discomfort index may be **(+ +)**, although there is no hazard. Allot about half an hour for everything, and perhaps some muscle soreness for a day or so.

Bottom Line: **(+ +)** They have discovered a way to make breathing tough.

Challenge Tests   These are procedures that attempt to simulate conditions that occur naturally and are thought to be responsible for your complaint. Therefore, if you think your complaint is a result of something that you have eaten, you might be asked to eat the offending food in a controlled setting—the doctor's office—so that if, indeed, you are right, and you do experience a reaction, it can be quickly and safely controlled. The same sort of challenge (sometimes called provocation) tests can be created for other concerns. Perhaps the reaction is caused by something that you breathe—take a breathing challenge. Perhaps it is something at work—simulate the experience. Perhaps it is due to excessive stress, perhaps to particular temperature conditions. Whatever it is, a test can usually be created.

A definitive evaluation is difficult because these tests are so individualized and varied. Suffice it to say that the allergist will be there and make every effort to diminish both the discomfort and hazard consistent with getting an answer.

Bottom Line: **(?)** These really test not only you but the ingenuity of the allergist.

CHAPTER

2

Go See a Cardiologist

A cardiologist is a physician who specializes in diseases of the heart and circulatory system. To assume this title, men or women spend three years after graduating from both college and medical school studying internal medicine and then two more years devoted only to those problems that affect the heart and circulatory system.

Heart disease in the adult falls into four major categories: ISCHEMIC, MYOCARDIAL, VALVULAR, and CONGENITAL. In ischemic disease, perhaps better known as CORONARY ARTERY disease, there is inadequate circulation of blood to the heart. Myocardial disease affects the muscles of the heart, the heart walls. Valvular conditions attack the specialized structures that separate the chambers of the heart from one another and whose openings and closings control and regulate the flow of blood. Congenital diseases result from some defect or defects in the development of the heart before birth.

Each major disease category is studied by procedures appropriate to its unique set of problems. Often the same examination or test is used in more than one category, and sometimes in all. Whatever the symptoms, a history will always be taken and a physical examination will always be performed. Additionally, although a particular form of examination (such as ultrasound imaging) will always seem the same to you, it can provide different information depending on the problem at hand.

For a detailed discussion of each examination, start with the accompanying table. It identifies the four major areas of investigation. Within each category are listed the tests that can be performed. Suppose the cardiologist said, "I'm recommending that you have a nuclear stress test to evaluate your

Cardiology

Disease Category/ Procedure	Discomfort* (−) to (++++)	Hazard* (−) to (+++)	Hospital (Incl. Short Procedure)	Special Prep.	Physician	Extras*	Informed Consent*	Exam Time* (Hrs.)	Bottom Line* (−) to (++++)	Exam Description (Page)
Ischemic (Coronary)										
Physical exam	(½+)	(−)	N	N	Y	N	N	½	(½+)	14
Laboratory tests	(+)	(−)	N	N	N	Y	N	¼	(+)	15
EKG: { Resting	(+)	(−)	N	N	N	N	N	¼	(+)	15
EKG: { Exercise	(+++)	(++)	N	Y	Y	N	Y	1	(++) to (+++)	16
Nuclear	(+++)	(+++)	N	Y	Y	Y	Y	4	(++) to (+++)	17
Ultrasound	(+)	(−)	N	N	Y/N	N	N	1	(+)	17
X-ray	(++++)	(+++)	Y	Y	Y	Y	Y	3	(++++)	17
Myocardial										
Physical exam	(½+)	(−)	N	N	Y	N	N	½	(½+)	18
Laboratory tests	(+)	(−)	N	N	N	Y	N	¼	(+)	19
EKG: { Resting	(+)	(−)	N	N	N	N	N	¼	(+)	19
EKG: { Ambulatory	(+)	(−)	N	N	N	Y	N	24	(+)	19
Nuclear	(+)	(−)	N	N	N	N	N	2	(+)	19
Ultrasound	(+)	(−)	N	N	Y/N	N	N	1	(+)	20
X-ray	(½+)	(−)	N	N	N	N	N	¼	(½+)	20

Cardiology—cont'd

Disease Category/Procedure	Discomfort* (−) to (+++)	Hazard* (−) to (+++)	Hospital (Incl. Short Procedure)	Special Prep.	Physician	Extras*	Informed Consent*	Exam Time* (Hrs.)	Bottom Line* (−) to (++++)	Exam Description (Page)
Valvular										
Physical exam	(½+)	(−)	N	N	Y	N	N	½	(½+)	20
Laboratory tests	(+)	(−)	N	N	N	Y	N	¼	(+)	20
EKG: Resting	(+)	(−)	N	N	N	N	N	¼	(+)	21
EKG: Ambulatory	(+)	(−)	N	N	N	N	N	24	(+)	21
Nuclear	(+)	(−)	N	N	Y	Y	Y	4	(++) to (+++)	21
Ultrasound	(+)	(−)	N	N	N	N	N	1	(+)	21
X-ray	(½+)	(−)	N	N	N	N	N	¼	(½+)	21
Congenital										
Physical exam	(½+)	(−)	N	N	Y	N	N	½	(½+)	21
Laboratory tests	(+)	(−)	N	N	N	Y	N	¼	(+)	22
EKG: Resting	(+)	(−)	N	N	N	N	N	¼	(+)	22
EKG: Ambulatory	(+)	(−)	N	N	N	N	N	24	(+)	22
Nuclear	(+)	(−)	N	N	N	Y	N	2	(+)	22
Ultrasound	(+)	(−)	N	N	N	N	N	1	(+)	22
X-ray	(½+)	(−)	N	N	N	N	N	¼	(½+)	22

* See Appendix, Table Details.

coronary arteries." Find this test under Ischemic (Coronary) and read across its entire line. There you'll find a quick synopsis of the pertinent data characterizing this study (these data are elaborated upon in the Appendix). The last item on the line is the page number where the study is described in detail.

And finally, after you have read about the particular examination that you are preparing for, reread pages xiv through xvi, General Events Common to All Adult Diagnostic Procedures.

Ischemic (Coronary Artery) Heart Disease

The heart is a most specialized hollow ORGAN whose muscular walls permit it to act as a marvelous pump to move blood throughout every portion of your body—a function known as *circulation*. In order for the muscular walls (known as the myocardium) to function, they must be supplied with blood. The blood that supplies the myocardium is brought to it by the coronary arteries, of which there are three. If any or all of these vessels should fail to deliver sufficient blood to the heart wall to satisfy its required need, the condition is known as ISCHEMIA. This is a very serious problem and results from a narrowing or actual blockage of the vessel—not unlike rust that forms on the inside of pipes. The "rust" in the coronaries is a consequence of increased CHOLESTEROL levels in the body. In the beginning, the narrowing is gradual and "silent"—that is, there are no real symptoms until the original LUMEN of the vessel has been reduced more than 60 percent. When this stage has been reached, symptoms may develop in some people, but not all. These symptoms, as a rule, are some type of chest pain.

It should be understood that the needs of a body part for blood are not always the same. They are dependent on the level of activity of that part. Thus, when you are sitting at a desk or "potatoing it" in front of the TV, the amount of blood required to "prime the pump" is far less than the amount you need when you're jogging, playing tennis, having sex, or even walking up stairs. So the diminished blood supply that could satisfy your needs when sedentary is suddenly found wanting when your activity heats up. When that occurs, pain may be experienced. All of this, in theory, is a logical progression of increased narrowing, increased episodes of circulatory insufficiency, and thus, increased frequency and severity of symptoms. But it isn't always that way. Sometimes without warning, or from minimal symptoms, that which was only a relatively small narrowing suddenly becomes complete. The blood supply is abruptly "turned off." That is what the headlines that read, "He suffered a sudden massive heart attack and died," are all about. The detection of the problem, and its correction before irreparable damage occurs to the walls, is the *raison d'être* for all of these studies, and to reword a phrase from the Good Book, "and a cardiologist shall lead the way."

The diagnostic procedures for ischemic heart disease include a physical examination, laboratory tests, an electrocardiogram (EKG)—resting, an electrocardiogram—exercise (stress tests), nuclear imaging, ultrasound imaging, and X-rays.

Physical Examination   You will be asked to disrobe completely from the waist up. Panties or shorts are permitted from the waist down. The handsome gown that you will don opens in the front. You will probably be seated on an examination table and the cardiologist will begin by just looking at your neck and chest for any obvious or unusual pulsations. That's called INSPECTION. This takes only a minute or two. No discomfort except conceivable embarrassment.

Next is AUSCULTATION. This is where the stethoscope is used. The doctor will place the appropriate ends into his or her ears and firmly place the other end on various points on your chest, listening intently for a moment or two over each area. You may be asked to hold your breath. You will probably also change your position several times. The whole thing takes 5 to 10 minutes, at most, and is free of discomfort or hazard.

Then your blood pressure will be taken. (Actually, the order of procedure is unimportant and variable.) The apparatus used for blood pressure determination is called a sphygmomanometer, and it consists of a strip of material about six inches wide and about two feet long that can wrap around your upper arm or upper thigh. Going into one end of the strip, or cuff, is rubber tubing attached to a bulb that permits it to be inflated. There is a gauge connected as well, that identifies the pressure to which the cuff has been inflated. The sphygmomanometer is usually applied above your elbow. The doctor applies the end of the stethoscope to the inside of your elbow and then pumps up the cuff. The pressure that is necessary to eliminate the sound of your blood flow (which had been heard through the stethoscope) is the upper value of your blood pressure (systolic pressure). Once this pressure is reached, the air in the cuff is then let out slowly, and the pressure at which your blood flow is again heard represents the lower value of your blood pressure (diastolic pressure). The same determination is usually obtained from your other arm and each leg. The evaluation is made in one to two minutes at each site and may invoke a (½ +) discomfort.

Next comes PALPATION. The doctor's hands and fingers will gently brush across your scalp, neck, chest, abdomen, and each of your arms and legs feeling for anything unusual—an irregular pulsation, an atypical vibration, an area too hot or too cold, or an organ that feels enlarged or irregular. It is rarely uncomfortable and rarely more than several minutes in duration.

Needless to say, there are multiple individual variations and sequences to the above description. Some will include PERCUSSION, some will have you strain, some will have you perform exercise, and so on. The overall examination is similar. The entire examination takes 15 to 20 minutes. There is essentially no discomfort, certainly no hazard, and no aftereffects.

Bottom Line: (½ +) Kinda fun.

Laboratory Tests There are a host of blood and urine examinations that are helpful. See Chapter 17.

Electrocardiogram (EKG)—Resting The ELECTROCARDIOGRAPH is an instrument capable of recording, usually in graphic form, the heart's function. It actually detects the heart's electrical activity. It provides accurate information on the organ's rate (the number of beats in a minute) and rhythm (the regularity of the beats), on its axis (the direction in which the electrical impulse moves and spreads throughout the heart), and on the presence of HYPERTROPHY and INFARCTION.

The resting study is performed with you in a lying position. No prepreparation is necessary. Your arms, legs, and the front of your chest must be bared. A technologist will prepare points on your wrists, ankles, and chest by rubbing each area briskly with a small piece of bandage to which a LUBRICANT is applied so that each spot is mildly red and coated with the "goo." A small metal disk (about the size of a quarter) is then affixed to each spot. These disks, called SENSORS or ELECTRODES, are capable of detecting the electrical impulses given off by the body. Each sensor is connected by a wire (lead) to the machine. It will detect electrical impulses that originate from you, and transmit them to the machine, where they will be analyzed and recorded in the form of a graph. The recording is usually on special paper tape that runs continuously and commonly spills out of the machine and onto the floor. The technologist will move a lead wire from one spot on your chest to another six different times. At each location a tracing will be made. As a rule, 12 individual recordings are obtained. The collection of the tracings causes you absolutely no discomfort. Except for the movement of the sensors, you'll have no awareness that anything is going on. There is no hazard. It takes about 15 minutes. Everything will then be removed; the grease will be wiped off, and you'll be freed. There may be residual redness or mild tenderness over the rubbed places for several days.

Bottom Line: (+) No big deal.

Electrocardiogram (EKG)—Exercise (Stress Test) This procedure can be performed alone or more effectively with nuclear medicine imaging. Its rationale is based on the well-known fact that significant narrowing of the inside diameter of coronary arteries can exist without necessarily producing symptoms if the heart muscle's demand for blood is not greater than that supplied by the impaired artery. It is known that the lumen of the vessel is often decreased greater than 60 percent of normal before any indication of disease becomes evident. It is this "quiet" narrowing that explains the almost daily news report of someone who had never been sick a day of his life experiencing a massive (and often fatal) HEART ATTACK.

The concept of the procedure is to increase the heart muscle's demand for blood through monitored exercise and to determine whether or not this demand can be satisfied. If it can, then the arteries can be considered to be free of significant disease. If the demand cannot be satisfied, the condition known as ischemia (inadequate blood supply to a part) exists, and the probability of coronary artery disease is sufficiently great to warrant further testing.

Such a study is called an exercise stress test. Stress is the word used to describe any force that increases demands on your physical endurance in such a way that it creates muscular tension, fatigue, and even exhaustion. In this case, the stress is initiated by carefully monitored exercise either on a treadmill (a stationary device with a slightly inclined moving floor on which you walk) or pedaling a stationary bicycle. In special situations in which an individual is incapable of performing physical exercise—perhaps someone with severe arthritis or missing a leg—increasing the heart rate can be achieved with special medication administered either by mouth or by injection.

Throughout the procedure, from the resting state to the peak of maximum activity, your heart is monitored by an electrocardiograph. This machine depicts your heart's electrical activity and provides accurate information of its rate and rhythm, usually in graphic form. The changes that occur from the resting to the stress state permit the trained observer to make accurate judgments regarding the status of the vessels. This assessment is accurate in finding any problem about 80 percent of the time when done alone. The sensitivity of detection improves to about 90 percent if at the peak of the exercise an ISOTOPE is injected into a vein. The isotope will be carried by your blood to your heart and remain within the muscle for several hours. If the arteries to the heart are normal the isotope will be distributed throughout the muscle uniformly. If, on the other hand, there is an abnormality in a vessel, the distribution of the isotope will reflect this deficiency. Images of the heart are taken immediately upon completion of the exercise and usually three hours later, when your heart rate has returned to a resting state. At the present time the isotope used is thallium-201. (When the isotope is added to the conventional exercise stress test the examination is called a thallium stress test; this procedure will be described more thoroughly in Chapter 19.)

Here is the technique: You will have been given a set of instructions by your cardiologist prior to arriving for the test. These will identify, among other things, those medications that must be discontinued. On the morning of this procedure you are not to eat. Dress in clothing that is comfortable for exercise—a sweat suit, a jogging outfit, shorts, sneakers, whatever. Your chest will be bared long enough for a technologist to apply the special electrodes that are connected to the electrocardiograph (see discussion of the application in the previous section, Electrocardiogram—Resting). You are now ready and will be asked to stand on the treadmill or sit on the stationary bicycle.

Enter the cardiologist, who will monitor your exercise (your stress). The extent of the exercising and its vigor is under that person's supervision, which assures your safety. How long you will "stress" is unpredictable—it may be only a minute or two or it could be as long as ten minutes. This depends on how you feel and what the EKG is showing. When the cardiologist decides that you have exercised sufficiently the procedure is terminated.

Bottom Line: (+) A long walk to nowhere.

Nuclear Imaging Besides the stress test images, two other nuclear studies are valuable. These are the infarction detection and wall motion studies; the wall motion test also permits the calculation of the heart's ejection fraction, which is the percentage of change in the size of a heart chamber between its being completely filled with blood at rest and its having discharged a volume of blood with its contraction. These may be helpful in detecting previous damage caused by infarction. See Chapter 19.

Ultrasound Imaging See Heart and Blood Vessels in Chapter 20.

X-rays When all of the other procedures have been done and there is enough data to suggest that there is disease of the coronary vessels, this impression must be confirmed by direct visualization of these arteries. All of the other stuff provides only inferential evidence. The time has come to finally answer the questions: What do the vessels actually look like? How bad are they? Is more than one involved? Is surgery a viable alternative?

The moment has arrived to invoke the gold standard—ANGIOGRAPHY, or more precisely, ARTERIOGRAPHY. This entire subject is presented—angiography as a whole, and arteriography, including the study of the coronary arteries—on page 194.

Myocardial Heart Disease

Myo refers to muscle. Cardium refers to heart. Put them together and it spells heart muscle. Except for the extras like the linings, the valves, and the blood vessels, that is what the heart mostly is—a special kind of muscle. This specially configured muscle behaves like any other muscle. It is subject to diseases that attack it directly, such as infections and tumors, and it is affected by other conditions that result in its working abnormally. It is the latter group that includes the more commonly encountered problems. A prime example is HYPERTENSION. This condition, unfortunately, is prevalent in large numbers of adults. Regardless of its underlying causes, of which there are many, its long-term effect on the heart is usually the same—the heart muscle works harder to do the same job. This results in the muscle becoming larger—a condition known as HYPERTROPHY—and ultimately weakening the heart to the point that it cannot perform its necessary function. This condition is known as circulatory or heart failure.

Symptoms are often sneaky, and may not exist until the problem has been present for a long period and circulatory failure has begun. Shortness of breath with mild exertion is common. Swelling of the legs may exist. There may be episodes of unexplained "faintness." The veins in your neck may seem "fatter." Or you look and feel "heavy," and indeed you have put on some weight. Whatever it is, *check it out!*

The diagnostic procedures for myocardial heart disease include a physical examination, laboratory tests, an electrocardiogram (EKG)—resting, an electrocardiogram—ambulatory (Holter monitor), nuclear imaging, ultrasound imaging, and X-ray.

Physical Examination The routine physical examination performed by the cardiologist has been described earlier in this chapter. See pages 14–15.

Laboratory Tests There are a host of blood and urine examinations that are helpful. See Chapter 17.

Electrocardiogram (EKG)—Resting The ELECTROCARDIOGRAM has been detailed earlier in this chapter. See pages 15–16.

Electrocardiogram—Ambulatory (Holter Monitor) Sometimes the resting EKG does not identify a problem that the cardiologist suspects may exist because of problems in your history. These might include: intermittent (not all the time) cardiac arrhythmia (irregular heart rhythm); changes in your heart function as a consequence of certain stressful or emotional factors that exist in your average day; or side effects from certain medications that you are taking. Since these problems might not be detected at a "one-time" resting EKG, a twenty-four-hour continuous monitoring is used. This study is commonly referred to as the Holter 24-hour monitor (Holter is the name of the company that makes the monitor).

All the principles discussed in the resting study pertain. The only change is that the ELECTRODES (5 of them) will all be affixed to your chest. (It is sometimes necessary to shave off hair to ensure a tight seal before the sensors are applied.) The wire leads run to a small box—about eight inches long and two inches wide—that contains the electrocardiographic device. This is the monitor, and it will either be worn at your waist with a belt, or looped over your shoulder on a strap. Either way it shouldn't cause any real discomfort since it is neither particularly bulky nor heavy. As with the conventional EKG, you will not be aware that tracings are being made. You will be asked to record, either by microphone into the monitor (if your particular unit is so blessed) or into a diary that you will keep, anything that occurs over the 24-hour period that you think is unusual or important, and the time that it occurred. You will return the monitor the next day. The tracings will be computer-analyzed for the doctor's review. It is expected that you will attempt to live an average and normal day. The only thing you may not do is shower or bathe. So—discomfort is (+), hazard is (−), and time is 24 hours.

Bottom Line: (+) You might even find you miss it after it is gone.

Nuclear Imaging Those studies that provide valuable contributions to the "workup" are found in the Heart and Blood Vessel section of Chest in Chapter 19.

Ultrasound Imaging   See Heart and Blood Vessels in Chapter 20.

X-ray   A conventional routine chest examination is indicated. See page 190.

Valvular Heart Disease

In the two preceding sections we have discussed the walls (myocardia) and blood supply of the big red machine. But you need to know a tad more: the heart is composed of four compartments called chambers. The chambers are separated from one another by "swinging doors" called valves. Blood enters the first chamber and remains there until the valve opens to permit it to enter the second—and so on until it leaves the heart. The correct opening and closing of these valvular "doors" is crucial to appropriate function.

Valvular disease may be CONGENITAL or acquired. The latter variety is frequently the consequence of infection, often occurring in childhood and commonly known as rheumatic fever, or as a consequence of longstanding HYPERTENSION. Often the problem is discovered on a routine physical examination during AUSCULTATION; your doctor says, "Something sounds funny. Do I detect a murmur?" Frequently symptoms appear only late in the disease when sufficient changes in the heart have occurred to affect its normal function. Then the same symptoms or physical changes as described in the myocardial section (see above) are complained of: shortness of breath, palpitations, irregular heartbeat, swelling of the lower extremities, faintness, fullness of the neck veins, and so on. Which symptom or which group of symptoms alerted you is no longer important. The important—top of the agenda—issue is to evaluate the nature and extent of the damage so a treatment plan can be formulated.

The diagnostic procedures for valvular heart disease include a physical examination, laboratory tests, an electrocardiogram (EKG)—resting, an electrocardiogram—ambulatory (Holter monitor), nuclear imaging, ultrasound imaging, and X-rays.

Physical Examination   The routine physical examination performed by the cardiologist has been described earlier in this chapter. See pages 14–15.

Laboratory Tests   There are a host of blood and urine examinations that are helpful; CULTURES are sometimes required. See Chapter 17.

Electrocardiogram (EKG)—Resting The ELECTROCARDIOGRAM has been detailed earlier in this chapter. See pages 15–16.

Electrocardiogram—Ambulatory (Holter Monitor) The procedure has been detailed earlier in this chapter. See page 19.

Nuclear Imaging Wall motion studies, which include the determination of the ejection fraction, are valuable contributions to the "workup." See Chapter 19.

Ultrasound Imaging See Heart and Blood Vessels in Chapter 20.

X-rays A routine chest examination is indicated. See page 190.

Congenital Heart Disease

It is beyond the scope of this primer to discuss the diseases of the infant, child, or adolescent. Therefore, only those CONGENITAL heart diseases that are encountered in adulthood will be detailed here.

Congenital refers to those diseases that result from some defect or defects in the development of the heart before birth. There are literally hundreds of documented anomalies and there is a tremendous variation in their consequence. Many prove incompatible with life either at birth or within childhood. Many, however, are compatible with life, and the sufferer may live to adulthood before the birth defect becomes manifest and demands investigation and attention.

The symptoms and physical signs may come late in the disease. They are indentical to those discussed in the previous sections on myocardial and valvular diseases. Or you may well be aware of the condition, having coped with it your entire life, but now find something new is happening that causes you sufficient concern to seek advice and attention.

Diagnostic procedures for congenital heart disease include a physical examination, laboratory tests, an electrocardiogram (EKG)—resting, an electrocardiogram—ambulatory (Holter monitor), nuclear imaging, ultrasound imaging, and X-rays.

Physical Examination The routine physical examination performed by the cardiologist has been described earlier in this chapter. See pages 14–15.

Laboratory Tests There are a host of blood and urine examinations that are helpful. CULTURES are sometimes required. See Chapter 17.

Electrocardiogram (EKG)—Resting The ELECTROCARDIOGRAM has been detailed earlier in this chapter. See pages 15–16.

Electrocardiogram—Ambulatory (Holter Monitor) The procedure has been detailed earlier in this chapter. See page 19.

Nuclear Imaging Wall motion studies, which include the determination of the ejection fraction, are valuable contributions to the "workup." See Chapter 19.

Ultrasound Imaging See Heart and Blood Vessels in Chapter 20.

X-rays A routine chest examination is indicated. See page 190.

3

Go See a Dermatologist

A dermatologist is a physician who specializes in diseases of the skin. To earn this title, a person, after graduating from both college and medical school, spends four additional years studying the vast array of diseases and disorders that afflict the skin.

The dermatologist must sort out these various conditions so that appropriate treatment can be instituted. The procedures that are employed in this sorting-out process are limited to two categories: physical examination and laboratory studies, of which the biopsy is the most important.

For a detailed discussion of each examination, start with the accompanying table. It identifies each of the procedures that are the usual province of this specialist. Suppose she or he said, "I'll have to take a small piece of tissue out of that lump on your forehead and sent it to a pathologist for examination." Find this procedure, biopsy, under Laboratory Tests, and read across its entire line. A quick synopsis of the pertinent data characterizing this study is listed. (These areas are elaborated upon in the Appendix.) The last item on the line is the page number where the study is described in detail.

And finally, after you have read about the particular examination that you are preparing for, reread pages xiv through xvi, General Events Common to All Adult Diagnostic Procedures.

Dermatology

Procedure	Discomfort* (−) to (++++)	Hazard* (−) to (+++)	Hospital (Incl. Short Procedure)	Special Prep.	Extras*	Informed Consent*	Exam Time* (Hrs.)	Bottom Line* (−) to (++++)	Exam Description (Page)
Physical exam	(+)	(−)	N	N	N	N	¼	(+)	25
Laboratory tests	(+) to (++)	(−)	N	N	N	N	¼	(+) to (++)	25

* See Appendix, Table Details.

Skin

The skin is the outer layer of your body. It is a tough but flexible cover that not only protects "all of the rest of you" from the outside but also helps to keep "all of the rest of you" inside. The skin is subject to many attacks: the sun and the other elements; all manner of irritants—soaps and other detergents, plants such as poison ivy, chemicals, and many, many more; stings (mosquitoes, bees) and bites; lumps and bumps—freckles, moles, and nevi (pigmented areas like birthmarks); infections from bacteria, fungi, and viruses. And more! It wards off these attacks remarkably well, but sometimes "things" just appear that weren't there before and require attention.

Diagnostic procedures for skin problems include a physical examination, a biopsy, and laboratory tests.

Physical Examination The examination performed by the dermatologist is usually confined to the area of your complaint. Although it would probably be better if your entire body were checked, many patients object to a total "strip down" simply because one of their fingernails "looks funny." The examination is composed of two parts—looking and touching, or INSPECTION and PALPATION.

Inspection is the big ticket. It employs the most sophisticated instrument in existence—the eyes. Magnifying lenses are often employed to improve the details. But basically inspection is concentrated looking. The whole thing takes perhaps 5 to 10 minutes. There is no discomfort unless being looked at causes you some embarrassment. There is no hazard. Clearly, there are no aftereffects.

Palpation: Often the "thing" will have to be felt. Is it firm, hard, or soft? Is it rough or smooth? Is it elevated? Does it hurt when touched? All of these questions are answered with a "once over lightly"—with gentle fingertips feeling the part. Total time is minutes. Total discomfort and hazard is zero.

Final Score: (+) Kind of boring.

Laboratory Tests Biopsy, which means the removal of tissue, cells, or fluids from the body so that they can be examined and their nature defined, is the most common procedure performed by the dermatologist. Almost all biopsies of the skin are of the excisional type. Other studies that may be ordered include those of the blood and urine and various types of CULTURES. All of these are discussed in Chapter 17.

4

Go See an Endocrinologist

An endocrinologist is a physician who specializes in diseases of the endocrine system. This person has graduated from both college and medical school. He or she has then spent three additional years studying internal medicine and after that, two more years devoted only to those problems that affect the endocrine system.

Endocrine refers to specialized tissues known as ductless glands that manufacture, store, and then secrete hormones—chemical substances that are discharged by a gland and which produce a specific and often regulatory effect on an organ or organs elsewhere in the body. The glands that compose the endocrine system are the pituitary, the thyroid, the parathyroids, the adrenals, the pancreas, the ovaries, and the testicles. Each manufactures and secretes one or more hormones.

Functional changes in one of the glands often result in changes in others, since they are very closely interrelated. Thus, your symptoms are frequently confusing; it can be hard to determine which gland originated the abnormal cycle and is essentially to blame. So, after listening carefully to your story, the endocrinologist must sift through and sort out the possibilities of cause and then validate these hypotheses (assumptions) by appropriate testing. All of the usual procedures that this specialist might recommend are divided into seven categories; each category corresponds to one of the seven endocrine glands.

For a detailed discussion of each examination, start with the accompanying table. It identifies the seven major areas of investigation. Within each category are listed the tests that can be performed. Suppose your doctor said,

Endocrinology

Endocrine Gland/ Procedure	Discomfort* (−) to (++++)	Hazard* (−) to (+++)	Hospital (Incl. Short Procedure)	Special Prep.	Physician	Extras*	Informed Consent*	Exam Time* (Hrs.)	Bottom Line* (−) to (++++)	Exam Description (Page)
Pituitary										
Physical exam	(½+)	(−)	N	N	Y	N	N	¼	(½+)	29
Laboratory tests	(+)	(−)	N	N	N	Y	N	¼	(+)	29
X-rays	(½+)	(−)	N	N	N	N	N	¼	(½+)	30
Thyroid										
Physical exam	(½+)	(−)	N	Y	Y	N	N	¼	(½+)	30
Laboratory tests	(+)	(−)	N	N	N	Y	N	¼	(+)	30
Nuclear	(½+)	(−)	N	Y	Y	Y	N	24	(+)	30
Ultrasound	(½+)	(−)	N	N	N	N	N	½	(½+)	31
Biopsy	(++)	(+)	N	N	Y	Y	Y	1	(++)	31
Parathyroids										
Laboratory tests	(+)	(−)	N	N	N	Y	N	¼	(+)	31
Nuclear	(+)	(−)	N	N	Y	Y	N	1	(+)	32
Ultrasound	(½+)	(−)	N	N	N	N	N	½	(½+)	32
Adrenals										
Laboratory tests	(+)	(−)	N	N	N	Y	N	¼	(+)	32
X-rays	(½+)	(−)	N	N	N	N	N	½	(½+)	32

Endocrinology—cont'd

Endocrine Gland/ Procedure	Discomfort* (−) to (++++)	Hazard* (−) to (+++)	Hospital (Incl. Short Procedure)	Special Prep.	Physician	Extras*	Informed Consent*	Exam Time* (Hrs.)	Bottom Line* (−) to (++++)	Exam Description (Page)
Pancreas										
Laboratory tests	(+)	(−)	N	N	N	Y	N	¼	(+)	33
X-rays	(½+)	(−)	N	N	N	Y	N	½	(½+)	33
Ultrasound	(½+)	(−)	N	N	N	N	N	½	(½+)	33
Ovaries										
Physical exam	(++)	(−)	N	N	Y	N	N	¼	(++)	34
Laboratory tests	(+)	(−)	N	N	N	Y	N	¼	(+)	34
Ultrasound	(½+)	(−)	N	N	N	N	N	½	(½+)	34
Testicles										
Physical exam	(++)	(−)	N	N	Y	N	N	¼	(+)	34
Laboratory tests	(+)	(−)	N	N	N	Y	N	¼	(+)	35
Ultrasound	(½+)	(−)	N	N	N	N	N	½	(½+)	35
Nuclear	(+)	(−)	N	N	N	Y	N	½	(+)	35

* See Appendix, Table Details.

"I'm recommending that you have a nuclear scan of your thyroid." Find this test under Thyroid, and read across its entire line. A quick synopsis of the pertinent data characterizing this study is listed. (These data are elaborated upon in the Appendix.) The last item on the line is the page number where the study is described in detail.

And finally, after you have read about the particular examination that you are preparing for, reread pages xiv through xvi, General Events Common to All Adult Diagnostic Procedures.

Pituitary Gland

The pituitary gland, often called the master gland, is indeed the puppeteer who pulls the strings that make all of the other GLANDS behave. It is a small, pea-shaped structure, located on the undersurface of the brain, about halfway back, and inside the skull. Most of the HORMONES that it produces act on the other endocrine glands and serve to regulate their function. The pituitary is also a primary controller of growth and is responsible for particular types of dwarfs and giants. Besides the symptoms caused by the altered glandular functions, certain types of headaches and visual changes are other clues that this organ is in trouble.

Diagnostic procedures for the pituitary gland include a physical examination, laboratory tests, and X-ray examinations.

Physical Examination   The examination will be a combination of parts of physicals as might be performed by a cardiologist (see pages 14–15), a neurologist (see pages 73–74), and an ophthalmologist (see pages 95–111). It will include close physical inspection of the entire body to observe in particular both hair and fat distribution. It will include PALPATION, particularly of the neck. It will include evaluation of the back of each eye. It will be tailored to the complaints that have been identified in your history.

There will be no true discomfort and no hazard. The exam usually requires about 15 minutes.

Bottom Line: (½ +) Ho-hum.

Laboratory Tests   There are a host of blood and urine examinations that are helpful. See Chapter 17.

X-ray Examinations The pituitary gland and the surrounding brain and skull can be seen quite well employing CT techniques. See pages 176–78 for a general description of CT examinations.

Thyroid Gland

The thyroid gland is located in the front of the neck at the level of the Adam's apple. The particular HORMONES that the thyroid produces regulate the body's METABOLISM. Alterations in thyroid function may cause widespread and diverse symptoms and problems. Underactivity (hypothyroidism) commonly results in weight gain, chronic fatigue, menstrual changes, and an intolerance to cold. Overactivity (hyperthyroidism) frequently results in weight loss, nervousness, irregular or rapid heart rate, excessive sweating, and an intolerance to hot weather. This gland is also particularly prone to irregular enlargement, a condition known as goiter, and to the formation of NODULES, some small percentage of which are malignant. Therefore, visualization of the gland when these changes are seen or felt is imperative.

Diagnostic procedures for the thyroid gland include a physical examination, laboratory tests, nuclear medicine procedures, ultrasound imaging, and biopsy.

Physical Examination Your neck must be bared. You will be sitting. The doctor will first visually INSPECT your neck and will ask you to swallow several times, sometimes while sipping water, sometimes "dry." He will then place the fingers of his left hand against the right side of your neck and gently feel the area. The same with the right hand and the left side of your neck. There is neither discomfort nor hazard. It will take only a minute or two. Then the doctor will walk behind you and repeat the same PALPATION. Total time: five minutes.

Bottom Line: (½ +) Boring.

Laboratory Tests There are many, but they are all initiated by a collection of either blood or urine. See Chapter 17.

Nuclear Medicine Procedures These will necessitate your going elsewhere since they are not done by an endocrinologist but by a physician skilled in nuclear medicine. See Neck in Chapter 19.

Ultrasound Imaging These, too, will probably necessitate going else-where since these procedures are the province of another medical specialist. See Neck in Chapter 20.

Biopsy Biopsy is the removal of tissue so that it may be examined micro-scopically by a pathologist, the medical specialist trained in these evaluations. There are different ways to perform this technique and the type selected depends on the location in the body from which the specimen is taken.

Since the thyroid is so close to the skin and the area of concern can be palpated, the biopsy, in this case called a NEEDLE ASPIRATION, is commonly performed by endocrinologists in their offices. On occasion, it may also be done by the nuclear medicine or ultrasound physician. The procedure using ultrasound assistance—which is not always required—is described in detail in Chapter 20, page 272.

Parathyroid Glands

The parathyroid glands are four small (pea-sized) bodies usually located in the front of the neck, but behind the thyroid. (See discussion of the thyroid above.) Sometimes they live elsewhere, often behind the breastbone, and then finding their true address is a real trick. The HORMONE that they produce regulates the body's calcium metabolism particularly as it affects the SKELETAL SYSTEM. Abnormalities in parathyroid function cause widespread and diverse symptoms and problems. These might range from vague complaints such as muscle twitching and spasms, lethargy, and headaches to severe symptoms associated with kidney stones and osteoporosis. Such alterations may be a result of noncancerous tumor growths that are known as adenomas. Thus, when dysfunction of these GLANDS is suspected it is imperative to determine whether or not adenomas are the cause. If they are, surgical removal will correct the problem. Imaging techniques have recently been developed that are highly accurate not only in the detection of parathyroid tumors, but also in pinpointing the exact location of the glands.

Diagnostic procedures for the parathyroid glands include laboratory tests, nuclear medicine procedures, and ultrasound imaging.

Laboratory Tests There are many, but they are all initiated by a collection of either blood or urine. See Chapter 17.

Nuclear Medicine Procedures These tests will necessitate your going elsewhere since they are not done by an endocrinologist but by a physician skilled in nuclear medicine. All parathyroid examinations utilizing nuclear imaging procedures are described in Chapter 19, page 230. Make sure you also read the section on bone density.

Ultrasound Imaging This modality, too, will necessitate going elsewhere since these procedures are the province of another medical specialist. See Chapter 20. The examination is identical to the procedure employed in examinations of the thyroid gland. See Chapter 20, page 278.

Adrenal Glands

Some parts of the body, regardless of their importance, just never get to be as well known as others. Take the appendix, for example. Almost everyone recognizes and respects it despite the knowledge that one can get along without it very well. But the poor adrenal glands live in relative anonymity, known by few, while serving us all. ("Let's hear it for the adrenals!")

The adrenals are very complex GLANDS located just above each kidney. They are about an inch long and are triangular in shape. The HORMONES that they make (cortisol and adrenaline are the best known) are essential to control water distribution in the body; they regulate the METABOLISM of sugar, proteins, starch, and fat; they regulate the production of insulin (a hormone manufactured in the pancreas and essential to the proper utilization of sugar); they reduce certain inflammatory processes; and they regulate blood pressure. Altered function of the adrenal glands results in a multiplicity of symptoms and conditions that include obesity, hirsutism (excessive body hair), marked fatigue and lethargy, severe HYPERTENSION, and even DIABETES.

Diagnostic procedures for the adrenal glands include laboratory tests and X-ray examinations.

Laboratory Tests There are many. They are initiated by a collection of either blood or urine. See Chapter 17.

X-ray Examinations The adrenal glands can be seen quite well employing CT techniques. See pages 222–23.

Pancreas

The pancreas (I have never heard a patient use a common name for this organ, but you may get it in a restaurant by ordering sweetbreads) is located just below and slightly behind the stomach. This organ, unlike any of the other components of the endocrine system, wears two hats. It has two major functions and belongs both to the DIGESTIVE SYSTEM and the ENDOCRINE SYSTEM.

We will discuss only its endocrine activities here. (The digestive role is cited in Chapter 5.)

The pancreas manufactures the HORMONE insulin, which is essential to the appropriate management of sugar in the body. Altered production results in the development of diabetes, a most serious illness with a host of symptoms and changes: obesity, increased thirst, increased frequency of urination, changes in circulation, changes in vision, and so on. Altered insulin production can also lead to a condition in which there is too little circulating sugar —hypoglycemia.

Diagnostic procedures for the pancreas include laboratory tests, X-ray examinations, and ultrasound imaging.

Laboratory Tests   There are a host of blood and urine examinations that are helpful. See Chapter 17.

X-ray Examinations   The pancreas can be seen quite well employing CT and angiographic techniques. See page 212.

Ultrasound Imaging   See Abdomen and Pelvis in Chapter 20.

Ovaries

The ovaries are small, plum-shaped ORGANS, two in number, found on each side of the uterus in women. The ovaries are responsible for the manufacture of the egg cell, or ovum. They also manufacture female HORMONES that are responsible for the changes that occur in the uterus in anticipation of the reception of a fertilized egg—the menstrual cycle—and in the maintenance and development of the fertilized egg—pregnancy. Additionally, these hormones are responsible for what are called the secondary sexual characteristics such as breast development. Abnormality in hormonal production will cause changes in the menstrual cycle, fertility, pregnancy, and general appearance.

Diagnostic procedures for the ovaries include a physical examination, laboratory tests, and ultrasound imaging.

Physical Examination   The physical examination of the ovaries is usually called a "pelvic" or an "internal." See Chapter 6.

Laboratory Tests   There are a host of blood and urine examinations that are helpful. See Chapter 17 for the description of how these are done. Additionally, the mucus that is present at the mouth of the womb may also provide valuable information. The technique used for obtaining this specimen is described on page 58.

Ultrasound Imaging   This has become the most useful imaging modality to visualize these structures. See Pelvis section in Chapter 20.

Testicles

The testicles are the male ORGANS of reproduction. They are paired GLANDS, each about the size and shape of a small plum. They are found in a sac called the scrotum, just below the penis. They produce the male cells necessary for reproduction—the sperm. They also produce the hormone—testosterone—that is responsible for secondary sexual characteristics such as facial hair and depth of voice. (Testosterone is also produced to a far lesser degree by the adrenal glands in both men and women, and the ovaries in women.) Infertility is not uncommonly a result of altered sperm production, and changes in masculine characteristics may result from altered levels of hormone production.

Diagnostic procedures for the testicles include a physical examination, laboratory tests, ultrasound, and nuclear medicine imaging.

Physical Examination   This is an examimation that is part of the "routine physical." It is done by the gentle PALPATION of each testicle by the physician. The doctor will hold one of the testicles between the thumb and fingers of one hand while gently moving over its surface with the fingers of the other. Then the second testicle will be examined in the same fashion. This feeling and squeezing is **(+)** uncomfortable. There is no hazard. Time equals about two to five minutes.

Bottom Line: **(+)** What is there to say?

Laboratory Tests   The semen (the fluid that contains the sperm) can be studied. Additionally, there are a host of blood and urine examinations that are helpful. See Chapter 17.

Ultrasound Imaging   See Pelvis in Chapter 20.

Nuclear Medicine Imaging   See Chapter 19, page 264.

5

Go See a Gastroenterologist

A gastroenterologist is a physician who specializes in diseases of the digestive system. This person has graduated from both college and medical school. He or she has then spent three additional years studying internal medicine and after that, two more years devoted only to those problems that affect the digestive system.

The usual concerns that bring a patient to the gastroenterologist, and the usual procedures that are then performed to evaluate them, can be divided into four categories: problems of the upper gastrointestinal tract, problems of the lower gastrointestinal tract, problems of the gall bladder, and problems of the liver and pancreas.

For a detailed discussion of each examination, start with the accompanying table. It identifies the four major areas of investigation: upper GI, lower GI, gall bladder, and liver and pancreas. Within each category are listed the tests that can be performed. Suppose your doctor said, "I'm recommending that you have a biopsy of your liver." Find this test under Liver and Pancreas, and scan across its entire line. A quick synopsis of the pertinent data characterizing this study is listed. (These data are elaborated upon in the Appendix.) The last item on the line is the page number where the study is described in detail.

And finally, after you have read about the particular examination that you are preparing for, reread pages xiv through xvi, General Events Common to All Adult Diagnostic Procedures.

Gastroenterology

Disease Category/ Procedure	Discomfort* (−) to (++++)	Hazard* (−) to (+++)	Hospital (Incl. Short Procedure)	Special Prep.	Physician	Extras*	Informed Consent*	Exam Time* (Hrs.)	Bottom Line* (−) to (+++)	Exam Description (Page)
Upper GI										
Physical exam	(½+)	(−)	N	N	Y	N	N	½	(½+)	39
Laboratory tests	(++)	(−)	N	N	N	Y	N	2	(++)	39
X-rays	(+)	(−)	N	Y	Y	Y	N	½–3	(+)	40
Nuclear	(+)	(−)	N	Y	N	Y	N	2	(+)	40
Endoscopy	(+)	(++)	Y/N	Y	Y	Y	Y	2	(++)	40
Biopsy	(+)	(++)	N	Y	Y	Y	Y	3	(++)	42
Esophageal function	(+++)	(+)	N	Y	N	Y	N	3–24	(++) to (+++)	42
Lower GI										
Physical exam	(½+)	(−)	N	N	Y	N	N	½	(½+)	45
Laboratory tests	(+)	(−)	N	N	N	Y	N	¼	(+)	45
X-ray	(+++)	(+)	N	Y	Y	Y	N	1	(+++)	45
Endoscopy	(++)	(++)	N	Y	Y	Y	Y	4	(++)	45
Biopsy	(++)	(++)	N	Y	Y	Y	Y	3	(++)	48
Anal tonometry	(++)	(+)	N	Y	Y	Y	N	¼	(+++)	48

Gastroenterology—cont'd

Disease Category/ Procedure	Discomfort* (−) to (++++)	Hazard* (−) to (+++)	Hospital (Incl. Short Procedure)	Special Prep.	Physician	Extras*	Informed Consent*	Exam Time* (Hrs.)	Bottom Line* (−) to (++++)	Exam Description (Page)
Gall Bladder										
Physical exam	(½+)	(−)	N	N	Y	N	N	½	(½+)	49
Laboratory tests	(+)	(−)	N	N	N	Y	N	¼	(+)	49
Nuclear	(+)	(−)	N	Y	N	Y	N	2–4	(+)	49
Ultrasound	(½+)	(−)	N	N	N	N	N	½	(½+)	49
X-ray	(+)	(−)	N	Y	N	Y	N	½	(+)	49
Liver & Pancreas										
Physical exam	(½+)	(−)	N	N	Y	N	N	½	(½+)	50
Laboratory tests	(+)	(−)	N	N	N	Y	N	¼	(+)	50
Nuclear	(+)	(−)	N	Y	N	Y	N	2–4	(+)	50
Ultrasound	(½+)	(−)	N	N	N	N	N	½	(½+)	50
X-ray	(½+)	(−)	N	Y	N	Y	N	½	(½+)	50
Biopsy	(++)	(++)	Y	Y	Y	Y	Y	1	(++)	50

* See Appendix, Table Details.

Upper Gastrointestinal Tract

The upper gastrointestinal tract is just one division of a larger system, known as the DIGESTIVE TRACT, which deals with a major body function: digestion.

The tract is a long continuous tube that extends from the mouth to the anus. In different parts of the body it takes different diameters and different shapes according to the particular digestive function performed at that way station. It also takes different names in its journey. Let's start at the top—the mouth. Behind it, the pipeline through the neck is called the pharynx. When it reaches the chest it is known as the esophagus. Once it enters into the abdomen it assumes three major divisions: the stomach, the small bowel or intestine, and the colon or large bowel.

Back to the upper GI. For simplicity's sake, I have lumped all of the component parts from the mouth to the end of the small intestine (the ileum) under this heading. Almost all of the upper GI examinations performed apply to all of these component structures. Each is simply modified to accommodate to the uniqueness or the peculiarity of the particular part. As an example, X-ray examination of the upper GI can be described as a single study, although each component part is done individually as part of the whole. The exception to this approach is the esophagus. There are certain examinations that are unique to it, and these are considered separately.

Diagnostic procedures for the upper GI include a physical examination, laboratory tests, X-ray examinations, nuclear imaging, an endoscopy, a biopsy, and esophageal function studies.

Physical Examination The examination performed by the gastroenterologist will not differ substantially from that done by the cardiologist. See Chapter 2.

Laboratory Tests One particular study that is unique to this area is gastric juice analysis. It deserves a few explanatory lines.

Gastric juice is manufactured by the stomach and is an essential component in digestion. This fluid is a combination of chemical substances essential for proper digestion. One of the major components is hydrochloric acid. While too much of this stuff can cause ulcers, too little results in certain anemias and even contributes to the development of a certain type of cancer. So, if what you complained about up front, or what has been found already, in any way suggests that the "juice" may be the culprit, yep—you know the order: "Go have your gastric juice tested."

This procedure is described in Chapter 17 in the section Fluids—Intubation. Any other laboratory test that may be required is also found in Chapter 17.

X-ray Examinations   There are four common procedures used to investigate the upper gastrointestinal tract, as I have taken liberties to define it above. These are: deglutition, or swallowing study; examinations of the esophagus and the upper GI tract (the stomach and duodenum); and the detailed small bowel (jejunum and ileum) study. All of these are discussed in Chapter 18.

Nuclear Imaging   The two most commonly requested procedures are utilized because they are both highly accurate and "patient friendly" (easy on you). One, called esophageal reflux, is done to determine the presence or absence of hiatus hernia (a condition in which a portion of the stomach is within the chest cavity). The other, known as gastric emptying, is done to measure how long it takes for both the solids and the liquids that you swallow to actually leave the stomach. The description of these, and other less commonly employed procedures, can be found in Chapter 19.

Endoscopy   *End* is from the Greek, meaning "within." *Oscopy* refers to the direct visualization of a body cavity by a special optical instrument that is designed for the particular part it is to enter and see. Thus, "endoscope" is the term for an instrument that permits direct observation of structures within the body; in this case, the esophagoscope to see the esophagus or the gastroscope to see the stomach. Endoscopy is usually done if the X-rays are not definitive or if TISSUE is required for analysis because something was found, but it is not clear whether or not it represents a malignant process. Occasionally, particularly in problems of active bleeding where the patient is vomiting blood, the esophagus will be examined alone. However, the usual procedure when endoscopy is utilized is for the gastroenterologist not only to survey the esophagus, but to continue downward and visit the stomach and duodenum as well. The description that follows assumes that the entire upper GI will be looked at. (If only the esophagus is "scoped," cut the time that is given in half, and keep everything else the same.)

Preparation is necessary and consists of *nothing by mouth* after bedtime of the night before the examination. Although the study is commonly performed in a hospital, it does not require your being admitted. In all probability, you will be given medication that will make you unfit to drive, so if you do want to get home safely, bring a pal!

You will be asked to undress and don a hospital gown. (No reason not to bring your own robe if that would make you happier.) You will have to remove any dentures that move, so bring an appropriate container for them. A nurse will make you comfortable on some form of couch and a monitoring device, usually a blood pressure cuff, will be wrapped around your arm so that readings of both your pressure and your pulse can be made throughout the study. You will then be given some reasonably foul-tasting liquid to swish around your mouth, gargle, and then swallow. This is a local anesthetic, and within seconds things will begin to get numb. Next the gastroenterologist will give you some medication by vein. (The technique of an intravenous injection is described on page 160.) You'll experience a (½+) discomfort. This medication will make you very drowsy within a minute. You will not lose consciousness, but you will be amnesic (without memory) of the events that will follow. It is important that you discuss this phase with the doctor to be sure that this is acceptable to you. The alternatives are two: no intravenous medication and only the "local," which makes the procedure very difficult on both you and the looker, or more medication in the form of a general anesthetic, which imposes a higher risk factor on the study and necessitates your being admitted to the hospital either through the short procedure route (see the Short Procedure discussion on pages xvi–xviii) or for an overnight stay. If you go the #1 route (intravenous medication), which is really the easiest, or the #3 route (general anesthesia) you won't remember anything that will follow. If you tough out option #2 you will never forget it.

Here's what happens next. The doctor will have you lie on your left side with your mouth open. The gastroscope will then be introduced into your mouth, and then advanced down through your pharynx and into the esophagus. After appropriate inspection it will then be pushed further down into the stomach. Again, after what is to be seen has been seen, the instrument will be moved deeper, this time to enter the first portion of the small intestine, the duodenum. Often a specimen of the gastric or even the duodenal secretions may be obtained for later analysis by sucking some of the fluid back through the scope. It is also possible to remove (BIOPSY) a piece of any suspicious tissue that may be seen or that may have been noted on earlier X-rays. It is also possible to take direct photographs of the inside of the part through the instrument. The whole thing usually takes 10 to 15 minutes. The scope is withdrawn. You awake in another 10 to 15 minutes wanting to know when they are going to get started.

Discomfort rates a (+) unless you insist on no medication—then it is (++++); hazard is (++), since there is always the slight risk of poking the endoscope through the bowel wall and there is always the slight risk of serious bleeding, particularly if a biopsy is taken. Total time is two to three hours, when you add up everything, including the amount of time you'll want to rest after it is over before starting for home. You'll probably experience no remarkable aftereffects except feeling "kind of knocked out" for the rest of the day, and perhaps a mild sore throat for a day or two. (Remember not to eat until the anesthesia has completely worn off.)

Bottom Line: (+ +) Somehow you will think of it as a biggie but won't quite remember why.

Biopsy The entire subject of biopsies can be found in Chapter 17. As noted above, if any biopsy is to be taken it will probably be done at the time of endoscopy, and you will be unaware that it is occurring.

Esophageal Function Studies There are several different examinations that are performed on your esophagus for very specific reasons and with very specific findings. However, from your standpoint they will all seem like one long and moderately uncomfortable experience.

The esophagus is a flexible, predominately muscular tube, whose major function is to act as a conduit for the solids and liquids we take into our mouths as they move to our stomachs and intestines for digestion. It is appropriate that the movement is in only one direction—downward. Under normal conditions material, once reaching the stomach, should not reenter the esophagus.

This tube is not a simple rigid pipe. It has the ability to get larger (DISTEND) when we swallow, and to propel the swallowed material along by muscular action called peristalsis. Problems arise that affect this transit, and depending on their nature and severity, the swallowing act may become uncomfortable ("It seems hard for me to swallow solids; liquids are O.K."), difficult ("Food seems to get stuck right here"), or even impossible ("I vomit everything I eat"). All of these problems are grouped under the term DYS-PHAGIA.

Another common complaint that may require investigation is the sensation of pressure, discomfort, or actual burning, often, but not always, associated with eating, that is felt somewhere behind the breastbone in the chest. All of these various symptoms are grouped under the term heartburn.

And, finally, any chest pain that cannot be satisfactorily explained otherwise demands an esophageal evaluation.

Each of the various examinations has its own name: manometry, tensilon (edrophonium) test, acid reflux (Tuttle test), and acid perfusion (Bernstein test). They will all be described together.

Procedure 1 The studies will, in most instances, be performed in a hospital, but do not require your remaining there. The room will be "standard hospital" which means smallish, containing an examining table, cabinets, and a large machine that is the monitoring and recording device for the tests. There is prepreparation: nothing by mouth after midnight, not even medication that is being taken for diabetes or hypertension.

You will be asked to remove everything from the waist up, put on a gown, and sit on the examining table. The technologist will then spray a local anesthetic into one of your nostrils and your mouth. You will be asked to gargle some mildly unpleasant liquid which is also an anesthetic. Your mouth and throat will feel numb. You will then be asked to swallow a semi-rigid tube. (You may elect to pass it through your nose.) This tube or CATHETER will be gently pushed so that it eventually reaches your stomach. You will be asked to assist this passage by swallowing and relaxing by deep breaths until it is in position. Despite the anesthetic you will feel discomfort, and the procedure may cause some gagging. The degree of unpleasantness is highly variable but rates an average of (+ +). Relaxing, if at all possible, is the big trick—the less you fight, the less the tendency to gag. Slow and deep breaths are most helpful.

A wide belt will then be placed around your abdomen and a small metal disk will be placed over the front of your neck with a strip of tape. Both of these items are monitors that record various events such as the way you are breathing. They will cause you no discomfort. You are now ready! You will be asked to lie flat on the table, refrain from talking, and try to avoid swallowing except on command.

For the next hour or so you will be asked to do various things—all with that tube down your throat. You will be given water to swallow. You will be given medication by injection into a vein, probably in your arm. It is possible that this injection could cause you some short-lived problems such as blurred vision, lightheadedness, excessive tearing, sudden feelings of heat, or even numbness in portions of your body. Don't panic! If any of these events occur they are not dangerous, and will be gone in minutes. They could amount to a (+ +) misery.

Another event that could cause you discomfort is that a liquid will be injected into the catheter, causing symptoms that might replicate heartburn. You will be asked if you are experiencing such discomfort. If yes, another liquid will be put in to counteract the first.

Finally, one more message. Throughout the procedure the technologist will manipulate the catheter; he or she will push it deeper, pull it back, etc. Each movement will reactivate the discomfort and sensation of gagging. Unfortunately, they are all essential to get the job done. All that you can do is try to *relax*. Again, follow the slow and deep breathing suggestion. Figure that an hour is not forever, and then it will be over.

You shouldn't eat or drink anything until all of the numbness is gone— probably an hour or so. You may experience a sore throat for a day.

Bottom Line: (+ +) for most; if you are a "gagger" (+ + +).

Procedure 2 This is a 24-hour ordeal. It is done when your symptoms suggest that you are suffering with REFLUX but Procedure 1 failed to confirm the diagnosis. However, since it is well known that this problem is commonly intermittent it is possible that it just didn't occur during the first test. There-fore, to confirm or rule out the diagnosis, the problem is tested for over a 24-hour period.

It is almost the same as Procedure 1 as far as the start-up. A catheter will be positioned essentially as described above. But now the switch—the cath-eter will not be wired to the large monitor but to a small "black box" which will then be worn by you on a belt. Yes, you, the catheter, and the box are "one" for the next 24 hours. Because of the nature of the equipment and that thing down your throat you may be asked to remain in the hospital overnight.

Bottom Line: (+ + +) Especially if you are a "gagger" this is no joke.

Lower Gastrointestinal Tract

The colon or large bowel or large intestine makes up the lower half of the DIGESTIVE TRACT. The junction of the small and large bowel is normally in the lower right-hand corner of the abdomen. The large bowel then travels straight up until it bumps into the liver. This portion is the ascending colon. At the liver, it makes a sharp bend and moves across the abdomen from right to left (transverse colon) until it bumps into the spleen on the left side. It makes a sharp bend again, and heads straight down to the pelvis (descending colon). Here it makes an "S" curve (sigmoid colon) and ends at the rectum. The opening from the rectum to the outside world is the anus.

The colon is the final conduit of the system. All of the major digestive processes have already occurred higher up. The necessary food and fluids for the body have been absorbed and distributed. What is left must be eliminated, and this material is passed through the colon on its way out of the body. Some further processing, mainly reabsorption of fluids, occurs so that the waste product is normally in solid form.

The colon is particularly prone to tumor formation. In fact, in those over 50, direct examination of its last portion—the rectosigmoid—is recommended as a routine SCREENING evaluation every three years.

Diagnostic procedures for the lower gastrointestinal tract include a physical examination, laboratory tests, X-ray examinations, an endoscopy, a biopsy, and anal tonometry.

Physical Examination The examination performed by the gastroenterologist will not differ substantially from that done by the cardiologist. See Chapter 2.

Laboratory Tests The examination of the feces, known by laboratory folks as a stool analysis, is almost a routine request made by the gastroenterologist, who looks particularly for the presence of blood or evidence of infection. This and any other laboratory examinations that may be suggested are described in Chapter 17.

X-ray Examinations All of the usual examinations for the colon are detailed on page 209.

Endoscopy A general discussion about endoscopy appears on page 40. Endoscopy of the colon comes in three flavors: Bad, Badder, and Wow!

Procedure 1 ("Bad") This is called proctoscopy and views only the anus and rectum. Although this is an office procedure, it requires a moderate amount of preparation. These preps will vary but are all designed to have you arrive for study with the lowest portion of your bowel (the anus and rectum) empty. Sample prep: You'll be asked to take a laxative in the late afternoon preceding the day of study, and to have a light dinner that same night. You'll have a light breakfast and perform a cleansing enema an hour before the scheduled event.

The procedure itself goes like this: You will strip completely from the waist down. The assistant will position you on a table either on your left side with your knees drawn up to your chest or face down with your knees drawn up. The table may be tilted so that your head is lower than the rest of your body. The gastroenterologist will then expose your anus and may gently insert a gloved and LUBRICATED finger into your rectum to be sure there are no reasons not to insert the proctoscope. You may find this a (+) pressure. Then the proctoscope, a short, approximately 6-inch tube with a light will be inserted (sometimes, a simple rectal SPECULUM is used instead). The combination of the embarrassment, the awkward position, and the pressure of the instrument warrants a **(+ +)** discomfort. There is essentially no hazard and the examination takes only a few minutes. You may feel mildly uncomfortable the rest of the day.

Bottom Line: **(+ +)** This is one that, contrary to the usual, seems to get worse with reflection.

Procedure 2 ("Badder") The procedure called sigmoidoscopy views the sigmoid colon. This, too, is an office procedure, but it requires a slightly more demanding preparation than Procedure 1. These preps will vary but are all conceived to have you arrive for the study with the portion of the bowel that is to be examined empty. Sample prep: you'll have a soft diet the day preceding the study, have a liquid supper that night, and take an enema at bedtime. You'll then have a light breakfast and then a cleansing enema an hour before the scheduled event.

The procedure itself goes like this: You will strip completely from the waist down. The assistant will position you on a table on your left side with your knees drawn up to your chest. The gastroenterologist will then expose your anus and may gently insert a gloved and lubricated finger into your rectum to be sure there are no reasons not to insert the sigmoidoscope. You may find this a **(+)** pressure. Then the sigmoidoscope will be inserted. (There are two types of sigmoidoscopes—the rigid and the flexible. Demand the flexible, and don't take No for an answer unless there is a very compelling reason given why the rigid is necessary. There is a significant difference in the discomfort index between the two. The flexible is far easier to tolerate and it is also a better optical tool.) The flexible scope (I won't even describe the rigid) is about two feet long and about one-half inch in diameter. You will feel it "in you" but it is only a **(+)** discomfort. If it is necessary for the doctor to pump in air, as it commonly is, to obtain better visualization, add another **(+)**. The embarrassment factor, always a variable from one person to the next, warrants at least another **(½ +)**. There is a small but real hazard —**(+ +)**. With this type of examination there is always the risk of bowel PERFORATION and bleeding. Additionally, if the doctor sees anything that appears suspicious or demands further microscopic TISSUE evaluation, a BIOPSY can be performed through the scope. This does not, as a rule, add to the discomfort, but it does add to the hazard. For these reasons an informed consent will be required. The examination takes about 15 minutes. You may feel mildly uncomfortable and perhaps somewhat bloated the rest of the day.

Final Score: **(+ +)** It reads like it's worse than it actually is.

Procedure 3 ("Wow!") In this procedure, called colonoscopy, they examine "the whole thing." The procedure is performed by the gasteroenterologist either in the office or in a hospital, but hospitalization is not necessary. The instrument is called a colonoscope and it is always flexible. It is several feet long but only half an inch in diameter. The preparation of the entire colon is big time. The particular methods vary but the following is a representative sample: You have a low-residue diet (which consists of clear liquids, juices, clear soups, and gelatin products) for 2 days prior to the study. You'll take laxatives in the late afternoon of the day preceding, and one or possibly two enemas on the morning of the event. (An alternative to the 2-day "semi-fast" is taking an eight-ounce glass of a special liquid laxative every 15 minutes for 4 hours throughout the afternoon and evening preceding the colonoscopy, and the cleansing enemas on the morning of.)

The procedure starts like this: You will be asked to undress and don a hospital gown. An assistant will make you comfortable on some form of couch, and a monitoring device like a blood pressure cuff will be wrapped around your arm so that readings of both your pressure and your pulse can be made throughout the study. Next the gastroenterologist will expose your anus and gently insert a gloved and lubricated finger into your rectum to be sure there are no reasons not to insert the colonoscope. You may find this a (+) pressure. You will now be given some medication by vein, (½ +) discomfort. This injection will make you very drowsy within a minute. You will not lose consciousness, but you will be amnesic (without memory) of the events that will follow. It is important that you discuss this phase with the doctor to be sure that this is acceptable to you. The alternatives are no medication, which makes the procedure quite difficult on both you and the looker (because you will be tense and prone to move, which will increase the difficulty of the passage of the tube and in turn will increase your discomfort), or more medication in the form of a general anesthetic, which imposes a higher risk factor on the study and necessitates your being admitted to the hospital. If you go the Procedure 1 route (intravenous medication) or the Procedure 3 route (general anesthesia) you won't remember anything that will follow. If you elect option 2, you will never forget it.

Here's what happens next: The colonoscope will be introduced into your rectum and gently advanced up until the entire structure has been visualized. It is common to add air to help distend the LUMEN. Secretions may be ASPIRATED for later analysis. It is also possible to remove a piece of any suspicious tissue or even the entire abnormality, as in the case of small POLYPS that may be seen or that may have been noted on earlier X-rays. It is also possible to take direct photographs of the inside of the colon through the instrument. The whole thing takes about one hour. The scope is then withdrawn. You awaken in another 10 to 15 minutes wanting to know when they are going to get started.

Total time is three to four hours when you include how long you'll want to rest after it is over before starting for home. You probably won't experience any remarkable aftereffects, except feeling "knocked out" for the rest of the day—and even for the next day as well. Don't forget the rule of BAP—bring a pal! You may feel "gassy," which will last for hours. You may see some traces of blood in your bowel movements or on your underwear for a few days. If it is only a trace, it will pass. If the amount gets heavier, holler.

Bottom Line: (+ +) Somehow you will think of it as a biggie but won't quite remember why.

Biopsy   See Chapter 17. As noted above, if any biopsy is to be taken, it will probably be done at the time of endoscopy and you will be unaware that it is occurring.

Anal Tonometry   Anal refers to the anus, the last portion of the large bowel —the opening to the outside—and tonometry is the measurement of the tension of a part and is performed with a special instrument known as a TONOMETER. This is an examination that is not performed commonly, but in certain problems of constipation or fecal incontinence (the loss of voluntary control of bowel movements), it may be useful.

Procedure: Your lower bowel must be absolutely empty so that several enemas, which may be of any type, are required before you go for the test. You will then take everything below your waist off, and the doctor will ask you to lie on your side, facing away, and with your knees drawn up. He or she will then gently insert a lubricated gloved finger into your rectum to be sure it is empty. Discomfort equals (+). Time equals 30 seconds. If all is "go," a metal tube will then be gently inserted for a distance of about six inches—it is no worse than the finger. A second, thinner tube will then be slid through the first. This one has a special balloon at its end that will be slowly inflated. You will be asked to announce when you first become aware of its pressure. At this point, the response of the inside walls of your rectum to the expanding balloon are being measured. You will feel as if you have to have a bowel movement.

Total time is about 10 minutes, and you shouldn't experience any aftereffects.

Final Score: (+ +) It's mostly the indignity.

Gall Bladder

The gall bladder is another component of the DIGESTIVE SYSTEM. It is located in the upper right abdomen just below the middle portion of the last rib. The gall bladder works to concentrate and then store a liquid that is essential for the digestion of fats. This liquid is called bile. It is made in the liver and delivered to the gall bladder by tubes called ducts. When fatty foods are eaten, the bile is needed. The gall bladder contracts and pushes some bile into another set of ducts, which empty into the duodenum, where fat digestion occurs.

Prone to calculus (stone) formation, the gall bladder is also a frequent site of infection. Fortunately, it is an ORGAN that we can live without if it becomes necessary to remove it.

Diagnostic procedures for the gall bladder include a physical examination, laboratory tests, nuclear imaging, ultrasound imaging, and X-ray examinations.

Physical Examination   The examination performed by the gastroenterologist will not differ substantially from that done by the cardiologist. See Chapter 2.

Laboratory Tests   There is often need to determine the level of bilirubin (one of the components of bile) in the blood. How this sample is obtained, as well as information on other laboratory tests that may be required, can be found in Chapter 17.

Nuclear Imaging   See pages 263–64.

Ultrasound Imaging   See pages 283–84.

X-ray Examinations   See pages 210–11.

Liver and Pancreas

Both the liver and pancreas play a large role in digestion, but neither is concerned with this function alone. The techniques of examination for each are similar and can be described together.

The liver is the largest solid ORGAN in the body and perhaps the most complex. It lives in the upper right corner of the abdomen. Its primary involvement in digestion is that it makes the bile that is essential for the proper digestion of fats.

The pancreas is located just below and slightly behind the stomach. This organ wears two major "hats"—that is, it belongs to both the DIGESTIVE SYSTEM and the ENDOCRINE SYSTEM. The endocrine role is discussed in Chapter 4. Its "digestive hat" is the manufacture of ENZYMES needed in fat digestion.

Diagnostic procedures for the liver and pancreas include a physical examination, laboratory tests, nuclear imaging, ultrasound imaging, X-ray examinations, and a biopsy.

Physical Examination   The examination performed by the gastroenterologist will not differ substantially from that done by the cardiologist. See Chapter 2.

Laboratory Tests   See Blood Tests, Chapter 17.

Nuclear Imaging   There are no nuclear imaging procedures that are of any value for imaging the pancreas, but there are splendid studies for visualizing the liver. These are described in detail in Chapter 20.

Ultrasound Imaging   See Abdomen and Pelvis, in Chapter 20.

X-ray Examinations   All of the usual X-rays for the liver and pancreas will be found under their names on pages 206, 207, 211, 213.

Biopsy   The techniques of obtaining TISSUE suspected of being abnormal vary considerably and are dependent on where in the body the tissue is. Many BIOPSIES require the aid of imaging modalities such as CT, FLUOROSCOPY, or ultrasound. This is particularly true when the pancreas is the target, but is also the case if some particular defect has been found in the liver on an earlier imaging study. This subject is addressed in detail in the chapters on X-ray, ultrasound, and laboratory tests, which define the usual methods of approach.

Under very special circumstances the tissue sample may be obtained by inserting an instrument known as a laparoscope through the wall of your abdomen and into your abdominal cavity. This instrument permits both direct vision and also the ability to obtain a biopsy specimen. Once "in," it will be moved to the area of the liver to actually see the lower edge of that organ and choose the spot to obtain the tissue sample. This method of biopsy is far more common in gynecologic investigations than in problems of the gastrointestinal tract. If, however, it is recommended for your biopsy, a more detailed description of the technique can be found in Chapter 6, p. 63.

However, if there is laboratory evidence of liver disease or the organ is enlarged, a sample is taken from the liver without concern for an exact location. In these cases the biopsy consists of obtaining a specimen from the most accessible site—usually near the lower margin around the level of the last rib—and is usually performed by the gastroenterologist. No particular preparation is necessary, but you may have nothing by mouth after bedtime the night before the procedure. It is not uncommon, but not mandatory, that you will be given some type of medication, either by mouth or injection, about an hour before the study. This will reduce some of your natural anxiety and tension, but should not make you particularly sleepy. An assistant will expose your upper right abdomen and cleanse and drape it. The gastroenterologist will wear gloves and be gowned. He or she will feel the lower edge of your liver, select a spot, and inject a small amount of local anesthetic under the skin. There will be an instantaneous "burn" for a few seconds (+); then the area will be numb. The doctor will then take a somewhat larger needle attached to a syringe and firmly insert it into your liver. You will be aware of the pressure and even a dull pain (+). Once the needle is in place, the plunger of the syringe will be pulled back sharply, producing suction that will pull liver cells back into the syringe. The whole thing takes only a minute or two. The needle is then removed and pressure is applied to the puncture site for several minutes. That's it.

You will have to hang around for several hours being checked periodically to make certain there is no bleeding. You can then go home. There may be dull pain around your abdomen or even in the region of your right shoulder for the next few days. You will be advised to "take it easy," avoiding any strenuous lifting or exercises for a few days.

Final Score: (+ +) "Kind of scary, but not too bad."

6

Go See a Gynecologist

A gynecologist/obstetrician is a medical specialist who manages those diseases that are unique to women (gynecology) as well as another condition unique to women, pregnancy, in both its normal and its complicated states (obstetrics). To earn this title a man or woman, after graduating from both college and medical school, spends an additional four or five years studying how to recognize and manage these problems and conditions. Some practice both disciplines, while others limit themselves to one or the other. For our purposes we will divide the two and devote an individual chapter to each. This chapter is limited to subjects of gynecologic concern.

The problems that bring women to the gynecologist are many and varied and, for the most part, are age determined. Younger women suffer with abnormalities of menstruation, possible infertility, infections, and pain in the abdomen, pelvis, and breasts. In the middle-aged group, the changing pattern of menstruation, the beginnings of menopause, and concern about tumors arise. In the older group, tumors of both the breasts and the pelvic organs are paramount.

The usual procedures that are performed by this medical specialist can be divided into three categories of problems: breasts, pelvic organs, and fertility.

For a detailed discussion of each examination, start with the accompanying table. It identifies the three major areas of investigation—breast, pelvis, and fertility. Within each category are listed the tests that can be performed. Suppose your gynecologist said, "I'm recommending that you have colposcopy." Find this test under Pelvis, and scan across its entire line. A quick synopsis of the pertinent data characterizing this study is listed. (These

Gynecology

Disease Category/Procedure	Discomfort* (−) to (++++)	Hazard* (−) to (+++)	Hospital (Incl. Short Procedure)	Special Prep.	Physician	Extras*	Informed Consent*	Exam Time* (Hrs.)	Bottom Line* (−) to (++++)	Exam Description (Page)
Breast										
Physical exam	(+)	(−)	N	N	Y	N	N	¼	(+)	55
Mammography	(++)	(−)	N	?	N	N	N	½	(++)	55
Ultrasonography	(+)	(−)	N	N	N	N	N	½	(+)	56
Biopsy	(++)	(−)	N	N	Y	Y	N	½	(++)	56
Pelvic Organs										
Physical exam	(++)	(−)	N	N	Y	Y	N	¼	(++)	57
Pap	(++)	(−)	N	N	Y	Y	N	¼	(++)	58
Colposcopy	(++)	(−)	N	N	Y	Y	Y	1	(+++)	59
Cervical biopsy	(+++)	(+)	N	N	Y	Y	Y	1	(+++)	59
Hysteroscopy	(+++)	(+)	Y/N	N	Y	Y	N	¾	(+++)	60
Endometrial biopsy:										
Suction	(+++)	(+)	Y/N	N	Y	Y	Y	¾	(+++)	61
D&C	(++++)	(++)	Y	N	Y	Y	Y	1	(+++)	61
Culdocentesis	(+++)	(+)	Y/N	N	Y	Y	Y	1	(+++)	62
Laparoscopy	(+)	(+)	Y	Y	Y	Y	Y	1	(++++)	63

Gynecology—cont'd

Disease Category/Procedure	Discomfort* (−) to (++++)	Hazard* (−) to (+++)	Hospital (Incl. Short Procedure)	Special Prep.	Physician	Extras*	Informed Consent*	Exam Time* (Hrs.)	Bottom Line* (−) to (++++)	Exam Description (Page)
Fertility										
Laboratory tests	(+)	(−)	N	N	N	Y	N	¼	(+)	65
Physical exam	(++)	(−)	N	N	Y	Y	N	¼	(++)	65
Hysteroscopy	(++)	(+)	Y/N	N	Y	Y	N	¾	(++)	65
Endometrial biopsy (D&C)	(+++)	(++)	Y	Y	Y	Y	Y	1	(+++)	65
Laparoscopy	(+)	(+)	Y	Y	Y	Y	Y	1	(+++)	65
Cytology	(++)	(−)	N	N	Y	Y	N	¼	(++)	65
Ultrasonography	(+)	(−)	N	N	N	N	N	½	(+)	65
X-ray	(++)	(+)	N	Y	Y	Y	N	1	(++)	65
Cervical mucus	(++)	(−)	N	Y	Y	Y	N	½	(+)	65

* See Appendix, Table Details.

data are elaborated upon in the Appendix.) The last item on the line is the page number where the study is described in detail.

And finally, after you have read about the particular examination that you are preparing for, reread pages xiv through xvi, General Events Common to All Adult Diagnostic Procedures.

The Breasts

Diagnostic procedures for the breasts include a physical examination, mammography, ultrasonography, and biopsy.

Physical Examination Prepreparation is rarely demanded. Some doctors prefer that the study be made in the middle of your menstrual cycle, and others request that you refrain from ingesting caffeine, of any sort, for several weeks prior to examination. But they are the exception. This examination is not unlike that which you may (or *should*) be doing yourself. It will vary somewhat from one examiner to the next, but all will include both looking at and feeling your breasts—usually with you in both sitting and lying down postures. You will be asked to sit up straight with your hands in your lap; to lean forward from the waist; to raise your arms up over your head; to lie on your back; to lie on one side and then on the other. The doctor will gently glide his or her fingers over the entire surface of one of your breasts and then place your breast between each hand and press into it with his or her fingers. The nipple will be squeezed for evidence of discharge. This procedure will be repeated for your other breast. Your armpits will also be felt for any unusual lumps. There may be slight discomfort from the pressure—particularly if tenderness is your complaint. There may be an even greater discomfort—embarrassment. So score the discomfort category (+). There is no hazard. The most thorough of studies requires less than 10 minutes. There should be no aftereffects.

Bottom Line: (+) I hope you are finished and don't need more.

Mammography This is an X-ray examination of your breasts. At one time it was reserved only for those who had a positive finding on physical examination. Now it is recognized as the most sensitive detector of early disease—often well before it becomes evident to you or your doctor. The American Cancer Society, the National Cancer Institute, and the American College of Radiology all recommend that a baseline mammogram be obtained on all women between the ages of 35 and 39 years, and then every one to two years between the ages of 40 to 49, and then yearly thereafter. For those who have "high-risk" family histories—a mother, sister, or other close relative who has had breast cancer—mammography should be done annually after the age of 35. See Chapter 18.

Ultrasonography This study is reserved for those who have had a mammogram and the findings are inconclusive as to whether the "lump" seen is CYSTIC (which is usually BENIGN), or solid (which has a higher risk of being MALIGNANT). If the examination clearly finds the "lump" to be cystic, that usually ends the concern. On the other hand, if the images identify it to be solid, further study may be indicated. See Breasts under Chest section in Chapter 20.

Biopsy For BIOPSIES of the breasts two common techniques are performed and are described separately: ASPIRATION and INCISION.

Aspiration The general procedure for all aspiration biopsies is described in Chapter 17.

Incision *Incision* means "cutting into." This technique is often referred to as "open biopsy." It is resorted to when the LESION in question is solid and there is a suspicion that it could be malignant. If the mass was an accidental discovery on a screening mammogram and is so small or so deeply placed within the breast that it cannot be felt, it must first be localized (a technique employing X-ray guidance, which is described on page 192). If localization is not necessary, because the mass can be felt, then you will skip the second trip to X-ray and make arrangements for the surgical procedure. More times than not it can be done as an "in and out," or short procedure. That means that the deed will be done in a hospital but that you don't necessarily have to remain there as a patient. (Review the section describing the short procedure experience on pages xvi–xviii.)

On the morning of the surgery you will report to the hospital having had nothing by mouth for at least 10 to 12 hours. You will be taken to a hospital room, undressed, and given a hospital gown. The anesthesiologist will then inject some medication into your upper arm—(½ +) discomfort—that will make you sleepy, or at least, less tense. Usually within a half hour or so of your arrival a gentleman wearing a hospital uniform and driving a hospital carrier will arrive, help you aboard, and chauffeur you to the surgical suite. Here you will again meet the anesthesiologist, be taken into an operating room, and be prepared for the procedure. However, before they get very far, you will fade out. When you awaken, you'll be back in the room that you started in and there will be a dressing (bandage) over your breast. If you are to go home, be sure that someone is there to help you get home. You won't feel like driving. You may not feel like doing anything for a day or two— anesthesia just tires you out. If you can—it is not absolutely essential, but certainly desirable—take an extra day or two to relax. Your breast will be sore and discolored for several weeks. You will have to return on a prearranged schedule to see your gynecologist. (Hopefully just to get the stitches out, since the incision was undoubtedly closed by SUTURES, and not to discuss going back for more surgery or other treatments because they "found something.")

Bottom Line: (+ +) or (+ + +) I hope you worried for nothing!

The Pelvic Organs

Diagnostic procedures for the pelvic organs include a physical examination, a Pap smear, a colposcopy, a cervical biopsy, a hysteroscopy, an endometrial biopsy, culdocentesis, and laparoscopy.

Physical Examination This examination is commonly referred to as a "pelvic" or an "internal," and it goes like this: After you have completely disrobed from the waist down and have emptied your bladder, you will be asked to lie on your back on the examining table, which will have been draped with a sheet. You will then be asked to bring your knees up and place your heels into the STIRRUP on either side of the end of the table. (Some stirrups are built so that the backs of your knees rest in them.) This will cause you to be exposed, so a sheet or towel will be placed over your drawn-up knees. The labia (lips of the vagina) will then be separated and the vagina will be exposed. The gynecologist will insert one or two gloved and LUBRICATED fingers of one hand into your vagina while placing his or her other hand over your lower abdomen. Each hand then tries to reach the other, thereby feeling the size, shape, and position of your ovaries and uterus, and anything else that might be within your pelvis. This maneuver, called a bimanual, is mildly uncomfortable, usually only a (+), but sometimes a (+ +). This takes two to three minutes, as a rule. Next a SPECULUM that has previously been lubricated will be gently inserted into your vagina, in the closed position, and then opened so that the inside of the vagina and the cervix (the opening of the uterus, located at the back of the vagina) and its os (mouth) can be viewed. This, too, takes only a few minutes. This part of the procedure is known as the specular examination. It rarely causes more than a momentary pressure. When everything that can be seen has been seen, the speculum is closed and withdrawn. Now the last part—the rectal examination. When the speculum has been removed the gynecologist will again insert a gloved finger into your vagina and another gloved finger into your rectum. Again these fingers will seek each other out and thus feel anything abnormal that may be between them. This is another (+) or (+ +) discomfort and (−) for hazard. It takes about two minutes. Then it is over! You will be given a sanitary napkin, because the procedure may initiate some staining for a day or two.

So, although there is undoubtedly some embarrassment, and possible feelings of indignity or other negative emotions, the actual physical discomfort is only (+) to (+ +), and there's no hazard. A quarter-hour is all the exam takes.

Bottom Line: (+ +) Add this to your already-long list of "Why it's easier to be a man"!

Pap Smear   This examination is really a particular form of BIOPSY known as SCRAPING. (See Chapter 17.) However, it is so much a part of the gynecologic experience that it is described here in detail.

This procedure is probably the most frequently performed screening study for the detection of cancer of the uterine cervix. It is a procedure developed by Dr. George Papanicolaou, which consists of obtaining a sample of the cells that are on the surface of the cervix or which line the canal that extends from the cervical os to the inside of the uterus. Depending on whose statistics you read, the number of "Paps" done each year in the United States alone varies from 25 to 50 million. The American College of Obstetrics and Gynecology recommends that a Pap smear first be obtained at age 18 or earlier if the woman is sexually active, and then yearly thereafter. The results are reported in one of five diagnostic categories. Classes I and II rule out malignancy. Classes IV and V are of sufficient concern to warrant immediate attention. Class III is a maybe—maybe yes, maybe no—and should be repeated at least once before a final decision is made.

The examination: The procedure can be done any time except during your period. Although not absolutely essential, it is preferable that for the 24 hours before the study you avoid vaginal medication of any kind, douching, tub bathing, and/or vaginal intercourse. The exact same procedure identified as "specular" in the above description of the pelvic or internal examination is repeated. At the point where the cervix is visualized the doctor will insert a small applicator which has a special end appropriate for scraping (a SPAT-ULA) through the open SPECULUM and gently rub it against the surface of the cervix, and sometimes just inside the os as well. The spatula is then removed and rubbed onto some glass slides—the smear. There is no additional discomfort or hazard by this addition to the physical. So give the Pap exactly the same scores as noted above.

Colposcopy and Cervical Biopsy *Note:* These two procedures can be considered together, because if a biopsy is to be done it will immediately follow the colposcopy.

Colposcopy (*colpo* refers to the vagina, and *oscopy* identifies a visual examination) is an examination performed using an instrument called a colposcope, which is a short telescope that can be looked into like binoculars, and is positioned on an adjustable stand that has wheels. It is moved up to the mouth of the speculum that is dilating the vagina. It has its own light source and permits the examiner to see the surface of the cervix magnified as much as 40 times its normal size. Colposcopy is performed when there have been two or more abnormal Pap smears.

The examination: It begins like the specular examination that is described above. At the point at which the cervix is seen the colposcope is wheeled into place. It does not touch you. The gynecologist looks through it to better study your cervix and to try to locate the abnormality that resulted in the positive Pap. The first thing that may be done is to obtain a more substantial specimen from the os (or just inside it) than that which was gotten by the spatula at the time of the original Pap. A sharper instrument, called a curette (a loop or ring-shaped tool with sharp edges which is attached to a rod), may be used. This will be inserted through the speculum and just inside the cervical os. (It does not go up into the uterine cavity.) It will be moved in and out in a scraping motion. It will hurt (+ +)! This procedure can cause mildly severe cramping for several minutes. The cramps will subside in intensity but may persist for as long as an hour. The curetting takes only a few minutes. The major time is spent meticulously examining the entire surface of the cervix. This can take 10 to 15 minutes, but it does not add to the discomfort. Sometimes the examiner will "paint" the surface with a special dye that may improve the detection of abnormality. When all the looking and all the scraping is finished, a final application of a mustard-like material is made, both to diminish the bleeding that the CURETTAGE and maneuvers may have initiated and to decrease the possibility of subsequent infection. This may induce a momentary stinging.

Finally, observe the orders that you will be given—known as the "vaginal rest period." It prohibits anything, including tampons, douches, tub bathwater, and sex, from entering the vagina for two weeks.

Bottom Line: (+ + +) It's cold shower time again.

If the above inspection uncovers an area or areas of suspicion then a biopsy will be performed.

Cervical biopsy is the collection of a sample of TISSUE from an area of suspicion. Once such an area is identified at the time of colposcopy, the gynecologist will insert a biopsy forceps—a scissors-like tool with a special cutting end—through the speculum and to the area of concern. A small "nip" will be made and *felt*. The sensation is often described as a menstrual type cramp that is a (+ +) and lasts only seconds. A minimum of three specimens is obtained, frequently more. Each one has its own "pinch." When completed, all of the instruments are removed.

At this point, you're almost finished,—but there's a bit more: Because of the curetting and the biopsy there will be bleeding. Besides the blood there will also be some of the dye that may have been used, plus the final "mustard application." These latter products will change the color of the discharge and may even make it somewhat "lumpy." Therefore, do not panic! The bloody discharge should never be excessive (you shouldn't need more than one pad every few hours) and should taper off and be gone after a few days. If not—call the person who did the biopsy and find out whether you should be seen.

The ratings are about the same as the colposcopy alone, except add another (+) to the discomfort score, and give this a (+) for hazard as a result of the biopsy samples. Don't forget your pal and prepare for the "rest."

Hysteroscopy (*Hystero* means "uterus"; *oscopy* means a visual examination) is the technique that permits the inside of the uterus to be directly visualized. It is a procedure that is gaining in diagnostic popularity among gynecologists for evaluation of abnormal uterine bleeding and for problems of fertility. It may be used in conjunction with other procedures such as a D & C (dilatation and curettage, described below) to ascertain that these studies are thorough and nothing has been missed.

The examination can be done in an office but it is more commonly performed in a hospital as part of a more extensive pelvic evaluation which frequently includes both endometrial biopsy and laparoscopy (both described below). If it is part of the latter group then you will be asleep after having been given a general anesthetic. If, however, hysteroscopy is to be done without anesthesia you will experience the following: it begins, like almost all pelvic studies, by first exposing the cervix. (See Physical Examination, page 57.) A TENACULUM, a long forceps with a special end that looks like small prongs or teeth, will be passed through the speculum and will be used to grasp the cervix. The "grasp" is equal to a (**+ +**) ouch! It is necessary since it permits the operator to steady the uterus for the next step, which is the gentle insertion of the hysteroscope, a thin tube-like optical instrument, through the os and canal, and into the uterine cavity. This may add a (½ +) to the discomfort score. There is always the potential that it may be inserted too far and PERFORATE the uterus. So give hazard a (**+**). The total "look" takes about 10 minutes, and then all the instruments come out. You will be given a pad and told to watch for anything greater than mild bleeding for the next day or two. (*Note:* Often a thick and sticky liquid is put into the uterine cavity to separate its walls and permit better visualization. If that is the case, then the bloody discharge may also be somewhat tacky as well. So, if things are a bit different than you are used to, that's why.) You will also be advised against sexual activity for at least a week.

Bottom Line: (**+ + +**) Further reinforcement of an earlier conclusion: "It's easier to be a man."

Endometrial Biopsy The *endometrium* is the name of the lining of the inside of the uterine cavity. Sometimes a piece of it is necessary for analysis. It may be because cancer is a concern, because unusual changes in the menstrual cycle have been noted, or because of infertility. The procedure used to obtain this tissue is dependent on how much of a sample is required. If small, it can often be obtained by a suction technique that is reasonably simple, safe, and does not ordinarily require hospitalization. If more extensive sampling is deemed essential, then the procedure is more involved, has a true hazard factor, may require general anesthesia, and commonly demands a night away from home. This method of tissue collection is called a D & C (dilatation and curettage).

Suction Technique Review the technique used in performing hysteroscopy above. In this procedure the same steps are taken except instead of the scope being inserted, a fine hollow tube called a cannula is passed through the os and cervical canal into the uterine cavity—a distance of an inch or so. Suction is then applied to the cannula and pieces of endometrial tissue are sucked out. The suction does not usually cause a discomfort problem—it is most frequently described as a mild tugging sensation. There are several modifications to this procedure, but all are essentially similar.

Dilatation and Curettage Reread the section on the physical examination, up until the point at which the cervix is sighted. As with the suction method, the cervix must be grasped. Now the difference: A larger instrument will be used to obtain the tissue—an instrument that has a cutting edge, and is called a curette. However, the curette is too thick to pass up the cervical canal, so the canal must be dilated first. This is accomplished by gently inserting a series of flexible but solid metal rod-like instruments into the canal. These rods or dilators come in graded thickness. Obviously, the first to be inserted is only minimally larger than the diameter of the canal. This is followed by the next larger one, and so on—each serving to enlarge the opening. Finally, the canal is sufficiently dilated to permit the passage of the curette. The dilatation takes only a few minutes and is only minimally uncomfortable. The curettage also requires only a few minutes, but it is truly uncomfortable. The discomfort is such that more often than not the procedure is performed under general anesthesia. If general is refused, local anesthesia can be used. This requires the injection of anesthetic material around the cervix, a procedure known as a paracervical block. At least four injections are necessary, and each is at least a (+) hurt. And after these have been done, you will still have a good (+ +) for the rest because you will still feel a good deal of the scraping. Regardless of anesthetic choice the procedure carries a definite hazard (+ +), due to the possibility of uterine perforation and the possibility of excessive bleeding. Have a pal available for getting home.

The rules for after the test are the same as for similar procedures—two weeks of "vaginal rest." Holler if anything unusual happens that you weren't warned to expect.

Bottom Line: (+ + +) You'll be glad you brought a pal.

Culdocentesis *Culdo* is from the name of the space that is just behind the vagina, and *centesis* is the term used to describe the technique of draining off abnormal fluid from a body CAVITY. This procedure is invoked when other tests—usually ultrasound—suggest that there is free fluid in the cul-de-sac. This condition may be a result of a ruptured ECTOPIC pregnancy or as a result of PID (Pelvic Inflammatory Disease).

The procedure begins like almost all of the ones described above (see Physical Examination), when the cervix is visualized and grasped. The cervix is then pulled up and a thin needle is pushed through the back wall of the vagina. Yes, it hurts! It rates a (+ +) or (+ + +), but it lasts only for a few seconds and this explains why it is usually done without anesthesia. (Injecting a local in this area hurts about the same. Using a general anesthetic is considered "overkill." But you can insist if that is your desire.) Sometimes medication is given before the procedure. This helps, but will make you sleepy.

So, bring a companion. Be aware, however, that your potential escort may be going home alone, because if the free fluid that this procedure is all about turns out to be blood, you are going to go into surgery, right now! There is some potential hazard (+) and some places will demand an informed consent. The total time may be as long as an hour. You may experience mild staining for a day.

Bottom Line: (+ + +) Hard to rate this one—kind of a tossup between a big ouch and a white-knuckler.

Laparoscopy The prefix *lap* means the anterior (front) of the abdomen, and the suffix *oscopy* means the use of an optical instrument. Put them together and we get a procedure using a very special viewing tool that permits the gynecologist to see the outer surfaces of those organs found in the abdomen and pelvis.

The examination is employed after other procedures have failed to answer what is causing that pain low down in your pelvis, why your menstrual cycle is so "screwed up," or why after being on treatment for infertility for over a year you still can't become pregnant. In the past, the "final solution" to such questions was a laparotomy (an exploratory operation to "see"). Now doctors can usually "see" in without needing to subject you to a major surgical adventure.

Laparoscopy is now characterized as a short procedure. (See pages xvi–xviii.) You will come to the short procedures floor of the hospital having had nothing by mouth, including water, for the last 10 to 12 hours. Here you will disrobe completely and be given a hospital gown. Someone will take your blood pressure and check your pulse. You will then receive an injection into your arm (or elsewhere). This will be a medication to relax you for the main event. Someone will appear pushing a lovely carrier, invite you to hop on, and wheel you to the operating room. Here you will reunite with the anesthesiologist that you met when you registered for the procedure and your gynecologist. You will be moved into an operating room, which will have a table in its center and a large light fixture above it, plus all the other stuff that you can hardly focus on now. You'll be placed on your back on the table, with your legs up in stirrups. Nurses will hover about getting you ready. At the same time, you will probably have a needle positioned into a vein on the inside of one of your elbows by the anesthesia-giver. That may be all that you will remember because once you get some of their "good stuff" it's bye-de-bye time.

But, even as you sleep, here is what is happening: Your abdomen will be cleansed with an antiseptic agent and draped with sterile towels. The gynecologist will make a small INCISION about one-half to one inch long in or around your umbilicus (belly button). A tube will be inserted into your abdomen and a gas—carbon dioxide—will be run in. This causes your abdomen to DISTEND, which serves to reduce the hazard of the instrument's injuring any of the abdominal or pelvic contents. The laparoscope itself is a short tube that has highly sophisticated lenses and lights that permit the trained observer to make an accurate assessment of the condition of many of the ORGANS. In particular, the ovaries, tubes, and uterus are scrutinized.

Although the procedure is primarily employed to find out what's wrong, it can be used to correct certain problems as well. When this is appropriate, and you have given prior permission that this may be done, it could save a major surgical intervention. When all has been accomplished the scope is withdrawn and the small incision is closed. The closure is usually made with a type of thread that is eventually absorbed by the body so that it won't be necessary to have it removed. A small dressing is applied. *Finis.*

You will awake to find yourself in a different area, the recovery room. This space is usually a large holding area occupied by stretchers with folks like you on them, recovering from their surgical adventures. Skilled nurses monitor your condition until it is deemed stable. Meanwhile the anesthesia that you received earlier will have worn off and, although you'll be a mite groggy, you'll be taken back to the Short Procedures Unit for another short rest. Again you will be checked to make sure there is no bleeding or other surgical complication. When you can take water by mouth and are able to urinate, you'll be ready to leave.

From your arrival to final departure will be at least half a day or longer. Try to have someone there to help you get home. Although it won't be demanded of you, you will probably want to go to bed for the rest of the day. There may be some pain in your upper abdomen or even in the region of your shoulder blades. This would be from the gas they pumped in earlier. It is usually gone in a day. You probably won't have any significant abdominal complaints. You will be "kind of knocked out" for at least a day or two. If you must, you could go back to work and resume your normal activities the next day, but if you can arrange it, don't. Try to hang loose for at least another day or preferably two.

Bottom Line: (+ + +) This one is sneaky tough.

Fertility

Diagnostic procedures for fertility problems include laboratory tests of both blood and urine, a physical examination, hysteroscopy, endometrial biopsy (a D & C), laparoscopy, vaginal cytology, ultrasonography of the ovaries, hysterosalpingography, and a postcoital cervical mucus and sperm study.

Laboratory tests are described in detail in Chapter 17, and details of the physical examination, hysteroscopy, endometrial biopsy, and laparoscopy are described in the preceding section, The Pelvic Organs.

Vaginal Cytology   Cytology is the study of cells. Therefore, this is a procedure for collecting a sample from the vagina. It is performed like a Pap smear (see pages 58–59) except that the specimen is taken from the vaginal wall and not from the cervix.

Ultrasonography of the Ovaries   The ovaries are the ORGANS that produce the egg (ovum) cells necessary for reproduction. The ovaries undergo a cyclic change each month in the preparation of the ovum and its discharge. These changes can be partially monitored using ultrasound techniques. See the Pelvis section in Chapter 20.

Hysterosalpingography   This is an X-ray procedure that is used to evaluate the size and content of the uterine (hystero) cavity and to determine if the salpinx or fallopian tubes are open. See pages 215–17.

Postcoital Cervical Mucus   A sample of postcoital (after sexual intercourse) cervical mucus is collected shortly after intercourse; it provides an excellent method to evaluate the admixture of sperm and mucus at the mouth of the uterus. The sperm are examined for both number and movement. The mucus is subjected to tests to make sure it is normal.

The procedure is best served if intercourse occurs a day or two before your expected day of ovulation. There are methods you can use to establish when this occurs. The commonest is taking your oral temperature every morning before you get out of bed, and keeping an accurate record of it. Your family doctor or the gynecologist will instruct you how to interpret and use this data.

Intercourse should be performed without any lubrication, douching, or the use of a condom. The collection (performed like the Pap smear) must be obtained the same day by your gynecologist.

Bottom Line: (+) This is all business.

7

Go See a Nephrologist

A nephrologist is a physician who specializes in diseases of the kidneys. To earn this title, a person spends three years studying internal medicine after graduating from both college and medical school and then two more years devoted only to those problems that affect the kidneys.

Perhaps the largest group that seeks out this specialist are people with HYPERTENSION. Another major group consists of those who have significant abnormalities in their urine. The change that initiates the concern, uncovered on a routine analysis, is the presence of either blood or certain proteins that shouldn't be there. And there is also the group who experience a wide assortment of problems that, after initial investigation, seem to be secondary to prolonged and silent kidney disease.

All of the usual procedures that a nephrologist might perform or recommend are directed toward confirming or disconfirming the existence of kidney disease. Thus, all of these will be grouped under the one title Kidney.

Start with the accompanying table. It identifies each of the procedures that are the usual province of this specialist. Suppose the nephrologist said, "I'm recommending that you have a biopsy of your kidney." Find the procedure under Biopsy, and read across its entire line. A quick synopsis of the pertinent data characterizing this study is listed. (These data are elaborated upon in the Appendix.) The last item on the line is the page number where the study is described in detail.

And finally, after you have read about the particular examination that you are preparing for, reread pages xiv through xvi, General Events Common to All Adult Diagnostic Procedures.

Nephrology

Procedure	Discomfort* (−) to (++++)	Hazard* (−) to (+++)	Hospital (Incl. Short Procedure)	Special Prep.	Physician	Extras*	Informed Consent*	Exam Time* (Hrs.)	Bottom Line* (−) to (++++)	Exam Description (Page)
Physical exam	(½+)	(−)	N	N	Y	N	N	½	(½+)	68
Laboratory tests	(+)	(−)	N	N	N	Y	N	¼	(+)	68
Electrocardiogram	(+)	(−)	N	N	N	N	N	¼	(+)	68
Nuclear imaging	(+)	(−)	N	N	N	Y	N	1	(+)	68
Ultrasound	(½+)	(−)	N	N	N	N	N	½	(½+)	68
X-rays	(++)	(+)	Y/N	Y	Y	Y	Y	1–4	(++)	69
Biopsy	(++) to (+++)	(++)	Y	Y	Y	Y	Y	½	(++)	69

* See Appendix, Table Details.

Kidneys

The kidneys are paired ORGANS. Paired means we have two of them, one on each side. They live just below the ribs and in the back part of your abdomen, behind and below the liver on the right, and behind and below the stomach on the left. They are each about the size and general shape of a large fist. (Their shape is really closer to that of certain beans and certain swimming pools.) Leaving each kidney and heading south is a thin tube-like structure called the ureter, which ends up in a hollow organ located in the midline of the lowest part of your pelvis—the bladder.

The kidneys have many functions. Their primary task is the removal of certain waste products from the blood and the discharge of them in a liquid called urine—about a quart of it each day. Additionally, the kidneys are the regulators of a most critical bodily function called water balance. They also regulate the acid levels of the blood.

Diagnostic procedures for kidney problems include a physical examination, laboratory tests, an electrocardiogram (EKG)—resting, nuclear imaging, ultrasound imaging, X-rays, and biopsy.

Physical Examination The examination performed by the nephrologist will not differ substantially from that done by the cardiologist. See Chapter 2.

Laboratory Tests Urine testing is Numero Uno. Routine blood sampling is also essential. Additionally, there is one blood test that may be required in the workup that is unusual and done only in problems of unexplained hypertension. It is the evaluation of a particular substance that is made by the kidneys and called renin. In some situations the measurement is made from the blood as it leaves the kidneys—from the renal veins. This measurement requires a special procedure described on page 265. All other laboratory tests are described in Chapter 17.

Electrocardiogram (EKG)—Resting See Chapter 2.

Nuclear Imaging See Genitourinary section of Abdomen and Pelvis in Chapter 19.

Ultrasound Imaging See Abdomen in Chapter 20.

X-rays All of the usual examinations for kidney disease will be found under the headings Kidneys, Ureters, Bladder, and Urethra in Chapter 18. Also to be found in the same chapter, under the heading Heart and Arteries, are the discussion and description of the examination of the renal arteries.

Biopsy BIOPSY of the kidney is usually of the ASPIRATION type (see Chapter 17). Since the kidneys are rather deeply placed and often vary somewhat in their exact position, the study is usually performed with either X-ray or ultrasound guidance. You will have to remain in the hospital overnight following the procedure to be sure that it has not caused any harm, such as continued bleeding.

The usual procedure is as follows: You will arrive at the hospital on the morning of the study. Best not to eat breakfast. The aspiration can be done with local anesthesia, but instead you will probably be given a shot in your arm that will help you relax and will probably make you sleepy. The nephrologist or radiologist will perform the deed. You will be placed, stomach down, on a table in either an X-ray or ultrasound room. The side selected (either can be used but the right is more commonly chosen) is carefully cleansed and draped. A local anesthetic is injected into the skin over the site selected—a sharp prick and an instantaneous burn that lasts only for seconds—(+). This is followed by the insertion of a longer aspirating needle into the kidney. This *hurts*. It is a (+ +) or even a (+ + +), but lasts only for a minute or so. There is a small but real hazard (+) that there could be bleeding afterward; thus, an informed consent will be requested. Start to finish averages one-half hour. You will be monitored through the rest of the day and night for any evidence of bleeding. Although you will see blood in your urine initially, it should be gone by the next morning. Then you can go home. You will have a mild backache for several days and will be warned against strenuous exercise or exertion for the next week.

Bottom Line: (+ +) Rather tough.

8

Go See a Neurologist

A neurologist is a physician whose medical practice is limited to nervous disorders. This woman or man has gained this title only after graduating from both college and medical school and then devoting four more years to the study of diseases of the nervous system.

The neurologist is skilled in the diagnosis and treatment of ills that affect not only the brain and the spinal cord (known as the central nervous system) but also all of the other nerves in the body (known as the peripheral nervous system). Regardless of the symptoms, a history will always be taken and a physical examination will always be performed. Each major area—the brain, the spinal cord, and the peripheral nerves—is studied by procedures appropriate to its unique set of problems. Often the same examination, test, or procedure is used in more than one area, and sometimes in all. Although a particular form of examination, such as CT imaging, will always seem to be the same to you, it can provide different information depending on the problem at hand. Therefore, I will discuss all of the appropriate procedures commonly utilized by a neurologist in reaching a diagnosis.

For a detailed discussion of each examination, start with the accompanying table. It identifies each of the procedures that are the usual province of this specialist. Suppose the neurologist said, "I'm recommending that you have an MRI of your brain." Find this test and read across its entire line. A quick synopsis of the pertinent data characterizing this study is listed. (These data are elaborated upon in the Appendix.) The last item on the line is the page number where the study is described in detail.

And finally, after you have read about the particular examination that

Neurology

Procedure	Discomfort* (−) to (++++)	Hazard* (−) to (+++)	Hospital (Incl. Short Procedure)	Special Prep.	Physician	Extras*	Informed Consent*	Exam Time* (Hrs.)	Bottom Line* (−) to (++++)	Exam Description (Page)
Physical exam	(½+)	(−)	N	N	Y	N	N	½	(½+)	73
Laboratory tests	(+)	(−)	N	N	N	Y	N	¼	(+)	74
Spinal tap	(+++)	(+)	Y	N	Y	Y	Y	1	(+++)	74
X-ray	(+) to (+++)	(−/+)	Y/N	N	Y/N	Y	Y/N	1	(+) to (+++)	75
MRI	(+)	(+)	N	N	N	?	N	1	(+)	75
Nuclear	(+)	(−)	N	N	N	Y	N	1	(+)	75
Ultrasound	(½+)	(−)	N	N	N	N	N	½	(½+)	75
Ocular plethysmography	(++)	(−)	N	N	N	Y	N	½	(++)	75
Neuro-ophthalmologic	(++)	(−)	N	N	Y	Y	N	1	(++)	76
Electroencephalogram	(++)	(−)	Y/N	N	N	Y	N	1–8	(++)	76
Electromyogram	(+) to (+++)	(−)	N	Y	Y	Y	N	1	(+) to (+++)	78
Nerve conduction	(++)	(−)	N	Y	Y	Y	N	1	(++)	78
Evoked potentials	(+) to (+++)	(−)	N	N	N	Y	N	1–8	(+) to (+++)	80

* See Appendix, Table Details.

you are preparing for, reread pages xiii through xvi, General Events Common to All Adult Diagnostic Procedures.

Central and Peripheral Nervous System

The brain is the original personal computer; it was there eons before IBM and Apple came out with their inferior substitutes. It is a remarkably complex ORGAN, composed primarily of nervous TISSUE, which effectively initiates and controls most of the body's sensations and functions. It lives above and behind your face in a bony box—the skull—that protects it. It is only recently that the first real glimmerings of true understanding of how the brain works have begun to appear. It is subject to most of the ills that befall other parts of the body: infection, tumors (either originating in the brain itself or spreading to it from some other source), injuries, degenerative diseases often attributed to aging, and many more. Brain disease affects any and all of our senses—vision, hearing, smell, taste, and touch. Disease also affects our state of consciousness and awareness, our motor activities (movements), and so on.

The spinal cord is a collection of special nervous tissue that extends from the brain and travels south to the base of the spine. The spinal cord passes down through the center of a series of small bony boxes—the vertebrae, or spinal column—that protect it. It serves as the "telephone wire" that delivers messages from the brain to nerves throughout the body, and also delivers messages from these same nerves back to the brain. It, too, is subject to a variety of evils, not unlike those besetting the brain. Problems here, however, reflect losses of sensory (relating to sensations; for example, pain and numbness) and motor (relating to muscle function; for example, twitching, weakness, and paralysis) capacities of the body rather than those functions that are controlled solely by the brain.

All of the nerves other than those found in the brain and spinal cord supply messages to the rest of the body and are considered the peripheral (located away from the center) system. It is these nerves that tell you that you have just touched a hot oven or that you have stubbed your toe and it really hurts. The peripheral nerves are also part of that system that the brain tells to activate the muscles in your hand to get it off that hot plate, now! Problems at this level are localized to a particular part of the body.

Diagnostic procedures for problems in the central and peripheral nervous system include a physical examination, laboratory tests, a spinal tap, X-ray studies, MRI examinations, nuclear imaging, ultrasound imaging, ocular plethysmography (OPG), neuro-opthalmologic examinations, an electroencephalogram (EEG), an electromyogram (EMG), and evoked potentials.

Physical Examination You will be asked to disrobe completely from the waist up. You will probably be seated on an examination table and the neurologist will begin by looking at your head, neck, and chest for any obvious or unusual pulsations. That's called INSPECTION. This will be followed by having your blood pressure taken and having your heart and each side of your neck listened to by the examiner using an instrument called a stethoscope. (A detailed discussion of AUSCULTATION can be found in Chapter 2.) It will take a minute or two for both.

Next you will be asked to stand up, put your feet together and your hands at your side, and then shut your eyes. This takes a moment and is to see if you sway significantly or even fall.

Then you'll be seated again, and a short series of cursory eye tests will be done. (If any are even possibly abnormal, you will be referred to a neuro-ophthalmologist for more detailed and sophisticated testing. See Chapter 11.) The doctor will ask you to look straight ahead as a pencil flashlight is shined into each of your eyes. Then you will be asked to follow the examiner's finger with just your eyes as it moves closer and then further away from you. The same finger will start somewhere in left field and slowly move toward you. You must identify when you first detect the wiggling digit. Then, without so much as a warning, a wisp of cotton will be touched to the corner of each eye to see if you feel it. Finally, the doctor will look into the back of your eye with an instrument called an ophthalmoscope.

You will be asked to touch the tip of your nose with the tip of your right index finger, and repeat the same action with the left. Then you'll have to repeat the whole thing with your eyes closed. Again with your eyes closed, you will be asked to bring the tips of your index fingers around to the front of you so that they touch. You will be asked to extend your arms with the palms up; then instructed to turn each hand over so that the palms are down; and then told to repeat this "up-down" turning as quickly as you can, to determine if both hands end up (or down) in the same position. A coin will be placed in your hand and you will be asked to identify both what it is and even its denomination. You will be asked to extend your tongue. You will be asked to show your teeth. Something will be whispered into your ear, and you will be asked to repeat what was said. A tuning fork will be placed on the middle of your forehead and then behind each ear. Questions will be asked. Answer to the best of your ability—this is no time to "take the Fifth."

Next your REFLEXES will be tested with a rubber hammer. The most common site of attack is the inside and outside of each elbow, the side of each thumb, the front of each knee, and the back of each ankle. Each takes but a second and really is more fun than uncomfortable. The doctor will test your other reflexes by stroking the front of your abdomen on either side of the umbilicus (belly button), and the sole of each foot with a fine wooden stick or similar object.

You'll also be tested for strength. The doctor will place his or her hands on your shoulders and lean down with slight pressure as you raise your shoulders up. Similar movements will be requested testing your ability to move other parts (arms, legs, etc.) against some mild resistance.

By now you will probably be lying flat on the examining table. Delicate touches on different parts of your body will be made with a cotton wisp to determine whether or not there has been any loss of sensation. Then the doctor will use a straight pin to gently poke you in different places, sometimes with the point, sometimes with the flat end. With each poke you are to respond with "sharp" or "dull," as you perceive the sensation. The old tuning fork will come out again and you will be asked whether or not you feel vibration over the spot on which it has been placed. You may even be touched hither and thither with tubes containing both hot and iced water. Guess what you will be asked to respond. Right! "Hot" or "cold," as the case may be.

Finally, your large toe will be wiggled up and down and you will be asked its position when the motion stops.

That about does it. There may be a maneuver or two that is added or subtracted. The whole exam takes about 30 minutes to perform. There is neither discomfort nor hazard. There are no delayed effects.

Bottom Line: (½ +) Kind of fun in a nervy way.

Laboratory Tests Certain blood and urine evaluations may be helpful. CULTURES of the spinal fluid for infection may be required. See Chapter 17.

Spinal Tap Although listed as a procedure unto itself because it is so special, it actually is only another laboratory examination performed by a neurologist. (Often the doctor is an orthopedist, a radiologist, an anesthesiologist; any physician carefully trained in this technique.) This was once a fairly common procedure, but now, thanks to other modalities such as CT and MRI, which can supply similar data in a far friendlier way, it is reserved almost exclusively for those situations in which there is concern that infection exists. See Chapter 18 in the section on the spine for its description.

X-ray Studies See pages 178–88 under the section Head and 203–6 under the section Spine. There are no X-ray studies that evaluate the peripheral nerves.

MRI Examinations See Chapter 21.

Nuclear Imaging See the section on the head in Chapter 19.

Ultrasound Imaging The procedure most applicable to neurologic problems is the evaluation of the state of the arteries that carry blood to the brain —the carotid arteries. The study is described in the section on the neck in Chapter 20.

Ocular Plethysmography (OPG) *Ocular* is from the Latin word for "eye," and *plethysmo* is from the Greek for "increase." Thus, the term refers to any instrument that can measure changes in the size of an organ or limb, particularly with respect to the amount of blood present or passing through it. This examination further evaluates the condition of that portion of each carotid artery that is located in the head. (See ultrasound, above, which measures these arteries directly, in the neck.) This measurement is really of the blood pressure in each ophthalmic artery (a branch of the carotid artery that carries blood to the eye). OPG can detect STENOSIS, or narrowing, of these vessels of 50 percent or more. The procedure is routinely performed in patients who have suffered a stroke or who have experienced transient ISCHEMIC attacks (TIA) or dizziness (vertigo). It also is done as part of a complete neuro-ophthalmologic examination (see Chapter 11).

You will be seated in an examining chair which has a headrest and a back that can be lowered to an inclined position. After your blood pressure has been taken in each arm and EKG leads (see Electrocardiogram in Chapter 2) have been placed on your chest, the chair will be semireclined. Anesthetic drops will be placed in each eye—an instant of sting with a (½ +) discomfort. Then the technologist who performs this test will gently place a tiny plastic cup into the corner of each eye. (The cups are attached to wire leads that go back to a special machine, the plethysmograph, that supplies both the energy that produces the suction on the eye and also measures the eye's pressure, which is then recorded in the form of a graph.) The cup placement won't bother you because you have had drops. You will now be ready.

The doctor will instruct you to keep your eyes open and to fix your stare on the ceiling so that you don't move your eyes—*no matter what!* The "what" will be a sudden sensation of pressure in each eye, which is interpreted differently by different patients. Some say they see "lights"; others "snow-flakes"; still others "flashes" or "blurring." The pressure lasts no more than 20 seconds. Sometimes it has to be repeated, particularly if you move your eyes or blink. There is a wide discomfort index, (+) to (+ + +). There is no hazard. The procedure requires about half an hour to perform. No aftereffects once the anesthesia wears off except for occasional redness.

Bottom Line: (+ +) The eyes definitely have it.

Neuro-ophthalmic Examinations These are very specialized studies of the eye and are indicated when there are any abnormal or even questionable findings on the neurologic physical. These procedures are described in detail in the Neuro-ophthalmic Diseases Section in Chapter 11.

Electroencephalography (EEG) *Electro* refers to electrical impulses, *encephalo* to the brain. This is a study that detects and records the electrical impulses that originate in the brain. By placing SENSORS at carefully determined locations around the face and head, the impulses (often referred to as brain waves) from these various locations can be analyzed. The determination is performed for a variety of reasons, and there are slight modifications in the placement of the sensors and even in the duration of the procedure depending on the complaint being investigated. Perhaps the greatest value of the EEG is in the diagnosis of seizure disorders (the sudden onset of loss of consciousness, with or without convulsions, or muscular contractions, for any duration of time); but it is also useful following head injury, and in the presence of confusional states and many other suspected brain problems. Of growing interest is its special use in sleep problems and in the evaluation of impotence (the inability of a male to achieve an erection).

The routine first: No preparation is required. Comfortable clothes and time are all that you need bring. The technologist will take you into a room that has a chair and bed. You will be seated in the chair and for the next half hour or so it will be like being at a special kind of beauty salon. Some 16 to 22 very carefully selected sites around your head, including your forehead, the corners of your eyes, the bridge of your nose, and behind each ear will be marked by a skin pencil and then gently cleansed. Then the ELECTRODES, which have been prepared with a special paste, will be pressed firmly onto your skin and scalp. Each of these sensors has a lead wire that runs back to the instrument that will make the recordings—the electroencephalograph. Then the EKG leads (see Chapter 2) are placed on your chest. That's the "setup," and it is mildly uncomfortable (+) because there has been both rubbing and pressing. The rest is easy. You will be asked to lie down comfortably on the bed. For some of the time you will simply lie there with your eyes closed—many fall asleep. For some of the time you will be asked to take deep breaths on command. For some more of the time you will be asked to open and close your eyes, also on command, while a strobe simulator (flashing light) is activated. The frequency of the light pulses is adjusted and changed some 5 or 10 times, but all you do is "open and shut." That is the whole thing, and it takes about one and a half to two hours start to finish. The discomfort is (+). There is no hazard. The aftereffects are getting all that glop off your scalp.

In some cases in which the routine study is normal the neurologist may decide to perform a 24-hour observation, since a more prolonged search is often rewarding. You will be prepared in essentially the same way as above except that all of the electrode leads will be secured to a small monitor, about the size of a paperback book, that will be worn on a belt around your waist. You can go home when everything has been applied. The only thing you can't do is shower or bathe. The next day you return and they take everything off. The end. Give another (+) to the discomfort score because of the nuisance of the whole thing, and because you will miss your nightly bubble bath. Otherwise everything is the same as the routine described above.

Bottom Line: (+) for Routine; (+ +) for 24-hour. It's like the old way of getting a permanent wave.

Special situations call for special EEGs:

Sleep Problems This misery comes in two varieties—too little (insomnia), and too much (narcolepsy). These difficulties, particularly the insomnia type, have different causes that may be clarified by EEG testing. Apnea, a common breathing disorder that may occur during sleep, may be the culprit. Or certain muscular disorders may be the cause. Some cases are of a psychological nature. Monitoring by EEG helps to clarify the situation and direct treatment.

This examination demands that you spend at least one night—occasionally a second and even third are necessary—in the "Sleep Lab," which is a specially equipped room in a hospital. The setup of the electrodes is essentially the same as described above, except there are a few more, and they are more carefully secured in place so that they won't come off while you sleep. Another difference is that a nose clip like a clothespin is applied to your nose so that you must breathe through your mouth. And when everything is in place—it may take as long as two hours to get it all together—they say "Sleep!" (They seem to have forgotten it was this problem that got you to the lab to begin with.) For the tedium and "hands-on" of the electrode placement the discomfort is a (+ +). There is no hazard. It will cost you only one night, if you are lucky, more if they deem it essential. Except for fatigue there are no delayed effects.

Bottom Line: (+ +) Whatever it was that Hamlet said about sleep you will agree to completely.

Impotence Men usually achieve one or more erections during sleep. If there is something physically wrong, because of previous surgery or certain medications, for example, then sleep erections are affected. But if, as in most cases, the problem is of an emotional nature, the nighttime penile tumescence (swelling or erection of the penis) will not be affected. This test will document whether or not you had an erection while you were sleeping.

This procedure is conducted for three nights in a row. It is exactly like the routine, except that two sensors, each loop-shaped, are placed on the penis—one around the head and one around the base. The lead wires are attached to a monitor that is strapped around your thigh. The loops are only minimally uncomfortable, but many patients add a (+) for discomfort due to embarrassment. There is neither hazard nor aftereffects.

Bottom Line: (+ +) This is like adding insult to already-existing injury.

Temporal Lobe Seizure This is a very special type of problem that is caused by an abnormality in a specific location of the brain—the temporal lobe. When this problem is suspected, the EEG is performed exactly like the routine model described above, except that sensors are placed in each nostril.

Final Score: (+ +) With all the rest of the stuff going on, you will hardly be aware of the nose job.

Electromyogram (EMG) and Nerve Conduction Studies (NCS) These studies are about muscles and the nerves that supply them. Muscles work by contracting and then relaxing on orders given to them by nerves. A problem can be due either to the muscle itself or to the nerves that supply the stimulus to that muscle. When the nerve stimulus is to blame, that problem again may be due to the nerve itself—the peripheral nervous system—or to a cause that comes from the central nervous system—the spinal cord or brain. These procedures test for each possibility and are performed when the complaints are either motor (relating to muscle) or sensory.

The tests are best done in a special room that is copper-lined to eliminate any outside electrical interference. There is a bed and an examining chair for furniture. There is always a monitor, commonly large enough to resemble the console of the Starship Galactica. It will house a thousand or so switches and plugs (or so it seems), a TV screen, an audio system and heaven only knows what else. There is a technologist who monitors the monitor and a neurologist who tends you. You will have been advised to discontinue any medication that might be considered a muscle relaxant or an anticoagulant, and to stop using any body lotions for several days before testing. Each procedure is tailored to the area of your complaint; the whole body is rarely examined.

Testing the Muscle The electromyogram or EMG measures the electrical potential of a muscle. Under normal conditions there will be no potential if the muscle is relaxed. The electrical impulse develops only when the muscle works—when it is contracting. The doctor first attaches a small metal electrode—about the size of an aspirin—to your skin close to where you have the problem. Then the skin over the muscle that is in trouble is carefully cleansed. Another electrode or sensor in the form of a very fine needle is then inserted directly into the muscle. This insertion provokes a (+) to (+ + +) discomfort response which lasts for one to two minutes. The needle sensor and the skin electrode each have lead wires that return to the console monitor. Measurements of the electrical activity are made while you relax the muscle and while you contract it both gently and more vigorously. The needle position is then changed slightly—the needle is not withdrawn but merely repositioned. Another (+) to (+ + +). Measurements are repeated, relaxed and flexed. This can be repeated three, four, or even more times in the same muscle. The "ouch" just gets louder with each. The measurements take a wave form that can be printed out like a heart tracing (EKG) or be displayed on the TV monitor. An audible recording that sounds like a loud corn popper is another common method of analysis.

The "stick and measure" may be repeated in multiple locations—it is entirely dependent on your complaint. Over an hour is about average. The discomfort is highly variable, from (+) to (+ + +). The acute pain is gone in one to two minutes; the duller nag lasts three to six hours. There is no hazard. You will have both the doctor and technologist for company. It is not uncommon to have small "black and blue" spots (ecchymoses) over the sites of insertion that will last for a week or more. It is not uncommon to have a mild aching in the muscle for about the same length of time.

Bottom Line: (+ +) to (+ + +) Sometimes they really "stick it to you."

Testing the Nerve The nerve conduction study or electroneurogram is performed primarily to measure the speed of transmission of an electrical impulse across a nerve and the speed of response of a muscle to this stimulus. Electrodes are affixed to the skin over a muscle where the nerves are being tested. This sensor may be held in place by adhesive or it may take the form of a ring that can slip over a finger or toe. The nerve that is in question is then given a very mild electric shock with a small instrument (held by the neurologist) that is like a miniature cattle prod. The sensation is worth a (+) or perhaps a (+ +) discomfort score—no more. The impulse travels down the course of the nerve and when it reaches the muscle, the muscle responds by contracting. This feels like a strong twitch—(+). The electrode over the muscle measures the time taken from the initiation of the impulse to the nerve to the response by the muscle. The intensity of the response is also recorded. This "shock and measure" maneuver may be repeated multiple times and in multiple locations. Almost always a corresponding area on your nonaffected side is tested as well, to serve as a comparison. Each "shock" imparts a (+) or (+ +) sharp sting or burn that lasts only as long as the current. There is no hazard. There may be some latent twitching of the muscle that was stimulated that could last for several hours. Nothing more.

Final Score: (+ +) Here they "shock" it to you.

Evoked Potentials (EP)   The term *evoked potential* refers to the electrical response of sensory pathways of the nervous system when an external stimulus is applied to it. Three common procedures are performed:

Visual Evoked Potential   This is a test to evaluate the response of the retina (the back of the eye; see Diseases of the Retina in Chapter 11). The technologist begins by applying electrodes to the scalp in the manner described above under Electroencephalography. However, for this study only four electrodes are necessary. Once the electrodes are in place, you are seated in front of a TV screen. The room is darkened. A patch is placed over one eye. A picture appears on the screen that resembles a checkerboard—rows of black and white squares. This image is quickly replaced by another checkerboard that is identical to the first except that it contains one small red square. The pictures are made to alternate rapidly. This goes on for one to two minutes. Then the whole thing is repeated with the other eye. That is Part 1. Part 2 is also done with the head electrodes in place and with each eye alternately patched, as before. Now instead of looking at a TV screen, you are asked to place your head inside the opening of a large globe. There is a chin rest to support you. Inside the globe a flickering light goes on and off two times each second. You just look with each eye for about one to two minutes. Neither procedure produces any real discomfort and there is no hazard. Elapsed time, mostly because of the setup of the electrodes, is about a half-hour. You may experience "after flashes" for a few hours.

Bottom Line: (+) Boring.

Brainstem Auditory Evoked Potentials This procedure is performed when certain types of tumors (located either in the portion of the brain known as the brainstem or in the region of the inner ear) are suspected, or in certain types of hearing loss. Again there is a setup of electrode placement. An electrode is positioned with an adhesive paste on the midportion of your scalp, on each earlobe or behind each ear, and in the middle of your forehead. Earphones are then placed over each ear and you are asked to lie down on the bed. A series of tones, more like clicks, are then delivered to each ear separately. It is like "white noise." The room is darkened and you are encouraged to take a snooze. If you are like most, you will probably fall asleep because of the tranquilizing effect of the noise and out of sheer boredom. The test requires an hour of monitoring. There is no discomfort except in the application of the electrodes, no hazard, and no aftereffect.

Bottom Line: (+) Zzzzz . . .

Somatosensory Evoked Potential *Somato* relates to the body; *sensory* relates to the reception and transmission of induced sensations. These studies measure the condition of the nervous pathways from the peripheral nerves to the spinal cord, and from the spinal cord to that portion of the brain that recognizes the message—the somatosensory region. For example, suppose you are walking barefooted and you stub your toe. There is a nerve in that toe that is stimulated by the "stub." It starts a message going that moves upward from your periphery (the toe, in this case) until it gets to the big relay station —the spinal cord. Nerves in the cord then move the "stub" along the highway heading north until it gets to the end of the line—the somatosensory center. Then, suddenly, you both feel the pain and' exclaim *ouch!* That transmission and the time it took can be measured and are important to evaluate in certain problems that may affect both muscles and nerves, particularly injuries or diseases of the spinal cord.

The study is performed by again applying electrodes. As in the other studies, some are attached to the scalp. Five individual sensors are affixed to the spine, from top to bottom. Other sensors are placed in accordance with the area that is to be tested. Using the previous example, let us assume that after you stubbed your toe, the "ouch" was never felt. Was it because the "toe nerve" never sent the message, or was the message lost somewhere along the way? Sensors are positioned and stimuli are given along the entire pathway. The precise location of the breakdown will be established.

Each area evaluated requires at least 30 minutes, so that the entire examination may take many hours. Each area stimulated evokes its own degree of discomfort, ranging from ($\frac{1}{2}$ +) to (+ + +). There is no hazard. The only aftereffects are occasional twitching in the muscles of the parts studied.

Bottom Line: (+ +) to (+ + +) Let us hope that this does not evoke your potential for anger.

CHAPTER

9

Go See an Obstetrician

An obstetrician/gynecologist is a doctor who has chosen to specialize in pregnancy in both its normal and its complicated states (obstetrics), as well as in the recognition and management of diseases that are unique to women (gynecology). This title is appropriate only after the woman or man has graduated from both college and medical school and then has spent an additional four or five years studying how to recognize and manage these conditions and problems. Some of these physicians practice both disciplines, while others limit themselves to one. For our purposes we will divide the two and devote this chapter to obstetrics.

The obstetrician always hopes that your opening lines will be "I am pregnant. I am fine. Take care of me" and that the words "pregnant" and "fine" portend a normal progression to a happy ending. But often the progression is not normal. "Fine" changes to such problems as bleeding, cramping, unusual weight gain, or significant blood pressure elevation. The happy ending is then in serious jeopardy. The cause or causes of these events must be ferreted out so that appropriate corrections can be made. The ferreting constitutes the procedures that the obstetrician will employ.

For a detailed discussion of each examination, start with the accompanying table. It identifies each of the procedures that are the usual province of this specialist. Suppose your obstetrician said, "I'm recommending that you have an amniocentesis to make sure that your baby does not have a genetic disorder." Find this test under Ultrasound, and read across its entire line. A quick synopsis of the pertinent data characterizing this study is listed. (These

Obstetrics

Procedure	Discomfort* (-) to (++++)	Hazard* (-) to (+++)	Hospital (Incl. Short Procedure)	Special Prep.	Special Physician	Extras*	Informed Consent*	Exam Time* (Hrs.)	Bottom Line* (-) to (++++)	Exam Description (Page)
Physical exam	(+)	(-)	N	N	Y	N	N	½	(+)	85
Laboratory tests	(+)	(-)	N	N	N	Y	N	¼	(+)	86
Ultrasound:										
Routine	(+)	(-)	N	N	N	Y	N	½	(+)	87
Amniocentesis	(++)	(+)	N	N	Y	Y	Y	½	(++)	87
Chorionic villus sampling	(++) to (+++)	(++)	N	N	Y	Y	Y	½	(++) to (+++)	87
High-risk (special tests):										
Nonstress	(+)	(-)	N	N	N	Y	N	½	(+)	88
Oxytocin stress	(++) to (+++)	(+)	Y	N	Y	Y	Y	1	(++)	88
Fetal monitoring	(++)	(-)	Y	N	Y	Y	N	?	(+)	88

* See Appendix, Table Details.

data are elaborated upon in the Appendix.) The last item on the line is the page number where the study is described in detail.

And finally, after you have read about the particular examination that you are preparing for, reread pages xiii through xvi, General Events Common to All Adult Diagnostic Procedures.

Pregnancy

Unlike almost every other medical specialist, the obstetrician is sought out for a condition that is *normal*—the state of pregnancy. When this condition proceeds without event the physician's role is monitoring the progression and reassuring the mother-to-be that all is well. When the incubation and maturation period has run its natural course this same physician assists the mother in delivering her child.

However, when in the course of fetal events something unexpected and untoward arises, either during the pregnancy or at delivery, or both, this physician is skilled in meeting these challenges. The first step is usually to find out what is wrong.

Diagnostic procedures for pregnancy include physical examinations; laboratory tests; ultrasound imaging as a routine and for special procedures known as amniocentesis and chorionic villus sampling; possibly an MRI; and special tests for high-risk situations.

Physical Examination The physical examination, like almost all of the other procedures that will be performed during the nine-month period throughout which you will visit this specialist, will depend on the stage of your pregnancy and your general condition. Thus, the examination is best described in two parts: the first visit, and thereafter.

The first visit, which takes place when you may not even be certain that you are really pregnant, will probably result in your most thorough and comprehensive physical. It can be considered as a "two-fer." It will be similar to the exams that are done by a cardiologist and a gynecologist. Both of these examinations are detailed in their respective chapters. (See Chapter 2 and Chapter 6.)

All subsequent visits will also be of the "two-fer" variety, but this time one is for you and the other is for the boarder with the nine-month lease. The evaluation (presuming that this is a simple, routine, scheduled visit and all is well) will consist of checking your blood pressure, your heart, the condition of your breasts, and the size of your abdomen. The boarder will be checked by feeling for its size and position and monitoring its heart rate once that becomes possible. To do this, the obstetrician places a stethoscope over your lower abdomen—the part that is getting bigger—finds the baby's heart, and listens.

The total time for your first visit could be an hour. The thereafters average about 15 minutes each. There is no true discomfort except for the (+) of the "internal." There is never a hazard.

Bottom Line: (+) Let's hope the stethoscope is warm.

Laboratory Tests These, like the physical, are routine and geared to the stage of the pregnancy, and whether or not any problems exist. They are also geared to evaluate both you and your little friend. Most of these procedures are performed on urine and blood. There is one blood test that is quite special and that you may be told you are going to have. It is called MSAFP—Maternal Serum Alpha Feto Protein—and concerns the substance made by the baby that enters both the amniotic fluid (the bag of water that surrounds the fetus) and your blood. Its level can predict with high accuracy the possibility of a neural tube defect (the neural tube is the portion of the embryo that will develop into the brain and spine), Down's syndrome, and other similar CHROMOSOMAL abnormalities. But from your standpoint, this test is like any other blood test—someone will collect blood from a vein in your arm. What is done to that sample happens in the laboratory, a long way away from you. See the appropriate sections in Chapter 17.

Ultrasound Imaging Ultrasound has become the Numero Uno of pregnancy procedures. Because the images can be obtained without producing any hazard to either you or the baby, as was the case when X-rays were used, it has almost completely replaced all other modalities in monitoring the progress of the baby's development. As the technology continues to improve (see Chapter 20), more and more information can be obtained—and it can be obtained at earlier and earlier stages of development. Ultrasound may also uncover problems in the fetus that can be solved, saving some otherwise-threatened pregnancies or improving conditions until the baby is born. For example, blood transfusions can be given to the baby if tests suggest that there is such a need, and its bladder may be emptied if there is evidence of a developmental deformity that prevents the baby from urinating, which it must do normally.

Routine Imaging Ultrasound inspection will be a common and oft-repeated study throughout your pregnancy. The frequency and intervals along the way vary from one obstetrician to the next. Ultrasound will identify whether the pregnancy is single or multiple and it is thus used to monitor the size and development of the baby or babies. It is also of invaluable aid in assessing the amount of fluid that surrounds the fetus, and in determining the position and development of the placenta (the organ that forms in the mother's uterus during pregnancy and joins her to the baby). And there is an extra plus to this procedure. Every time it is done you can visit with your baby, because you can see what the doctor is seeing! The details of this procedure are described on pages 286–88.

Amniocentesis Amnion is a tissue or MEMBRANE that envelops the fetus. This is a one-time special procedure that is done when there is any reason to suspect that developmental or hereditary abnormalities might exist. When the indications for the examination are present, it will be done at about the fourteenth to eighteenth week of the pregnancy. If a caesarean section is contemplated, this procedure can clarify any uncertainty as to the exact age and/or maturity of the fetus. When this is the reason for the examination, it is done later in the pregnancy. See page 288.

Chorionic Villus Sampling This study is performed for the same reasons that send you for an amniocentesis. This procedure has an advantage over the "amnio" in that it can be performed as early as the eighth to the twelfth week of the pregnancy, and its results can be obtained in a far shorter period of time. Thus, if any abnormality is discovered it can be resolved so much sooner, and if everything is normal, peace of mind can also begin so much sooner. However, there is concern among some obstetricians that this procedure may be more hazardous than the "amnio." Those who perform chorionic villus sampling with regularity and have become skillful in its technique feel that this concern is unwarranted. (As of this writing the final word is not yet in.) See page 288.

MRI Since MRI can obtain exquisite images without using radiation it may not present any hazard to the baby, and therefore might be most helpful in certain problems that are not fully solved by other techniques. However, there has not yet been sufficient time to study any other hazards that its use might evoke. Thus the (?) as to its place in this area of diagnosis. See Chapter 21.

Special Tests for High-Risk Situations When the pregnancy is considered to be at high risk, whether due to a maternal history of diabetes, hypertension, heart disease, substance abuse (alcohol and/or drugs), obesity, anemia, previous difficult pregnancies (including delivery by caesarean section), previous stillborn delivery and/or spontaneous abortion, prolonged labor, or maternal age of under 16 or over 35, additional procedures may be performed.

Nonstress Testing This procedure is not one for the heart. It evaluates the function of the placenta and the extent of fetal movements and heart rate and is done routinely by some obstetricians throughout the last three months. It is done by having you lie flat on your back with your abdomen exposed. A wide rubber belt that is wired to a particular type of ultrasound device is placed around your "belly." When the baby moves or kicks, its movements will be transmitted to your abdomen and thence to the monitoring belt. The baby's heart rate will also be recorded and correlated to its movements. The measurements are made over a 20-minute period. They are neither uncomfortable nor hazardous—just boring.

Bottom Line: (½ +) How could nine months seem so long?

Oxytocin Stress Test Oxytocin is a hormone that initiates uterine contractions. This test is also performed to evaluate placental function and fetal well-being, and is done late in the pregnancy when there might be a decision required as to whether the delivery should be normal or by surgery. It, too, requires the use of the ultrasound monitoring belt around your abdomen. (See Nonstress Test, above.) A small amount of oxytocin will be injected into one of your veins. Almost immediately you will experience some cramping in your abdomen. This is your uterus contracting in response to the medication. Each contraction will be of short duration and not remarkably painful. The number, intensity, and relationship of these contractions to the baby's heart rate will be recorded and the status of the pregnancy decided. The discomfort could be (+ +) to (+ + +) and there is a (+) hazard that the test could initiate true labor. The effects of the injection last only about 15 minutes.

Bottom Line: (+ +) It's like a preview of coming events.

Fetal Monitoring It is becoming common practice to monitor the fetus at the time of labor and delivery to correlate the frequency and intensity of the uterine contractions with the fetal heart rate. When this is done the method may be identical to that described above under Nonstress Test—a simple external belt may be placed around your abdomen. There is another monitoring system, however, that is thought to be more accurate. In this method, detectors are passed through your vagina and into your uterus to be attached to the baby's scalp and the inside of the uterus. The placement of these probes is not any more uncomfortable than the internal examination that you know, and the actual monitoring is without sensation. Indeed, while this is happening you will also be in labor, so that your attention might be somewhat diverted to other happenings.

Bottom Line: (+) "As long as it's healthy . . ."

10

Go See an Oncologist-Hematologist

An oncologist-hematologist specializes in the recognition and treatment of cancer in all of its forms and in the recognition and treatment of diseases of the blood. To warrant this title men and women study for at least five years following graduation from both college and medical school, three years in internal medicine, and two or more after that devoted only to cancer and blood disorders.

Almost all patients seen by the oncologist-hematologist arrive with an established diagnosis of either some form of cancer or with some form of blood disease. However, an ultimate management plan cannot be formulated until this medical specialist knows just how extensive the problem really is. And, to answer that question, additional procedures are invoked. All of the usual examinations are grouped under one title: staging.

For a detailed discussion of each examination, start with the accompanying table. It identifies each of the procedures that are the usual province of this specialist. Suppose your doctor said, "I'm recommending that you have your liver biopsied to see if your disease has spread." Find this test under biopsy, and read across its entire line. A quick synopsis of the pertinent data characterizing this study is listed. (These data are elaborated upon in the Appendix). The last item on the line is the page number where the study is described in detail.

And finally, after you have read about the particular examination that

Oncology-Hematology

Procedure	Discomfort* (−) to (++++)	Hazard* (−) to (+++)	Hospital (Incl. Short Procedure)	Special Prep.	Physician	Extras*	Informed Consent*	Exam Time* (Hrs.)	Bottom Line* (−) to (++++)	Exam Description (Page)
Physical exam	(+)	(−)	N	N	Y	N	N	½	(+)	92
Laboratory tests	(+) to (+++)	(−)	N	N	N	Y	N	¼	(+) to (+++)	92
Nuclear	(+)	(−)	N	N	N	Y	N	4	(+)	92
Ultrasound	(½+)	(−)	N	N	N	Y	N	½−1	(½+)	92
X-ray	(+)	(−)	N	N	N	Y	N	1	(+)	92
MRI	(+)	(−)	N	Y	Y	Y	Y	1	(+)	92
Biopsy	(++) to (++++)	(++) or (+++)	Y	Y	Y	Y	Y	?	(++) to (++++)	93

* See Appendix, Table Details.

you are preparing for, reread pages xiii through xvi, General Events Common to All Adult Diagnostic Procedures.

Staging

Unlike almost every other medical specialty—in most cases, the practitioner deals only with a particular ORGAN or organ system—oncology tends all forms of MALIGNANCY, which can attack any organ or organ system. Additionally, cancer has its own unique set of circumstances: each type begins differently; each has its own symptom complex; each spreads in its own manner; each is treated individually. Thus when you are told to undergo a particular procedure necessary in the staging process, you must find the particular study required under the specific body part or system in the general category of the examination. If, for example, you are ordered to have a bone scan, you will be told that it is a nuclear imaging procedure, and you will be able to find the detailed description by going to Chapter 19 and finding Bone Scan under Skeletal System in its table.

Diagnostic procedures for staging include a physical examination, laboratory tests, nuclear imaging, ultrasound imaging, X-ray, magnetic resonance imaging (MRI), and a biopsy.

Physical Examination   The examination performed by the oncologist will not differ substantially from that done by the cardiologist. (See Chapter 2.)

Laboratory Tests   There is one blood test that is unique to the workup of these problems and that is bone marrow sampling. This particular procedure is always done by the oncologist-hematologist rather than in the laboratory by a technologist. The techniques are described in Chapter 17.

Nuclear Imaging   See Chapter 19.

Ultrasound Imaging   See Chapter 20.

X-rays   See Chapter 18.

MRI   See Chapter 21.

Biopsy   General discussions of the procedures of BIOPSY are found in several chapters, including Chapter 17. There is, however, a special procedure that technically fits under the category of excisional biopsy but is really a "big-time" surgical procedure. This is called a splenectomy (removal of the spleen, an organ found in the upper left part of your abdomen) and is done as a staging procedure in certain malignancies of the LYMPHATIC SYSTEM. (The lymphatic system is described in Chapter 19 in the section Abdomen and Pelvis; see pages 268–69). It requires hospitalization for several days and is a full-blown surgical experience under a general anesthetic. You will have a lovely scar of over six inches on your left side under your ribs, and a recovery period of perhaps a week. Be sure to talk to both the surgeon and anesthesiologist who will attend you for further details. (This procedure is further detailed here because a major surgical procedure is not commonly done for diagnostic purposes. When it is, the doctors performing the surgery may have their own specific directions that will be relayed to you at the time.)

Final Score: (+ + + +) As with any major surgical procedure, you will not easily forget it.

CHAPTER

11

Go See an Ophthalmologist

An ophthalmologist is a physician who has spent four years after graduating from both college and medical school studying the characteristics and treatment of the vast array of diseases that may affect the eyes.

Opthalmology is no different from other branches of medicine where subspecialties have developed because increasing knowledge of the subject and its complexities makes it impossible for one person to be proficient in the whole field. Among ophthalmologists, there are those who are concerned with general eye problems, such as vision that will improve with corrective lenses (glasses), and who correct any condition that affects the transparency of the lenses, such as cataracts; those who deal only with diseases of the cornea (the colorless front of the eye); those who deal only with a most serious, and unfortunately common, disease called glaucoma, which, if uncorrected, leads to blindness; those who specialize in neuro-ophthalmology and concern themselves with problems of the optic nerve, including multiple sclerosis, myasthenia gravis, hyperthyroidism, and certain tumors; and those who concern themselves with diseases of the retina (the eyegrounds).

Each category of specialization has its own list of examinations. Many of the studies are similar, while others are specific to one area of concern.

For a detailed discussion of each examination, start with the accompanying table. It identifies the five major areas of investigation—general, corneal, retinal, glaucoma, and neuro-ophthalmic. Within each category are listed the tests that can be performed. Suppose your doctor said, "I'm recommending that you see an eye doctor and have a thorough checkup." Find General, and note the various procedures that can be performed. Then scan across each entire line. A quick synopsis of the pertinent data characterizing this study is listed. (These data are elaborated upon in the Appendix.) The last item on the line is the page number where the study is described in detail.

And finally, after you have read about the particular examination that you are preparing for, reread pages xiv through xvi, General Events Common to All Adult Diagnostic Procedures.

General Diseases of the Eye

The practitioner of general ophthalmology is the "Family Doctor" of the eye. This doctor is usually seen first with any complaint. He or she will determine why things have gotten "blurry" or why your arms have gotten either too long or too short when you read. That person deals with pain, itching, tearing, injuries, funny kinds of headaches that your friend said were due to "eyestrain," and any and all things that relate to the eyes.

Diagnostic procedures for general ophthalmology include a visual acuity examination, refraction, color defectiveness ("color blindness") determination, a muscle integrity evaluation, pupillary reflex response, a slit-lamp examination, intraocular pressure determination, and a retinal examination.

Visual Acuity Examination This examination is performed either by the ophthalmologist or that person's assistant. You will be seated, facing a distant wall. On that wall is a chart of letters or numbers or sometimes both. You will be asked to cover one eye (often you'll be supplied with a small plastic paddle on a stick) and read as many of the letters as you can see. When you have reached your limit, the examiner will have you switch the paddle to your other eye and the same chore is performed. The total time is minutes, and total discomfort or hazard is zero.

Bottom Line: (½ +) Nothing like knowing one's ABCs.

Refraction This procedure follows Visual Acuity 101, whether you flunked or passed. Something in your vision requires correction by glasses. You are still sitting and facing that chart. A rather heavy pair of metal "spectacles" called a trial frame will be put on your face. These spectacles are really only frames without lenses. Or your ophthalmologist will use a phorometer, which is essentially the same as a trial frame, but it is not put on you. It is a large

Ophthalmology

Disease Category/ Procedure	Discomfort* (−) to (++++)	Hazard* (−) to (+++)	Hospital (Incl. Short Procedure)	Special Prep.	Physician	Extras*	Informed Consent*	Exam Time* (Hrs.)	Bottom Line* (−) to (++++)	Exam Description (Page)
General										
Visual acuity	(½+)	(−)	N	N	N	N	N	¼	(½+)	95
Refraction	(½+)	(−)	N	N	N	N	N	¼	(½+)	95
Color "blindness"	(½+)	(−)	N	N	N	N	N	¼	(½+)	99
Muscle integrity	(½+)	(−)	N	N	N	N	N	¼	(½+)	99
Pupil reflex	(½+)	(−)	N	N	N	N	N	¼	(½+)	100
Slit-lamp	(+)	(−)	N	Y	Y	Y	N	1	(++)	100
Intraocular pressure	(½+)	(−)	N	Y	Y	Y	N	¼	(½+)	101
Retinal exam	(++)	(−)	N	Y	Y	Y	N	1	(++)	102
Corneal										
Visual acuity	(½+)	(−)	N	N	N	N	N	¼	(½+)	102
Refraction	(½+)	(−)	N	N	N	N	N	¼	(½+)	102
Pupil reflex	(½+)	(−)	N	N	N	N	N	¼	(½+)	103
Tear test	(½+)	(−)	N	Y	Y	Y	N	¼	(½+)	103
Slit-lamp	(+)	(−)	N	Y	Y	Y	N	1	(++)	103
Keratometry	(½+)	(−)	N	N	N	N	N	¼	(½+)	103
Retinal										
Visual acuity	(½+)	(−)	N	N	N	N	N	¼	(½+)	104
Refraction	(½+)	(−)	N	N	N	N	N	¼	(½+)	104

Ophthalmology—cont'd

Disease Category/ Procedure	Discomfort* (−) to (++++)	Hazard* (−) to (+++)	Hospital (Incl. Short Procedure)	Special Prep.	Physi-cian	Extras*	Informed Consent*	Exam Time* (Hrs.)	Bottom Line* (−) to (++++)	Exam Description (Page)
Color "blindness"	(½+)	(−)	N	N	N	N	N	¼	(½+)	104
Muscle integrity	(½+)	(−)	N	N	N	N	N	¼	(½+)	104
Pupil reflex	(½+)	(−)	N	N	N	N	N	¼	(½+)	105
Slit-lamp	(+)	(−)	N	Y	Y	Y	N	1	(++)	105
Intraocular pressure	(½+)	(−)	N	Y	Y	Y	N	¼	(½+)	105
Retinal exam	(++)	(−)	N	Y	Y	Y	N	1	(++)	105
Ultrasound	(+)	(−)	N	Y	N	Y	N	½	(+)	105
Photography	(+)	(−)	N	Y	N	Y	N	½	(+)	105
Fluorescein	(+)	(−)	N	Y	N	Y	N	½	(+)	106
Electroretinogram	(++)	(−)	N	Y	N	Y	N	1	(++)	106
Amsler test	(½+)	(−)	N	N	N	N	N	¼	(½+)	107
Glaucoma										
Visual acuity	(½+)	(−)	N	N	N	N	N	¼	(½+)	108
Refraction	(½+)	(−)	N	N	N	N	N	¼	(½+)	108
Pupil reflex	(½+)	(−)	N	N	N	N	N	¼	(½+)	108
Visual field	(½+)	(−)	N	N	N	N	N	¼	(½+)	108
Slit-lamp	(+)	(−)	N	Y	Y	Y	N	1	(++)	109
Intraocular pressure	(½+)	(−)	N	Y	Y	Y	N	¼	(½+)	109
Retinal exam	(++)	(−)	N	Y	Y	Y	N	1	(++)	109

Ophthalmology—cont'd

Disease Category/ Procedure	Discomfort* (−) to (++++)	Hazard* (−) to (+++)	Hospital (Incl. Short Procedure)	Special Prep.	Physician	Extras*	Informed Consent*	Exam Time* (Hrs.)	Bottom Line* (−) to (++++)	Exam Description (Page)
Neuro-ophthalmic										
Visual acuity	(½+)	(−)	N	N	N	N	N	¼	(½+)	110
Refraction	(½+)	(−)	N	N	N	N	N	¼	(½+)	110
Color "blindness"	(½+)	(−)	N	N	N	N	N	¼	(½+)	110
Muscle integrity	(½+)	(−)	N	N	N	N	N	¼	(½+)	110
Pupil reflex	(½+)	(−)	N	N	N	N	N	¼	(½+)	110
Exophthalmometry	(−)	(−)	N	N	Y	N	N	¼	(½+)	110
Corneal reflex	(+)	(−)	N	N	N	N	N	¼	(+)	110
Visual field	(½+)	(−)	N	N	N	N	N	¼	(½+)	111
Slit-lamp	(+)	(−)	N	Y	Y	Y	N	1	(++)	111
Intraocular pressure	(½+)	(−)	N	Y	Y	Y	N	¼	(½+)	111
Neurological	(½+)	(−)	N	N	Y	N	N	½	(½+)	111
Retinal exam	(++)	(−)	N	Y	Y	Y	N	1	(++)	111
Electroretinogram	(++)	(−)	N	Y	N	Y	N	1	(++)	111
Amsler test	(½+)	(−)	N	N	N	N	N	¼	(½+)	111

* See Appendix, Table Details.

disk with two empty holes that is positioned in front of your face. In either case, one eye is covered and again you will be asked to read from the chart. When things get blurry, a small lens, which looks like an old-fashioned monocle, is slipped into the frame or disk. The blur is lessened. Now the fun begins. It's a game called "Better this way or that way?" The tester will keep changing the lens and with each variation will ask the question. The point of the exercise is to find the combination that permits you to see best. (After a while it is sometimes hard to know which is better.) The same is done for the other eye. It only takes 15 to 30 minutes and is neither uncomfortable nor hazardous.

Bottom Line: (½ +) The happiest answer is "it's better because it's over."

Color Defectiveness (a.k.a. "Color Blindness") Determination Some 6 percent of men and some 0.6 percent of women are born color-defective— with a condition in which they cannot distinguish between certain colors— almost always reds and greens (the popular term "blind" is not strictly accurate since there is not a total loss of perception). Sometimes, the problem develops later in life. There are a host of different tests to evaluate the existence of this condition. The commonest is a series of cards, each bearing an array of colored dots. Within the seemingly random pattern on each card, those who do not suffer a color defect will be able to find a number. The sufferer will see only the dots, being unable to find the number. Other techniques for identifying color "blindness" are usually reserved for those who acquire this condition later in life as a consequence of other problems, frequently of the retina. Therefore, these procedures are described under Diseases of the Retina. The test takes about five minutes, and has neither discomfort nor hazard.

Bottom Line: (½ +) This explains why you've been wearing two different-colored socks.

Muscle Integrity Evaluation The movements of your eyes are performed by a group of muscles called the extraocular muscles. Each of these muscles has a particular function that is invoked by such commands as "Look right" and "Look left," and more generally in all acts of vision. Impairment of one or all results in a subsequent impairment of function, and sometimes vision. Testing the condition of these structures is relatively simple and quick. You will be asked to respond to commands such as the ones noted above, plus others of equal difficulty ("look up, look down"). The discomfort and hazard index is zero. The elapsed time is almost zero.

Bottom Line: (½ +) The test could best be performed at a tennis match.

Pupillary Reflex Response The pupil is the name given to the "black hole" that is in the center of the colored portion—the iris—of the eye. The pupil controls the amount of light that enters the eye by enlarging when the lighting is dim or "scrunching down" in bright sunlight. It is imperative to normal vision that this REFLEX be preserved. It is affected by many different entities, primarily those that affect the nervous system. Testing the pupillary reflex is a quick and easy procedure. You look straight ahead. The tester shines a light, usually from a penlike flashlight, at your eye, and watches what happens to the size of your pupil. The procedure is repeated several times for each eye, and may be done both in a dark and a lighted room. Rate the discomfort a (½ +) for the bright light, the hazard (−). The time? Perhaps as long as a minute.

Bottom Line: (½ +) All tests should be this easy.

Slit-Lamp Examination The slit-lamp is an apparatus that is composed of a high-intensity light source that can be focused to shine as a "slit" and an optical instrument called a biomicroscope, which is similar to a microscope with two eyepieces. The whole thing sits on one of the shelves on a pole next to your chair, and when the moment of truth is "now," the shelf is swung over in front of you. A chinrest and forehead rest are built in so that when you lean forward your head is comfortably supported. The examination is performed in two acts with one thirty-minute intermission.

Act I (performed before your pupils are DILATED): The assistant starts the action. With due warning, he or she touches the side of each of your eyes with a fine strip of paper that is stained with an orange-colored dye called fluorescein. This will provoke an instantaneous blink, and then it's over. The dye will stain the front of your eye and will significantly improve the sensitivity of the examination that is about to ensue. (The stain will be washed out by your tears and you will never even know it was there.) The ophthalmologist then sits down in front of you and looks deeply into your eyes through the biomicroscope. Your eyelids, the white parts (sclera), the colored parts (iris), the membranes that line the lids and white parts (conjunctiva), the transparent tissue that covers the iris (cornea), and the lens that lies behind it will all be carefully studied. Except for the (+) discomfort from the bright light, you won't feel anything. This part of the study takes about three minutes for each eye.

The second part of the examination is done after your pupils have been dilated. This is accomplished by special drops that are instilled into each eye and require 20 to 30 minutes to do their duty. Intermission. You will undoubtedly be escorted back to the waiting room. Bring something to do or read, even though toward the end things start to get blurry. The effect of the drops lasts for at least four hours, so bring a pal if driving is the way home—and bring sunglasses because glare from the sun, the light of day, and even head-lights at night can be most uncomfortable.

Act II: Back into the chair with your head on the chinrest and forehead rest. The ophthalmologist looks deeply into your eyes—like before, only deeper. Now the back portion (retina) is being inspected. The only thing that is different is that the discomfort is up a notch because with your pupils dilated the light seems more intense. This examination takes another three to five minutes. There is no hazard, but there is at least a four-hour delay until you can see well again. Remember your pal.

Bottom Line: (+ +) Really rather boring.

Intraocular Pressure Determination   *Intra* means "within" and *ocular* means pertaining to the eye. A most serious condition may develop, usually after the age of 40, in which the pressure within the eye begins to become intolerable. It occurs more often in those suffering with diabetes and in blacks. If undiscovered or identified too late, blindness will ensue. This con-dition is called *glaucoma*. The procedure that tests for this problem (that measures the pressure) is called TONOMETRY. There are two techniques that are commonly employed. Since it is impossible to predict which you will have, I will describe each.

Each begins with the instillation of a drop or two of a local anesthetic in each of your eyes. This will instantaneously cause a sting that is over in an instant. The effects of the anesthetic drops last for some 15 to 20 minutes and easily permit the examination to be performed without discomfort. Each is performed by the ophthalmologist or the assistant and takes less than a minute to accomplish. Neither is associated with real hazard nor will result in later nuisance symptoms. One of the exams employs an instrument called a tonom-eter that resembles a thin tire gauge. It is a pen-like tube with a very small tip which, when touched, moves back into the tube. The simplest technique involves gently placing the tip of the instrument against the front of each of your eyes. That's it. You will feel nothing or only the gentlest of pressure for only a few seconds. The other technique is reserved for situations in which there is an existent problem that makes it a good idea not to touch the front of your eyes at all. In these situations an instrument brought up close to your eyes emits a steady flow of an invisible gas like air. The gas moving against your eyes causes some detectable change that can be measured. Except for a slight hiss that can be heard, you feel nothing.

Bottom Line: (+) Easier and lots faster to have done than to read about.

Retinal Examination Lastly, the retina, the back of your eyes, will be studied. An instrument that looks like a fat flashlight with a disk at its end, called an ophthalmoscope, is used. The room will be darkened. The doctor places the disk portion, which houses small but powerful magnifying lenses, close to one of your eyes, turns on the light and looks through your pupil into the back of your eye. Except for the mild discomfort of the light there is no other sensation. There is no hazard, and it only takes a minute or two. This is known as the direct ophthalmoscopy. If your initial complaints or the results of the direct study demand a more extensive evaluation, the indirect technique will be used. Here, you might be placed in a reclined position. The doctor will use a light source from a headband that he or she will don. A special hand lens permits a much wider and more detailed "look." This causes **(++)** discomfort, not only from the tugging and pressure that could be applied to your eyelids to get a better exposure, but also, particularly, from the intensity of the light—it's like looking into the sun. There is no hazard from the indirect ophthalmoscopy and it takes only minutes, although it often feels longer. Final last words: Don't forget the pal or your sunglasses.

Bottom Line: **(++)** Not really a biggie, but often tedious.

Diseases of the Cornea

The cornea is the transparent covering of the iris and the pupil. (It is the part that a contact lens fits over.) It is remarkably sensitive and will really, really hurt if injured. It is subject to injury since it is way up front, and it is also prone to infection. Often problems begin because there is a decrease in the normal production of tears—"dry eyes." Often the problem is a consequence of aging. The TISSUE undergoes thinning and alteration in shape, which can greatly affect vision. So, testing is appropriate to determine the cornea's condition.

Diagnostic procedures for diseases of the cornea include visual acuity examination, refraction, pupillary reflex response, tear test, slit-lamp examination, and keratometry.

Visual Acuity Examination This study has been described above under General Diseases of the Eye.

Refraction This study has been described above under General Diseases of the Eye.

Pupillary Reflex Response This study has been described above under General Diseases of the Eye.

Tear Test Tearing is an essential component of the well-being of your eyes. Certain conditions result in excessive tearing, while some result in too little. The latter produces a complaint of "dry eyes," which among other things can result in serious damage to the cornea. The amount of tearing can be measured. A specially prepared sterile strip of paper will be carefully placed to "hook" over the border of a small section of your lower eyelid. It will remain there for about five minutes and then be removed. The amount of tearing that you do will be reflected on how wet the strip has become in the time allotted. The test is best done with local anesthesia so that it will not be uncomfortable and you won't tear excessively. (½ +) for discomfort. There is no hazard. There are no late aftereffects.

Bottom Line: (½ +) It's so easy you could cry from joy.

Slit-Lamp Examination This study has been described above under General Diseases of the Eye.

Keratometry *Kerat* refers to the cornea, and *ometry* is "the measurement of." This is an examination of the anterior (front) surface curvature of the cornea using a special instrument called a keratometer. The study is performed in conjunction with the slit-lamp examination. The keratometer is on another one of the swivel shelves on the pole beside the chair you sit in. It will be brought into place, a light will be shone into each of your eyes, and the machine will measure the angles of reflection that result. The study takes minutes.

Bottom Line: (½ +) A real nothing.

Diseases of the Retina

Lest we get too deeply mired in the description of the retina—a most complex structure—I have compressed the enormous subject into some simplistic generalities that should see us through.

The retina, often called the eyegrounds, is composed of a host of specialized structures: the rods and cones, the macula, the optic disk, nerves, blood vessels, and many, many more. Put them all together and they spell vision! Problems in this portion of the eye stem from a large menu of troubles:

HYPERTENSION, DIABETES, certain medications, certain aging problems that cause the degeneration or breakdown of the macula, and separations and tears that occur spontaneously or from a blow to the head.

The visual problems occur without pain. They vary, but flashes of light, floating blobs, cobwebs, and just plain blurring of vision are the most common. Diagnostic procedures for retinal diseases include visual acuity examination, refraction, color defectiveness ("color blindness") determination, muscle integrity evaluation, pupillary reflex response, a slit-lamp examination, intraocular pressure determination, a retinal examination, an ultrasound examination, photography, fluorescein angiography, an electroretinogram, an Amsler test, and miscellaneous procedures.

Visual Acuity Examination   This study has been described above under General Diseases of the Eye.

Refraction   This study has been described above under General Diseases of the Eye.

Color Defectiveness (a.k.a. "Color Blindness") Determination   The color plates with the dots described earlier (see page 99) are used routinely. However, there are situations in which a more sensitive and accurate indicator is necessary. For instance, your family might have a history of hereditary color deficit, but you might have no obvious manifestation, as yet. Or sensitive testing may be deemed essential to further refine an already established diagnosis of retinal disease. When such testing is indicated, the ophthalmologist has several techniques to choose from. All are similar in that you will be asked to work with colored materials in a way that will expose any deficit that may exist. One of these requires that you labor in a designated space called a color booth. You will be asked to wear gloves and an eyepatch. Four boxes containing about 25 small color disks each will be the materials for your examination. You must arrange the disks such that all units of the same color to include graded hues of that color are put together. None of these variations on the color theme cause discomfort or impose hazard. The time depends on you.

Bottom Line: (½+) Let's hope you find this a colorful experience.

Muscle Integrity Evaluation   This study has been described above under General Diseases of the Eye.

Pupillary Reflex Response   This study has been described above under General Diseases of the Eye.

Slit-Lamp Examination   This study has been described above under General Diseases of the Eye.

Intraocular Pressure Determination   This study has been described above under General Diseases of the Eye.

Retinal Examination   This study has been described above under General Diseases of the Eye.

Ultrasound Examination   The principles and techniques of ultrasonic examinations are discussed and described in Chapter 20. However, the eye is so special its examination is described here. The examination room contains a large comfortable chair with a headrest. The chair both reclines and swivels. There is a large pole next to the chair with shelves that can be moved in front of the chair. You are seated in the chair, and if you have not already received local anesthetic drops, you will get them now. A drop in each eye, a second of smarting, a tear or two, and you are ready. The room is darkened. The shelf containing the equipment will be swung around to face you. On it is also a chinrest and forehead support so that your head is held in a secure and comfortable position. The technologist will gently touch the front of your eye with a transducer (a thick pen-like instrument that sends out sound waves and then receives their echo). It might feel a mite sticky because of the goo that is put on its end. You will barely perceive its pressure. You will feel nothing else. When the first eye has been "sounded" the same procedure will be repeated on the second. The examination time, for both eyes, takes 10 minutes. Your eyes will come "back to life" in about half an hour.

Bottom Line: (+) Sounded like it would be more.

Photography   Yes, photography, but you needn't smile. Your pupils have been dilated. You will be seated in a chair with your chin and forehead supported as in previous examinations. Pointed at you, or more precisely, focused on your retina, is the long lens of a very nifty camera capable of rapid flash exposures. And away it goes. Multiple sequential pictures are taken of each retina. It is uncomfortable (+) because your pupils are wide open and the flashes are mighty bright. But the whole experience lasts less than five minutes. There is no hazard. There may be some afterimages (you will think you are still seeing the flashes) for a short time afterward. Remember that your pupils will remain dilated for the next four hours, so mobilize that old pal who will help you get home. Take a pair of sunglasses.

Bottom Line: (+) You can order both black-and-white and color prints.

Fluorescein Angiography   Fluorescein is an orange-colored dye. It is the same dye that was mentioned earlier when the slit-lamp examination was described. ANGIOGRAPHY is a method of taking pictures of blood vessels. This procedure is performed when information is required about the blood vessels in patients (often those suffering with diabetes) suspected of having vascular OCCLUSION and who may be candidates for laser therapy. It may also be suggested when tumor is a consideration. In concept it is similar to getting images of blood vessels elsewhere in the body. Usually these techniques are performed using X-rays and iodine as the "DYE." (See Angiography, Chapter 18.) However, the retinal vessels can be visualized without X-rays and without iodine—both of which carry an inherent hazard. These vessels can be seen quite well by the technique discussed above in Photography. There is one additional step—the addition of fluorescein. (Just as photography takes the place of X-ray, fluorescein dye is substituted for iodine. Neither imposes the hazards of the other, more conventional techniques, although a small group of people may exhibit a mild reaction to this dye such as nausea or hives.) This dye material must be injected into an arm vein. It will then be carried around until it reaches the vessels of your retina. These vessels will then take on a bright orange hue and cry out to be photographed. Actually, the picture taking begins simultaneously with the dye injection. Images are obtained every one to two seconds for about a minute. Pictures are again made some 20 minutes later, this time without dye. Figure about an hour for the whole procedure. Remember the dilated pupils, so bring a pal and a pair of "shades." Don't be concerned if your skin or the whites of your eyes look a tad yellow for about an hour. This discoloration will disappear. Also, don't panic if your urine is greenish or orangish for a day or two.

Bottom Line: (+) If you've had an X-ray angiogram, you know what a "snap" this has been.

Electroretinogram   This is a sophisticated procedure that provides detailed data on the functional status of certain structures within the retina, particularly the optic nerve and the rods (specialized cells that detect light) and cones (specialized cells essential to color vision). It requires that the eyes be totally dark-adapted (adapted to the dark to the point where you can see). After you have received drops to dilate your pupils, you will be seated in a darkened room with patches over each eye for the next 30 minutes. Then a technologist will apply ELECTRODES to each side of the front of your head, and in the midline from front to back of the top of your head. These small circular SENSORS are about the size of a dime and are attached with an adhesive paste. Then a contact lens is fitted over each eye and an electrode with wires is attached to each lens. Some people find these lenses to be particularly uncomfortable—(+ +). When all this suiting-up has been accomplished you are led to a rather large box that will admit your head. When you are comfortably seated, you put your head in the box, look straight ahead, and the show begins. The show is a series of sequential light flashes. These may go on for 10 to 15 minutes. There is no plot, there is no music. Then it is over. Out of the box, off with the sensors, out of that room—free at last!

There are no "aftershocks," except that your eyes will be dilated for at least the next four to six hours, so again bring sunglasses and a pal.

Bottom Line: (+ +) For some: The total existential experience. For most: The total bore of all time.

Amsler Test   (Amsler is the name of a person.) After all of the above, this little number seems anticlimactic. You will be given a small piece of graph paper. In the center of the sheet there will be a black dot. You will be asked to describe what you see. Does everything look all right? Are there lines missing? Are there any distortions? That's it! (−) for discomfort and hazard. Two minutes for time.

Bottom Line: (½ +) Why, oh why, can't they all be like this?

Miscellaneous Procedures   There are several other tests that may be used in very specialized situations. They are all quite similar to those that have just been described, so that from your standpoint there should be no remarkable events that you are not ready for. Well, I hope not, but I know that as I write this somebody out there is dreaming up a new test. We can only hope that he or she will be kind.

Glaucoma

Glaucoma is a disease of the eye that is a characterized by an increase in its pressure. Briefly, the eye is a globular structure that contains a large volume of fluid known as the aqueous humor. This fluid must circulate freely within the various chambers of the globe. When there is impairment or blockage to this movement the intraocular (inside-the-eye) pressure builds up. As this occurs, damage results to parts of the eye, and this in turn affects vision. Without appropriate management, blindness will ensue. Glaucoma is most prevalent in those over 40 years of age, in those suffering with diabetes, and in blacks. Routine SCREENING—perhaps once every two years—is urged for those 40 years old or older since the initial ravages of this condition are notoriously silent (without symptoms). By the time you are aware that you seem to be "blurring," or that there are funny lights or halos around lights, you may already have suffered serious damage. Diagnostic procedures for glaucoma include a visual acuity examination, refraction, pupillary reflex response, visual field measurement, a slit-lamp examination, intraocular pressure determination, and a retinal examination.

Visual Acuity Examination   This study has been described above under General Diseases of the Eye.

Refraction   This study has been described above under General Diseases of the Eye.

Pupillary Reflex Response   This study has been described above under General Diseases of the Eye.

Visual Field Measurement   The term "visual field" describes the entire area of one's vision. What does that mean? Well, if you stare straight ahead and don't move your eyes at all, you will still be able to see things above, below, and on either side of that direct line of sight. That circle of vision is the field. It is essential to ascertain that it is as large as it is supposed to be. A simple measurement of its condition is to have you sit and look straight ahead. The examiner will ask you to say "yes" when you become aware of his or her finger intruding on your field of view. Then that person will point his or her index finger and start bringing it toward you from each of four directions: from above, down; from below, up; from the right side in; and from the left side in. The distance from your eye at which you detect the invader will be recorded.

   There is a more accurate and sophisticated version of the same test. Here you sit in front of a large globe-shaped machine that has a front opening that you can put your face into and a place where you can rest your chin. One eye will be patched. You will be asked to fix your attention to a dot in the back center of the globe. You will also be asked to press a buzzer whenever a dot of light comes into your field of view. The technologist substitutes a spot of light for the wagging finger and each buzz creates a mark on a special graph paper.

The end result is a dot-to-dot connection of the marks—an outline of your visual field. The test takes about 15 minutes to perform. There is neither discomfort nor hazard. There are no aftereffects.

Bottom Line: (½ +) Easy but tiring.

Slit-Lamp Examination This study has been described above under General Diseases of the Eye, but it contains one additional feature not commonly performed except in glaucoma patients. Contact lenses are applied to each eye either before or after dilation (or both). This is to visualize the aqueous drainage channels and parts of the retina. For you it is only a minor inconvenience. Your eyes are already anesthetized so the lenses won't be a big deal. This adds about another minute to the procedure. So, all ratings are essentially the same.

Bottom Line: (+ +) Long and dull.

Intraocular Pressure Determination This study has been described above under General Diseases of the Eye.

Retinal Examination This study has been described above under General Diseases of the Eye. Note that as in the slit-lamp examination, lenses may be placed over each eye as an added component of the examination, and as before, it does not change the total experience.

Neuro-ophthalmic Diseases

There are literally dozens of different PATHOLOGIES whose nature is to attack many areas of the body simultaneously, often including the eyes. When the eyes are thus affected the most usual target is their neural (NERVOUS SYSTEM) component. The list is long and varied: diabetes, various tumors, hyperthyroidism, hypertension, multiple sclerosis and myasthenia gravis. The complaints offered are equally variable. Many of these have also been noted. Add to the symptoms list such miseries as migraine headaches, transient visual loss, double vision, and any changes in vision that affect only one eye. Any of the above, as well as certain abnormalities discovered on examinations performed by any of the other ophthalmologic specialists, may bring you to a neuro-ophthalmologist. Diagnostic procedures for neuro-ophthalmic diseases include a visual acuity examination, refraction, color defectiveness (a.k.a. "color blindness") determination, a muscle integrity evaluation, pupillary reflex response, exophthalmometry, corneal reflex response, visual field measurement, a slit-lamp examination, intraocular pressure determination, a neurologic examination, a retinal examination, an electroretinogram, an Amsler test, and miscellaneous procedures.

Visual Acuity Examination   This study has been described above under General Diseases of the Eye.

Refraction   This study has been described above under General Diseases of the Eye.

Color Defectiveness (a.k.a. "Color Blindness") Determination   This study has been described above under General Diseases of the Eye.

Muscle Integrity Evaluation   This study has been described above under General Diseases of the Eye.

Pupillary Reflex Response   This study has been described above under General Diseases of the Eye.

Exophthalmometry   *Exophthalmos* is the medical term for "bulging of the eyes" (or eye). When both eyes seem to protrude or be more prominent than average the cause is most frequently found in an overactive thyroid. When the bulge is one-sided, there is a real possibility that a tumor may exist behind that eye. In any event, the degree of the protrusion should be measured to confirm or deny that it is truly abnormal—and if it is, to establish a baseline so that changes can be monitored. The measurement is most simple: A ruler is placed along the side of your head. A measurement is taken from the corner of your eye to the most forward portion of your eyeball. That is exophthalmometry!

Bottom Line: (–) all the way!

Corneal Reflex Response   As has been described earlier, the cornea is the transparent membrane that covers the iris in the front of the eye and it is extremely sensitive. Anything that touches it evokes a loud "ouch!" and an immediate protective blink. This blink is the corneal REFLEX. Its presence ensures that the nerve supply to the cornea is O.K. Thus, the test is to touch your cornea with a wisp of cotton. If you feel it, you pass. If you don't, there is a problem that requires further investigation. The procedure is performed in seconds. There is a **(+)** discomfort, but no hazard.

Bottom Line: **(+)** It's over in a "twinkling of your eye."

Visual Field Measurement This study has been described above under Glaucoma.

Slit-Lamp Examination This study has been described above under General Diseases of the Eye.

Intraocular Pressure Determination This study has been described above under General Diseases of the Eye.

Neurologic Examination The detailed description of the complete neurologic experience can be found in Chapter 8.

Retinal Examination This study has been described above under General Diseases of the Eye.

Electroretinogram This study has been described above under Diseases of the Retina.

Amsler Test This study has been described above under Diseases of the Retina.

Miscellaneous Procedures There are several other tests that may be evoked in very specialized situations. They are all quite similar to those that have just been described, so that from your standpoint there should be no remarkable events that you are not ready for.

12

Go See an Orthopedic Surgeon

An orthopedic surgeon is a man or woman who, after graduating from both college and medical school, studies the vast array of techniques that are included under the umbrella of general surgery for three years, then spends an additional two years understanding the nature and correction (including surgery) of diseases of the spine and bones of the extremities and their joints.

The orthopedic surgeon is concerned with any problem that may arise because of injury, pain, tumor, infection, or any other cause that affects the spine or the arms and legs. A diagnosis of the cause must be established so that appropriate treatment can be initiated. To accomplish this goal, testing must be performed.

Each procedure that might be employed by the orthopedic surgeon is listed in the accompanying table. Suppose the doctor said, "I think you should have an MRI of your knee." Find MRI and read across its entire line. A quick synopsis of the pertinent data characterizing this study is listed. (These data are elaborated upon in the Appendix.) The last item on the line is the page number where the study is described in detail.

And finally, after you have read about the particular examination that you are preparing for, reread pages xiv through xvi, General Events Common to All Adult Diagnostic Procedures.

Orthopedics

Procedure	Discomfort* (−) to (++++)	Hazard* (−) to (+++)	Hospital (Incl. Short Procedure)	Special Prep.	Physician	Extras*	Informed Consent*	Exam Time* (Hrs.)	Bottom Line* (−) to (++++)	Exam Description (Page)
Physical exam	(+)	(−)	N	N	Y	N	N	½	(+)	114
Laboratory tests	(+)	(−)	N	N	N	Y	N	¼	(+)	114
X-ray studies	(++)	(+)	N	N	Y/N	Y/N	N	1	(+) to (++)	114
MRI	(+)	(−)	N	N	N	N	N	1	(+)	115
Nuclear imaging	(+)	(−)	N	N	N	Y	N	4	(+)	115
Ultrasound	(½+)	(−)	N	N	N	N	N	½	(½+)	115
Arthroscopy	(++)	(+)	Y	Y	Y	Y	Y	4	(++)	115

* See Appendix, Table Details.

Skeletal System

Skeletal refers to a skeleton, which is the name given to a supportive or protective structure or framework. When that framework is the human body, the structure is composed of bones and cartilage, and protects all of the softer parts, such as our internal organs, our brain, and our spinal cord. This complex of structures is prone to the same PATHOLOGIES as all of the other bodily systems: CONGENITAL defects, trauma, infection, metabolic disorders, tumors, and so forth. Some of the problems that develop may be treated by other specialists, particularly neurologists and rheumatologists. However, those that require surgical management are most often the particular province of the orthopedic surgeon. (Time out for the trivia buff: *Ortho* means straight, and *ped* refers to children. It is thought that the name "orthopedist" was originally given to physicians who were skilled in straightening the crooked spines of children.)

Diagnostic procedures for the SKELETAL SYSTEM include a physical examination, laboratory tests, X-ray studies, magnetic resonance imaging (MRI), nuclear imaging, ultrasound imaging, and arthroscopy.

Physical Examination The physical examination performed by the orthopedist is not unlike that done by the rheumatologist. See Chapter 15.

Laboratory Tests There are multiple blood tests that are remarkably helpful in differentiating many of the ARTHRITIDES from each other. There are other procedures that also provide very specific data. These include synovial fluid analysis and synovial membrane biopsy.

The *synovia* is the name of the special TISSUE or membrane that lines a joint. It is capable of producing a fluid—synovial fluid—which is necessary for normal joint function. However, various abnormal states stimulate the amount of fluid formed, and this is responsible, very often, for swelling that occurs. Analysis of this fluid is most helpful in determining the cause and type of the abnormality. This fluid can be obtained for study by ASPIRATION BIOPSY. The synovial membrane itself can be analyzed by employing the technique of EXCISIONAL BIOPSY to remove a small piece of tissue.

Both the biopsy procedures and the blood tests, along with any other examinations that may be ordered, are described in Chapter 17.

X-ray Studies See Upper and Lower Extremities and Spine and Bony Pelvis in Chapter 18.

MRI See Chapter 21.

Nuclear Imaging See Skeletal System in Chapter 19.

Ultrasound Imaging See Chapter 20. The procedure most applicable to orthopedic problems is the evaluation of whether or not a "lump or bump" in the region of a joint contains fluid or is solid. This type of study is described on page 278.

Arthroscopy *Arthro* refers to a joint; *oscopy* refers to the direct visualization of the inside of a body cavity. In this procedure, a specialized optical instrument equipped with lenses and lights, called an arthroscope, is used to study joints, particularly the knee, shoulder, ankle, elbow, and wrist.

The procedure does not require hospitalization but almost always requires anesthesia—either general, where you are put to sleep, or regional (often called spinal), where only the areas below the spine are affected and you remain awake. There are some patients who prohibit the use of either of these techniques and demand only local anesthesia. This can be done, but is not advised since there is still significant discomfort that almost always results in that person's moving which, in turn, diminishes the thoroughness and accuracy of the study. Most patients prefer general because after awakening (which does not take more than an hour) they can go home. Spinal is more "iffy" with respect to leaving the same day. So, because of the anesthesia, the examination is usually considered as a short procedure hospitalization. (Review Short Procedure Hospitalization on pages xvi–xviii.)

You will arrive at the hospital on the morning of the study having not eaten since bedtime the night before. You will be escorted to the short procedures area and the usual events that you just reviewed will occur. Then it's off to the operating suite where you will meet your anesthetist, who will put you to sleep.

Here is what will happen: The part to be examined (let us assume it will be your knee, since this is the joint most commonly studied, although the procedure is essentially the same for all), is scrubbed with an antiseptic soap. It is then draped—surrounded by sterile towels or sheets. The orthopedist, in full surgical gear, will make a small INCISION at the top part of your kneecap and insert a large plastic tube (CATHETER) into the joint. Fluid is run in through the catheter. A second, and smaller, incision through which the arthroscope is inserted and through which the fluid runs out is made lower down on your knee. The fluid makes seeing better and moving the instrument around easier. It also serves to wash out small fragments that may be present.

Then the orthopedist carefully looks. A half-hour to an hour may pass before the doctor feels that everything has been seen. The scope and catheter are then removed and the incisions sutured closed.

You will be carefully monitored until you recover from the anesthesia and are sufficiently aware of the world to go home. *You will need help,* so have a pal waiting.

Your knee will be swollen for at least three to five days and, depending on what was seen, you may be advised not to bear any weight for several days, but most patients are permitted to walk immediately. The only restriction is anything that produces pain—avoid it! It's a good idea, if you can arrange it, to take several days off from work. (Try to have the procedure done on a Wednesday or Thursday so you can get the benefit of the weekend.) Most people are back to their pretest status in about a week.

All of the above estimations are based on the condition that the procedure was purely diagnostic—that means that the orthopedist only looked and that no surgical corrections were performed. Be sure you know and have given appropriate permission for what actually will be done. Many orthopedists will argue, not without logic, that while they are "there," should they find something that is correctable, you should let them do what is appropriate rather than repeat the whole thing at a later date. If you say Yes, and a surgical correction is done, the period of recovery and restrictive activity will be far longer and greater than when only a diagnostic "look" is performed. So, if you say Yes, discuss all of the ramifications with the surgeon and make sure that this is the right time to have the surgery done.

Bottom Line: (+ +) This is a big-time study, but it won't seem too bad.

13

Go See an Otorhinolaryngologist

An otorhinolaryngologist (*oto* refers to the ear; *rhino* refers to the nose; *larynx* refers to a specialized structure in the throat that houses the vocal cords and is the organ of voice production) is known to friends as an ENT (E = ear, N = nose, T = throat) doc. This person, after graduating from both college and medical school, spent one year of a four-year post-doctoral program learning the basics of general surgery and the next three years concentrating on the problems of the ears, the nose, and the throat and their correction (including surgery).

I have divided otorhinolaryngology into three categories: problems of the ears, problems of the nose, and problems of the throat. Each category is studied by procedures appropriate to its unique set of problems. Often, the same examination or test is used in all. A history will always be taken and a physical examination performed. Additionally, a particular form of study, such as X-ray imaging, will always seem to be the same to you, but it can be made to provide different information depending on the problem at hand. Therefore, I will list all of the appropriate procedures commonly utilized by an ENT specialist in reaching a diagnosis under each of the parts to be considered.

For a detailed discussion of each examination, start with the accompanying table. It identifies the three major areas of investigation. Within each category are listed the tests that can be performed. Suppose the doctor said, "I'm recommending that you have X-rays of your larynx to evaluate your

Otorhinolaryngology

Disease Category/Procedure	Discomfort* (-) to (++++)	Hazard* (-) to (+++)	Hospital (Incl. Short Procedure)	Special Prep.	Physician	Extras*	Informed Consent*	Exam Time* (Hrs.)	Bottom Line* (-) to (++++)	Exam Description (Page)
Ears										
Physical exam	(+)	(-)	N	N	Y	N	N	¼	(+)	119
Laboratory tests	(+)	(-)	N	N	N	Y	N	¼	(+)	122
Audiogram	(½+)	(-)	N	N	N	N	N	¾	(½+)	122
Tympanogram	(½+)	(-)	N	N	N	Y	N	¼	(½+)	122
Electronystagmogram	(++)	(-)	N	Y	N	Y	N	1	(++)	123
Brainstem auditory response	(+)	(-)	N	N	N	Y	N	1	(+)	124
X-rays	(+)	(-)	N	N	N	Y	N	1	(+)	124
MRI	(+)	(-)	N	N	N	N	N	1	(+)	124
Nose										
Physical exam	(+)	(-)	N	N	Y	N	N	¼	(+)	124
Laboratory tests	(+)	(-)	N	N	N	Y	N	¼	(+)	124
X-rays	(+)	(-)	N	N	N	Y	N	1	(+)	124
Biopsy	(++)	(+)	N	N	Y	Y	Y	¼	(++)	125
Throat										
Physical exam	(++)	(-)	N	N	Y	N	N	¼	(++)	126
Laboratory tests	(+)	(-)	N	N	N	Y	N	¼	(+)	126
X-rays	(+)	(-)	N	N	N	Y	N	1	(+)	126
Biopsy	(++)	(+)	Y	N	Y	Y	Y	1	(+++)	126

* See Appendix, Table Details.

hoarseness." Find this test under Throat and read across its entire line. A quick synopsis of the pertinent data characterizing this study is listed. (These data are elaborated upon in the Appendix.) The last item on the line is the page number where the study is described in detail.

And finally, after you have read about the particular examination that you are preparing for, reread pages xiv through xvi, General Events Common to All Adult Diagnostic Procedures.

Ears

Not very much detail is necessary in discussing the ears, since we all know that they are responsible for one of the five major bodily senses—hearing. However, there is another, less well known function that is also their responsibility—the preservation of balance. Therefore, patients who complain of things like VERTIGO, walking "funny" (altered gait), and even inapppropriate falling, may be candidates for serious evaluation of the ears as well as those who have problems with hearing loss. TINNITUS is another rather common and annoying complaint that requires evaluation. Then, too, any pain or discharge from the ear demands attention.

Diagnostic procedures for the ears include a physical examination; laboratory tests; an audiogram; a tympanogram; an electronystagmogram; auditory brainstem response; X-ray examinations and magnetic resonance imaging (MRI).

Physical Examination The examination performed by the otorhinolaryngologist will always include the ears, nose, and throat, regardless of which of these areas may be the site of the chief complaint. Therefore, the description here includes the typical procedure for the physical evaluation of all of these areas.

Ears You will be asked to remove anything that can come off from your head and neck. This includes glasses, earrings, necklaces, and even teeth. You will sit in an examining chair that has a headrest. The doctor will first look at your ears to evaluate the skin. Then he or she will gently pull down on your earlobe while inserting an otoscope, which is a small hand-held instrument that is really a flashlight with a special endpiece; the endpiece is a small funnel-shaped plastic device positioned so that the light, when it is turned on, will pass through it and exit as a beam into the canal that is just inside the front of your ear. The narrow end of the funnel is what goes in. The doctor peers into the wide end of the funnel and thus is able to see all the way to the eardrum. The instrument will be moved in and out and your head may be turned slightly from side to side. The entire inspection lasts no more than one to two minutes. Then the whole thing is repeated on the other side.

On occasion, a more specialized tool, the pneumatic otoscope, will be used. This instrument is not significantly different in its appearance from the common variety but it does possess the ability to deliver puffs of air that will strike your eardrum. This injection of air will cause the normal drum to move, while the abnormal structure will not, or will at least seem stiff. Some believe it is a more sensitive detector of problems that include perforation of the drum. The "puffer" is slightly more uncomfortable than its nonbreathing cousin, but neither produces more than a (+) discomfort.

Still another sometimes-used method for evaluating the eardrum is the placement of a small vibrating instrument behind the ear and a small plug in the ear that is capable of recording the movement of the drum that is initiated by the vibrations. This device is called a tympanometer, and it is particularly effective in detecting the presence of fluid that might be behind the drum and therefore not otherwise detectable. This procedure requires only minutes to perform and is only minimally uncomfortable.

Finally, gross differentiation of hearing problems is performed. The differentiation is whether the loss is caused by a problem of the little bones in your inner ear or from conduction loss. (The nature of these differences is complex and beyond the scope of simple explanation here. This is a subject to explore with your physician.) The tests, however, are simple and utilize a tuning fork. In one examination, this instrument is made to vibrate and then is placed behind and then in front of your ear. You are asked which location produces the louder sound. A second variation is to cause the fork to vibrate and then to place it on the middle of your forehead. You will be asked whether you hear it better in one ear or the other.

The whole examination will take a total of perhaps 5 to 10 minutes for everything. Discomfort may reach (+). There is no hazard, and no delayed effects.

Bottom Line: (+) Just hope that your ears are clean.

Nose You will sit in the examining chair with your head tilted backward. The doctor will sit in front of you. The first step is usually to both decongest and desensitize the inside of your nose by gently inserting a small cotton plug that has been dampened with appropriate medication into each nostril for several seconds. Then a SPECULUM, a small hand-held instrument, is inserted into one nostril. This particular tool has at its end two short flat blades that touch each other unless the instrument's handle is squeezed. This action causes the blades to separate. Thus, when the blades are inserted into your nose in the closed position and then gently opened, the nasal cavity will be stretched, permitting the examiner a good look. The same "look" will be repeated on the other side. On occasion another tube-like instrument will be inserted through the open blades. This is an ASPIRATION tube that may be used to further improve visualization by removing any nasal secretions, such as mucus. It also is used to remove any secretions that need to be studied further in the laboratory. The suction is mild and produces no true discomfort. It may cause a noise because it is attached to a motor.

The examination causes a (+) discomfort and is a (−) hazard. Total time is two to three minutes. There is no delayed misery.

Bottom Line: (+) "The noes have it."

Throat The examination of the throat includes an inspection of the mouth as well. You will still be sitting in the examining chair. The doctor will still be sitting in front of you. First he or she will visually inspect your neck and will then feel for any lumps or bumps. Then the doctor will look into your mouth, using either the head mirror or a head lamp as a light source. He or she will use two tongue blades (those flat, round-edged pieces of whitish wood that doctors always stick down your throat when you have a sore throat to begin with and at the same time make you say "ah") to explore every nook and cranny. The blades are used to gently stretch and separate the gums from the cheek, the tongue from the gums, and the tongue from the floor of the mouth. The openings of the salivary GLANDS and the region of the tonsils are all checked. You will be asked not to swallow or gag. (That's a joke, but short panting breaths sometimes help.)

Now on to the throat. Out come the blades, and after the roof of your mouth and the back of your throat have been sprayed with a local anesthetic, in comes a small round mirror on a long thin metal handle that has been slightly warmed so as to prevent fogging. (It is like the mirror that dentists use.) This is slid to the back of your tongue and you are asked to say "E, E, E . . . ," and then to take in a deep breath. This sound makes your vocal cords move, and the breath makes the cords relax. The "look" at your vocal cords that is thus obtained is short and sometimes inadequate. For these reasons some ENT folks have abandoned the mirror in favor of either of two newer optical tools: the flexible laryngoscope (a thin, tubular optical instrument about one-half inch thick and about 10 inches long) or the laryngeal telescope (a short, rigid tube about one inch in diameter and six inches long that has a light source and magnifying lens). Each requires the use of a local anesthetic, which is applied by spraying. It is not unpleasant and the area becomes numb in seconds. The laryngoscope is passed through a nostril into the back of your throat and then farther down into the larynx. The telescope is inserted through the mouth. Either permits a more detailed examination. Neither "look" takes more than two or three minutes to perform.

The whole thing takes five minutes and is done by the ENT physician. Discomfort rates a (+ +). There is no hazard. Don't eat or drink anything until the anesthetic wears off—about a half hour. You may have a mild sore throat for several hours.

Bottom Line: (+ +) You will get the gag, but won't find it funny.

Laboratory Tests Testing for the types of infection that may be present can be accomplished by smears and CULTURES.

Audiogram *Audio* refers to hearing. The audiogram is a definitive evaluation and measurement of your hearing in each ear and both ears together. It is performed by a trained technologist. You will be asked to enter a telephone-booth-like chamber. (You will know it is not a real telephone booth because it is clean, comfortable, free of graffiti, and is soundproof.) You will be made comfortable in a chair. You will be told that when the test begins you will hear a series of different sounds and even words that change in both loudness and pitch. You will hear them in either one ear or the other—sometimes in both. Directions will be given as to how to acknowledge that you have heard the sound—sometimes you'll be told to raise your finger, sometimes to repeat the word you heard. Then earphones will be placed over each of your ears and adjusted so that they are both tight and comfortable. The technologist will leave the booth, and the fun will begin. The whole thing takes about 20 minutes. There is neither discomfort nor hazard. There are no aftershocks or sounds.

Bottom Line: (½ +) Kind of fun.

Tympanogram *Tympan* refers to the eardrum, a thin, special sheet of tissue called a membrane which separates the outer ear from the middle ear. It serves as a conductor of the sound that enters your outer ear and is transmitted to your middle ear. This is accomplished by the drum vibrating when it is struck by sound waves. If the drum is thickened because of previous infection, or if it is not whole because of previous injury ("perforated"), or if there is something behind it in the middle ear that can't be seen, like fluid, its movement will be abnormal. A detailed graph of its movement can be obtained by this procedure. (A similar procedure was described in the section above on the physical examination of the ear using a tympanometer. That study does not provide a written record.) The tympanogram is routinely made following the audiogram. A different headset is used. In this one a small rubber plug is inserted in one ear. A mild pressure is applied that you will feel. (If you have ever been in a plane or at particularly high altitudes you may have experienced the same feeling.) At most it is a ($\frac{1}{2}$ +). The same procedure is performed in the opposite ear. Total time for both is over five minutes. There is no hazard. There are no later effects.

Bottom Line: ($\frac{1}{2}$ +) Just a ho-hum.

Electronystagmogram This test is sometimes called ENG. *Electro* refers to the electrical impulses the body is capable of producing; *nystagmo* is from "nystagmus," a term that describes certain involuntary rapid movements of the eye, either up and down, side to side, or even rotary. Thus this test can measure and record the existence of such abnormal movements by detecting the electrical impulse such motion initiates. These eye drifts are frequently the result of some abnormality in the balance mechanism (known as the vestibular system) that is located in the inner ear. Patients who complain of dizziness must be evaluated for such problems that can arise from various causes—most commonly infection or tumor.

The test is best performed if you eliminate as many medications as your doctor will permit the day of the study, and avoid alcohol for at least 24 hours. Glasses and contact lenses should be removed. The procedure is done by a specially trained technologist. He or she will gently tape small metal disks, about the size of an M&M, just under each eye and on the bridge of your nose. These are SENSORS that will detect the electrical impulses. They are attached by lead wires to a special machine that will translate these impulses into graphs and measurements. You will be asked to look at, and follow only with your eyes, small lights that will be flashed on the wall in front of you. You will be asked to lie down, close your eyes, and turn onto each side. You will then be warned that water will be put into each of your ears in turn. The water at first will be cold, then warm. Any or all of these movements and particularly the water instillation can make you feel really dizzy and/or nauseous. These feelings can persist for hours. Therefore, it is a good idea to bring a pal to help you get home.

The discomfort ranges from (+) to (+ + +), but there is no hazard. Bottom Line: (+ +) "Stop the merry-go-round, I want to get off."

Auditory Brainstem Response See the section Brainstem Auditory Evoked Potentials in Chapter 8.

X-ray Examinations The examinations most appropriate for problems of the ears are described in the CT section of Brain on pages 179 and 187.

Magnetic Resonance Imaging (MRI) See Chapter 21.

Nose

As with the ears, most of us know about this body part, so it does not require too much explanation of why it hangs out there. The nose, like the ears, is involved with a major sense—smell. It, too, has other duties—primarily with respiration (breathing). Ideally, we take air into our bodies through our noses —yes, the mouth route will work, too, but it is really an alternate highway. The nose is also in direct association with several CAVITIES called sinuses that surround it and drain into it. Thus, problems of the paranasal (*para* here means "alongside or adjacent to") sinuses are considered along with problems of the nose. So, besides the common complaints of congestion (obstruction to normal flow or drainage), rhinorrhea (discharge from the nose), postnasal drip, and itching and sneezing, there are also the problems of facial pain, headaches (particularly over the eyes and top of the head), pain over the upper teeth, and unexplained fever, that may all arise from problems in the sinuses.

Diagnostic procedures for the nose include a physical examination, laboratory tests, an X-ray examination, and a biopsy.

Physical Examination The examination of the nose is part of the complete physical performed by the otorhinolaryngologist. See the section on the Ears.

Laboratory Tests Testing for the types of infection that may be present can be accomplished by smears and CULTURES. See Chapter 17.

X-ray Examinations Studies involve both the bony parts that might be the prime target in problems arising from injury, and the soft tissues that could be affected by infection, tumor, or other miseries. See Head in Chapter 18.

Biopsy The subject of BIOPSY and its general techniques are described in the section Cells and Tissues of Chapter 17. The specific techniques as they apply to problems of the nose and sinuses are ones of ASPIRATION and EXCISION.

Aspiration biopsy is performed to obtain secretions for culture and cell type. It may be necessary to insert a special type of needle known as a trocar into one of the sinuses. The approach is through the nose or upper gum of the mouth. Either requires the injection of a local anesthetic first. It will start like "at the dentist"—a small but painful (+ +) "stick" followed by a feeling of numbness. Dr. ENT will then insert the trocar. You will feel pressure, and perhaps a tiny "pop" when the sinus is entered. A tad more pressure when the secretions are aspirated, and then it's over. The total time is less than five minutes. The total discomfort is about (+ +). There is a small hazard of bleeding (+) that explains the request for informed consent. Expect mild pain in the area which will last for several days and which may require medication (usually aspirin or whatever you use that works like aspirin).

If something is seen within the nose that requires removal for cell type analysis, an excisional biopsy will be done. This will be almost like the aspiration described above. First the "local" will be administered and then a small piece of tissue will be removed with an appropriate instrument. All of the same scores and afterexpectations as above.

Bottom Line: (+ +) It's going to hurt, but you've had a lot worse.

Throat

The throat is the front part of the neck. It is the passageway from the nose and mouth to the lungs and points farther south. The Adam's apple—that bump in the front that bobbles up and down—is what interests us most. That bump is caused by a set of CARTILAGES that make up the outside of what is often referred to as the "voice box." Inside this "box" are the structures—primarily the vocal cords—that permit us to speak. So any problems with the voice—changes or hoarseness—will necessitate examination of this area. Additionally, any unexplained or protracted sore throat or difficulty in swallowing will call for an examination too.

Diagnostic procedures for the throat include a physical examination, laboratory tests, an X-ray examination, and a biopsy.

Physical Examination The examination of the throat is part of the complete physical performed by the otorhinolaryngologist. See the section on the ears.

Laboratory Tests Testing for the types of infection that may be present can be accomplished by smears and cultures. See Chapter 17.

X-ray Examinations All appropriate procedures for the examination of the larynx are described in Chapter 18 in the section Neck.

Biopsy The subject of biopsy and its general techniques are described in the section Cells and Tissue of Chapter 17. The specific technique utilized in this area is EXCISIONAL BIOPSY. It is usually initiated because "something" is seen at the time of the physical examination that demands further evaluation. As a rule the biopsy is performed under general anesthesia. It can now be done as a short procedure hospitalization (see discussion on short procedure hospitalization in the Introduction) which does not require overnight hospitalization, but does require careful monitoring for some hours. Since you will be "asleep" you will be unaware of the events. Actually, the biopsy is not too different from the laryngoscopic examination (described earlier, in the routine examination of the throat), except now a piece of tissue will be removed. There is always the potential hazard of bleeding, so you will be asked for permission and an informed consent signature. You will awake with a sore throat that will last for several days. Your voice will also be quite hoarse, and it is best to rest it for the same several days. Since you have had a "general" you will feel rather washed out and will probably go to bed after you get home. If you can arrange it—although it is not mandatory—take the next day off. Oh, yes, bring a pal to help you with things like getting home.

Bottom Line: (+ + +) It's a real pain in the neck.

14

Go See a Pulmonologist

A pulmonologist is a physician who specializes in diseases of the lungs. To assume this title a man or woman spends three years after graduating from both college and medical school studying internal medicine and then two additional years studying the nature and treatment of problems that affect the lungs.

Pulmonologists deal with any problem that affects the lungs. Often patients suffer from a prolonged disease that is the result of the inhalation of some toxic agent, such as cigarette smoke or asbestos dust. Often the problems are infection, either of the acute variety, such as pneumonia, or the chronic variety, such as longstanding tuberculosis. Sometimes a patient is seen because a possible tumor was noted on an X-ray of the chest. This must be aggressively investigated. If it is a tumor, surgery may be indicated. If surgery is called for, it is essential that the entire pulmonary (lung) status be known to ensure that the lungs that remain after the operation are sufficient to satisfy the patient's normal needs. Thus, the pulmonologist must first establish the diagnosis and determine the lung's functional capacity and then advise and counsel on the appropriate management.

All of the procedures to be described will be grouped under the title Lungs.

For a detailed discussion of each examination, start with the accompanying table. It identifies each of the procedures that are the usual province of this specialist. Suppose the pulmonologist said, "I'm recommending that you have a biopsy of that 'thing' they saw on your X-ray." Find this test and read across its entire line. A quick synopsis of the pertinent data characterizing

Pulmonology

Procedure	Discomfort* (−) to (++++)	Hazard* (−) to (+++)	Hospital (Incl. Short Procedure)	Special Prep.	Physician	Extras*	Informed Consent*	Exam Time* (Hrs.)	Bottom Line* (−) to (++++)	Exam Description (Page)
Physical exam	(½+)	(−)	N	N	Y	N	N	½	(½+)	129
Laboratory tests	(+)	(−)	N	N	N	Y	N	¼	(+)	129
Nuclear imaging	(+)	(−)	N	N	N	Y	N	1	(+)	130
X-rays	(½+) to (+++)	(−) to (+++)	Y/N	Y/N	Y/N	Y	Y/N	¼–3	(½+) to (+++)	130
Bronchoscopy	(+++)	(++)	Y	Y	Y	Y	Y	1	(+++)	130
Biopsy	(++)	(+++)	Y	Y	Y	Y	Y	1	(++)	132
Pulmonary function studies	(+)	(−)	N	N	Y	Y	N	¾	(+)	133
Cardiopulmonary exercise	(++) to (+++)	(++)	N	Y	Y	Y	Y	2	(+++)	134
Mediastinoscopy	(++)	(+++)	Y	Y	Y	Y	Y	1	(+++)	136

* See Appendix, Table Details.

this study is listed. (These data are elaborated upon in the Appendix.) The last item on the line is the page number where the study is described in detail.

And finally, after you have read about the particular examination that you are preparing for, reread pages xiv through xvi, General Events Common to All Adult Diagnostic Procedures.

Lungs

Our lungs come as a matched set of two. They are somewhat pyramidal shaped, and make their home on each side of the chest. They are separated from each other by the mediastinum, a compartment that lies in the middle and houses, among other residents, the heart. The top of each lung, known as its apex, ends just below each collar bone, while the bottom, or base, rests on a muscular floor, the diaphragm, that separates the chest from the abdomen. There is a series of passageways and tubes connecting the back of the mouth and nose to each lung—the pharynx, the trachea, and the bronchi. These structures serve as a two-way throughway for air—going in (inhalation), and moving out (exhalation).

The lungs are the "clearing house" for air. The air that we breathe in contains among other things a basic element, oxygen, that is also basic to life. The lungs are capable of extracting oxygen from the air and passing it through to the blood, which then distributes it to all of the cells of the body. On the other side of the RESPIRATORY coin is the product that results from the use of the oxygen—carbon dioxide—which must be gotten rid of. This chemical compound is also carried in the blood; it travels back to the lungs, where it is extracted and then expelled by breathing out.

So, when there is concern that something in the respiratory tract may be amiss, tests are required.

Diagnostic procedures for the lungs include a physical examination, laboratory tests, nuclear imaging, X-rays, bronchoscopy, a biopsy, pulmonary function studies, a cardiopulmonary exercise test, and mediastinoscopy.

Physical Examination   The examination performed by the pulmonologist will not differ substantially from that done by the cardiologist. See Chapter 2.

Laboratory Tests   Routine laboratory studies of the blood and urine are essential. But additional examinations are often required that are less routine.

These include obtaining arterial blood, sputum, cells, and other tissues. See Chapter 17.

Nuclear Imaging   See Lungs under the Chest section in Chapter 19.

X-rays   All of the usual examinations for Lung Disease will be found under the heading Heart: Conventional-Routine, CT, and Lungs, Trachea, and Bronchi in Chapter 18. Also to be found in the same chapter under the heading Arteriography is the discussion and description of the examination of the pulmonary arteries.

Bronchoscopy   *Broncho* refers to the bronchi, which are the part of the respiratory tract extending from the trachea to each lung. These are specially constructed tubes whose main function is to provide a conduit for the movement of air. *Oscopy* refers to the direct visualization of a part by a specially designed optical instrument. Thus, bronchoscopy is the procedure of passing an instrument into a bronchus and thereby permitting that structure to be examined visually. At the same time, samples of the bronchial and/or lung secretions can be collected. And, lastly, if there is need because of earlier X-ray findings or from what is directly seen, actual samples of tissue from the region of concern can be removed for analysis. This is known as a transbronchial or bronchial BIOPSY and it is discussed shortly, under Biopsy.

The trick is getting the bronchoscope down, because when the mighty laryngeal, tracheal, and bronchial engineers designed and built the first breathing prototype they said, "no bronchoscope is wanted here." So, they installed a safety valve called the "cough reflex." Anything other than air that enters the area will evoke vigorous coughing which will hopefully expel the invader. (Who has not experienced these paroxysms when food has gone down the "wrong way"?) Thus, getting the scope down requires a temporary disconnection of the coughing REFLEX. This is done by producing total anesthesia of the area.

The technique of accomplishing this state varies slightly from one performer to the next. The following is a standard routine: You will be asked to open your mouth. The pulmonologist will then spray a local or topical anesthetic into your mouth and the back of your throat. It will taste mildly bitter. In a moment your throat will begin to feel "thick." A thin metal tube called a cannula, about six inches long and shaped like a candy cane, will then be put into your mouth with the curved end placed over the back of your tongue. More anesthetic solution will be injected into the cannula and the "local" will run down your throat, through your larynx and trachea, and finally into

your bronchial tubes and lungs. The first few drops will induce severe coughing. But each subsequent few drops will cause less, until all coughing is gone.
Everything feels "thick." Finally, you will be asked if there is one side of your
nose that seems freer than the other. If yes, that nostril will be chosen; if no,
either will do. In either case, a jelly-like material will be inserted into your
nostril. This gel is also a local anesthetic and it will make it possible for you
to tolerate the insertion of the bronchoscope. Although this is the more
common route of entrance, the mouth is still sometimes used, particularly if
one has some nasal problem. At this point you will be ready for the scope.

The examination will probably, but not always, be done in a FLUORO-
SCOPIC room in the hospital X-ray department. (For a full discussion of the
various types of rooms in an X-ray suite and what happens in them, see the
introductory sections of Chapter 18.) You will probably be lying on your back
with your head propped up by pillows. The pulmonologist will stand next to
you and gently insert a thin flexible tube into your nostril (the one that has
been anesthetized) and continue to push the tube forward so that it passes
down into your throat and finally into a bronchus. I know this sounds gruesome, but remember, everything is numb and although you will feel the
pressure, it is only a (+) discomfort. Also, these folks are remarkably adept
at this thing and the whole passage is accomplished in seconds.

The tube is the bronchoscope. This instrument is truly a high-tech product, containing fiber optics, which means that the examiner can see to its
end even if the tube is not fully straight. This permits the scope to be flexible.
(In the past the tube had to be straight, or rigid. All of this translates into a
remarkable reduction of discomfort to you.) The instrument is about half an
inch wide and about two feet long. The end that remains on the outside has
a special eyepiece so that the examiner can look in. Additionally, the tube is
connected to various bottles that will be on a small table next to you. These,
in turn, are connected to a small motor that you may hear running. This
apparatus is a suction device that permits fluids that may be in your bronchi
to be sucked up and collected. The bronchoscope also has "side arms" that
are entrance ports that permit fluids to be "run in" in order to wash out the
area and aid in the collection of cells for later analysis by a PATHOLOGIST. It
is also possible to slide another, thinner CATHETER or wire, which may have
either a brush or small scissors-like apparatus at its end, down through the
scope. The bristle-ended wire permits cells to be "brushed" off the walls of
the bronchi. The scissors device permits small pieces of tissue to be removed.

So much for background. Now back to the ranch house—what will it be
like?

You will be aware of that thing down your throat! The first reaction is usually mild panic—"I won't be able to breathe." But you will, and quite well. Relaxing is the key. Breathe normally, except when ordered to do otherwise by the examiner. You will feel the pressure of the tube. It is certainly uncomfortable, but really not too bad—a (+). You may experience a sudden cough or two. This is a consequence of a spot or so being missed by the "local." More anesthetic will be added. You will be asked to change positions—"roll left," "roll right," whatever. You will be aware that the room lights have been dimmed and there is another physician, a RADIOLOGIST, in the act. He or she will move a fluoroscopic screen (see Fluoroscopy under Room Configuration in Chapter 18, page 176) over you and aid the pulmonologist in the exact positioning of the bronchoscope. You won't feel the fluoroscope. A biopsy may be taken, but that won't be felt either. After the scope has been removed they will probably take an X-ray of your chest, again, and compare it to the original (which in all probability is what indicated the need for the bronchoscopy in the first place), to be certain that there have been no observable changes produced by the procedure. That's it.

The total elapsed time is about one hour. The examination does carry some risk, particularly if a biopsy is performed. The hazard is (+ +). Therefore, many pulmonologists will insist on an informed consent from you, and may request that you go through the Short Procedures Unit (see short procedure routines on pages xvi–xviii) or even urge that you remain in the hospital overnight. This is for your protection, so say yes. Thus, the event will take at least the whole day. It might even be a good idea to arrange to stay at home the next day as well. Things to remember: You should take nothing by mouth for several hours after the procedure is over to permit the anesthetic to wear off; you may have a sore throat for a day or two; you may be mildly hoarse for several days; and you may cough or spit up some blood, also for a day or more. If any of the above are more severe than expected, particularly if you experience any real bleeding, get in touch with your doctor *immediately!*

Bottom Line: (+ + +) This one is big-time tough.

Biopsy Biopsy is the removal of tissue so that it may be evaluated and its nature determined. The technique of obtaining the particular specimen is dependent on where it is. When it is within the range of a bronchoscope, the biopsy will be done at the time of that examination, and is described above under bronchoscopy. When the tissue cannot be obtained this way, however, two other procedures are available: needle ASPIRATION and INCISIONAL biopsy. See Chapter 17, pages 167–68, and Chapter 18 under the heading Biopsy, pages 226–27.

Pulmonary Function Studies *Pulmo* refers to the lungs. These studies, of which there are four, are of utmost importance in distinguishing between two major categories of lung disease—restrictive and obstructive. Restrictive diseases are those in which the lungs are unable to expand properly or the lungs are unable to transfer oxygen to the blood. Obstructive diseases denote a narrowing or even a complete blockage of an air passageway. A partial list of the more important measurements includes: vital capacity (how much air can be forcibly exhaled after inhaling as deeply as possible); residual volume (how much air remains in the lungs after a forcible exhalation); tidal volume (how much air is expired with each normal breath); compliance (how well do the lungs stretch or distend with each breath in, and how well do they collapse or recoil with each breath out). From these evaluations the general nature of the problem, be it restrictive or be it obstructive, becomes known—a diagnosis. Can a treatment plan be far behind?

The individual pulmonary function tests (the "in" designation is PFT) are by name spirometry, lung volume, diffusing capacity, and airway resistance. From your standpoint they are all performed in the same manner, one after the next in sequence, and are therefore indistinguishable one from the next. Only the technologist and the computer that analyze the data know the truth. Here's how they are done.

No preparation is essential, although it might be well to empty your bladder and bowels before you start because there will be a lot of pushing down and straining as you attempt to take in the very deepest of breaths and attempt the very hardest of exhalations. Chances are good that you will already be in a gown because you will have had a physical examination. Now might be the time to put on that robe you brought from home because you are going to be busy for the next 30 to 45 minutes and you don't need the additional distraction of drafts.

The room in which the studies are performed may be chock full of different pieces of strange-looking equipment and computers. But rejoice, *none* of them will cause you any real discomfort or impose any real hazard. You will be escorted to what looks like a very mod phone booth. This is known as the "body box." It is shaped like a phone booth, but is larger. Within it is a chair that faces the wall that usually houses the phone. But in its place is a very special device that contains a mouthpiece that shortly you will have an affair with. The side of the booth that you face is a clear plastic panel, so you can see out. The door is also of the same material. Although you will eventually be enclosed because they will seal the door shut (the body box actually becomes a pressurized cabin) there is no significant "closed-in" feeling. Additionally, you will clearly see the technologist who is sitting in front of you, and will be able to hear his or her instructions.

When you are comfortably seated, you will be fitted with a nose clip that is just a fancy clothespin. It is placed securely on your nose, completely OCCLUDING your nostrils. Then a brand-new mouthpiece is brought out. It is a plastic flange-like thing with a hole in its center and two small bars on its inside—one above, and one below, the hole. It is fitted into your mouth so that the flange fits in front of your teeth and extends between the back of your lips and front of your gums so that air can only move in and out through the hole. You bite down on the bars. The technologist will then adjust the apparatus that is on the front wall so that its height just matches the hole in your mouthpiece. You will then be nudged forward so that the two are connected snugly. You will be asked to breathe normally until you become comfortable with these attachments and are convinced that you are getting enough air. If you are so inclined you can watch the TV screen that is next to the technologist. It is reproducing in graphic form the pattern that your breathing takes. The apparatus is recording it all.

When it is clear that you are comfortable the testing begins. You will be asked to perform a series of different breathing maneuvers on the commands of the technologist. Some begin with a deep breath in, others with a deep breath out, still others with short puffs. The entire battery of tests is completed in some 15 to 45 minutes. The only discomfort is the straining that you may invoke to satisfy the directions of the tyrant outside of the booth—once the friendly technologist—who is demanding greater and greater efforts. Except that you may feel that your eyeballs are going to pop out, or that you have developed a mild headache, there is no other misery. There are no hazards. There are no aftereffects.

Bottom Line: (+) Kind of fun.

Cardiopulmonary Exercise Test There are certain situations when the pulmonologist may not be certain whether your complaint—usually shortness of breath (dyspnea)—is being caused by some problem arising in the lungs, or from some heart condition. There is established data that can accurately predict the amount of physical activity, often called "work," one's body can perform after taking into account such factors as sex, age, height, and weight. This procedure is a form of stress test that will measure your "work" output. The findings will then be compared with standard tables of expectation and from this data a judgment can be reached as to whether the problem is of pulmonary or cardiac origin. (Sometimes it is neither—emotional causes may mimic organic disease—and that, too, is essential to identify.)

Preparation is necessary for this test. You need not stop any medication but you must refrain from cigarettes, caffeine, and alcoholic intake for a minimum of two hours before the procedure.

It will be necessary to obtain blood from an artery many times during the test so a needle is placed into an artery, usually on the inside part of your elbow. (See technique of arterial blood collection in Chapter 17.) A short piece of rubber tubing is then connected to the needle. The other end of the tubing is fitted with a valve that prevents bleeding. The tubing is taped to your upper arm. This procedure is called creating an arterial line and is accomplished in minutes. Samples of arterial blood can then be drawn at the appropriate times during the test by simply putting a syringe into the end of the tubing, opening the valve, and withdrawing the blood sample—all without any discomfort! Twelve samples will be obtained.

You will then be fitted with nose clips that will occlude your nostrils so that you can only breathe through your mouth. Then you will be fitted with a mouthpiece that will allow you to breathe only through its central hole. Finally, your mouthpiece will be hooked up to tubing that will capture all the air you breathe out while supplying you with as much of that good stuff as you need.

Additionally, the technologist will prepare points on your chest and back —thirteen in all—by rubbing briskly over each area with a small piece of bandage to which a LUBRICANT has been applied, so that each spot is mildly red and coated with the goo. A small metal disk (about the size of a quarter) is then affixed to each spot. These disks, called SENSORS or ELECTRODES, are capable of detecting the electrical impulses given off by your body. Each sensor is connected by a wire (lead) to a machine. The sensors will detect electrical impulses that originate from you and transmit them, via the wire leads, to the machine, where they will be analyzed and recorded in the form of a graph.

The pulmonologist will rehearse a series of hand signals that you are to use if there is need for you to communicate. (Remember, you will have the mouthpiece in and you won't be able to speak.) You will agree that thumbs up means O.K.; down means you are experiencing difficulty; and that you'll point to wherever you experience pain.

All systems are now "Go." You will be asked to ride a stationary bicycle or walk on a moving treadmill for a specified period of time—usually 10 to 15 minutes. You may find it difficult and often great effort is required to complete the desired end. But, give it your best shot! All the while you are working, various machines are recording your heart rate and rhythm, and your breathing efforts are being analyzed by a computer. If things get rough, "speak" with the agreed-upon hand signals. Hang tough and finish if it's at all possible. The pulmonologist and technologist will be watching and encouraging you. Rest assured that they will immediately terminate the study if any of the monitors suggest that you are in any danger.

When it is over the electrodes, nose clip, and mouthpieces will be removed. The needle will be withdrawn. (The technologist will apply firm pressure over the site for several minutes to control bleeding.) The whole thing takes about two hours. Any stress procedure is a (+ +) or (+ + +) discomfort if you give it your "all," and for the same reason it carries a (+ +) hazard. Good bet that you will be asked to sign an informed consent.

You will be tired! You will have some mild irritation from the electrodes on your chest for a few days. The area where the needle lived will also be tender for the same time. (It is a good idea to look at the spot occasionally to be sure that there is no bleeding under the skin.) After a good night's sleep you should be fine.

Bottom Line: (+ + +) You may think twice before the next "smoke."

Mediastinoscopy The mediastinum is a space that exists in your chest between your lungs. It is a condominium with such notable tenants as the heart, the esophagus, the trachea, the aorta, and a host of lesser-known celebrities, including lymph nodes. (See pages 223–25.) It is unfortunate, but true, that approximately one in every three lung tumors has spread beyond the lung by the time it is recognized. The spread is commonly to the lymph nodes of the mediastinum. If the tumor has spread, the treatment is markedly different than if this has not occurred. Thus, it is often most valuable to obtain such a node and determine its status. This is sometimes possible by the procedure known as mediastinoscopy.

This procedure is always performed in the operating suite of a hospital under general anesthesia. It is usually set up as a short procedure (see discussion of short procedures on pages xvi–xviii), which means that you can go home the same day. It is almost always performed by a chest surgeon, who will be recommended to you by the pulmonologist.

From your standpoint the experience will be essentially that which is described for any short procedure. Since you will be "asleep" during the actual event the only discomfort you will experience will be that of getting ready: being appropriately gowned, receiving preoperative medication about an hour before the big moment (which will both relax you and make you drowsy), and submitting to the transportation to the operating room for a reunion with the anesthesiologist and the surgeon. The procedure itself, begun only after you have been given general anesthesia, is the insertion of the optical instrument called a mediastinoscope through a small incision (about one-half inch) that is made in the front of your neck at the level of the top of the breastbone. The scope is moved down behind the breastbone until a lymph node is found. A small piece of its tissue is then obtained. Perhaps other samples will be taken as well. The scope is then removed and the incision closed with a stitch or two. The procedure itself takes about one hour. You will then be taken to the recovery area to be carefully monitored until you are fully awake. When this has occurred, you can go home.

Total discomfort is (+) at the startup, and (+) after it is over because of the incision, stitches, and events of the anesthesia and scoping; this will persist for several days. There is a (+ + +) hazard that is a combination of the anesthesia, the instrumentation, and the biopsy. An informed consent is required. Bring a pal to help you get home. Try to take the next day or two off because you will feel "punk."

Bottom Line: (+ + +) Hope the biopsy was negative.

15

Go See a Rheumatologist

A rheumatologist is a physician who specializes in the diagnosis and treatment of diseases that affect the musculoskeletal system—one's bones, joints, and muscles. This person, after graduating from both college and medical school, has spent two dedicated years studying this system and then three additional years studying internal medicine.

Rheumatology is concerned with the afflictions that our joints are prone to suffer. These afflictions, like the number of joints we each own, are many. Some are common, as in the older person who suffers with backaches and stiffness in the hips and knees and is often told by his or her doctor, "Don't worry about it because everyone at your age has arthritis." Some joint problems are rare and often masquerade as something else. Some are more common in women, and some more in children; some affect the same joints on each side of the body at the same time, and some only a single part; some begin with a sudden painful swelling, and some exhibit changes that develop without pain over long intervals; some can be treated and a cure obtained, and some can be treated with only the hope of providing comfort to the sufferer. And so on.

The rheumatologist is the medical specialist who sorts out the myriad complaints, signs, and symptoms and ultimately identifies the true diagnosis. This will be accomplished, in large measure, by the results obtained from different examinations. Fortunately, despite the multitude and variety of symptoms, the diagnostic procedures that are invoked are similar for all and thus can be described together.

For a detailed discussion of each examination, start with the accompa-

Rheumatology

Procedure	Discomfort* (–) to (++++)	Hazard* (–) to (+++)	Hospital (Incl. Short Procedure)	Special Prep.	Physician	Extras*	Informed Consent*	Exam Time* (Hrs.)	Bottom Line* (–) to (++++)	Exam Description (Page)
Physical exam	(½+)	(–)	N	N	Y	N	N	½	(½+)	141
Laboratory tests	(+)	(–)	N	N	N	Y	N	¼	(+)	141
X-rays	(+)	(–)	N	Y	N	Y	Y	1	(+)	142
MRI	(+)	(–)	N	N	N	?	N	1	(+)	142
Nuclear imaging	(+)	(–)	N	N	N	Y	N	1	(+)	142
Ultrasound	(½+)	(–)	N	N	N	Y	N	½	(½+)	142
Electromyogram (EMG)	(+) to (+++)	(–)	N	Y	Y	Y	N	1	(+) to (+++)	142
Nerve conduction studies (NCS)	(++)	(–)	N	Y	Y	Y	N	1	(++)	142

* See Appendix, Table Details.

nying table. It identifies each of the procedures that are the usual province of this specialist. Suppose your doctor said, "I'm recommending that you have an MRI of your knee." Find this test under Magnetic Resonance Imaging (MRI), and read across its entire line. A quick synopsis of the pertinent data characterizing this study will be listed. (These data are elaborated upon in the Appendix.) The last item on the line is the page number where the study is described in detail.

And finally, after you have read about the particular examination that you are preparing for, reread pages xiv through xvi, General Events Common to All Adult Diagnostic Procedures.

Joints and Muscles

Most people know about muscles. They are those specialized body TISSUES that are able to contract and by so doing make things move. Most, but not all of them, are under our conscious control. We "will" the cup on the table to reach our lips. We "will" the ball on the forehand side to be hit down the line. And, once these things are "willed," a series of muscular events (and other things, too) begins to happen. (Some muscles, like the heart, are not under our conscious control, but they nevertheless are being monitored, so that their function of contracting and relaxing is properly regulated.) Muscles must have strength to perform. A baseline strength exists normally in all, but appropriate usage can enhance this original power—check out the "ripples" on any weightlifter. Certain disease processes attack muscles and impair their power and thus their function.

Fewer people know about joints. Joints are the spaces that exist where two bones are coupled. This coupling provides the ability of these bones to move in more than one direction. Think of any of your joints—your knees, hips, elbows, ankles, shoulders, wrists, or fingers, for example. Each time you move them a whole set of activities occurs at that part. Over time this usage extracts a toll, commonly called "wear and tear" and medically designated "degeneration." This is the most common problem encountered—this is the arthritis of the elderly. But unfortunately there are many other afflictions that are the consequence of injury, infection, tumor, genetic factors, metabolic disturbances, and other diseases, to name only a few. Each is managed in a way appropriate to its cause. Thus, the sorting out by testing.

Diagnostic procedures for joints and muscles include a physical examination, laboratory tests, X-ray studies, magnetic resonance imaging (MRI),

nuclear imaging, ultrasound imaging, an electromyogram, and nerve conduction studies.

Physical Examination   You are asked to undress down to your basic underwear and to don a gown. The overall physical begins like most general physicals and is described in detail in Chapter 2. This is followed by a cursory
neurological examination; the complete neurologic is described in Chapter 8.

The rheumatologist adds to the above a definitive examination of all of
the joints: their appearance (are they swollen? red? deformed?); their range
of motion (do they move? appropriately? with restrictions?); tenderness (only
with movement? only on direct pressure? both?); the state of the muscles
surrounding the parts (are they relaxed? in spasm? exhibiting appropriate
strength?).

Each of your joints will be examined in turn—your fingers, wrists, elbows, shoulders, hips, knees, ankles, and toes. You will be asked to put each
of them through its normal range of motion. Depending on which particular
part is being tested, the examination will include bending it forward (flexion),
bending it backward, which often means simply straightening it (extension),
rolling it inward toward your body (adduction), and rolling it outward away
from your body (abduction). Each joint will be felt to determine whether or
not it is warmer than normal, swollen, or tender to mild pressure.

Next your spine will be checked, beginning with your neck—the cervical
spine. You will be asked to bend your head forward, backward, to one side,
to the other, and then to rotate it to the right and left. Then the rest of your
back—the dorsal and lumbar spine—will be examined. In the standing position with your knees straight you willl be asked to bend forward from your
waist. Then backward. Then to each side. Finally, to rotate in each direction.

The whole thing takes about 15 to 20 minutes. The examination itself
does not evoke any real discomfort, but since you are probably there because
something is hurting, when the doctor gets to examining that particular part
it probably will hurt worse. There is no hazard. There are also no lingering
effects.

Bottom Line: (+) Let's hope that none of your joints are found to be
"hot spots."

Laboratory Tests   There are multiple blood tests that are remarkably helpful in differentiating many of the different types of arthritis from one another.
Other procedures also provide specific data. These include ASPIRATION biopsy
of synovial fluid and excisional biopsy of both synovial membrane and muscle.
(See Chapter 17 under Blood and Biopsy.)

X-ray Examinations All studies that pertain to the joints are in the section Upper and Lower Extremities, pages 202–3. Also see Spine, pages 203–6, in Chapter 18.

Magnetic Resonance Imaging (MRI) See Chapter 21.

Nuclear Imaging The nuclear medicine procedures that are appropriate— bone and joint scans and tests to detect active infections—are described in detail in Chapter 19.

Ultrasound Imaging See Chapter 20. The procedure most applicable to rheumatic problems is the evaluation of whether or not a "lump or bump" in the region of a joint contains fluid or is solid. The study is described in the section entitled Neck.

Electromyogram (EMG) and Nerve Conduction Studies (NCS) These studies are about muscles and the nerves that supply them. See Chapter 8.

16

Go See a
Urologic Surgeon

A urologic surgeon is a man or woman who has graduated from both college and medical school, has studied the vast array of techniques that are included under the umbrella of general surgery for three years, and has spent an additional two years devoted to understanding the nature and correction of problems that affect the GENITOURINARY tract.

The urologic surgeon is concerned with any problem that may arise in men or women that impairs the free and normal elimination of the urine once it is properly manufactured in the kidneys; for example, calculi (stones) may lodge somewhere in the urinary tract and obstruct flow. Any pathologic condition requiring surgical correction, such as tumors of the kidney, ureters, or bladder, is also within the province of this specialist.

Additionally, urologic surgeons serve men in a manner analogous to the way women are served by gynecologists. They diagnose and then manage problems unique to men; examples include enlargement or tumor of the prostate gland, injury or tumor of a testicle, and evaluations of possible infertility.

But first—always first—there must be a diagnosis. What is the nature of what is wrong? To reach this conclusion, examinations, tests, and procedures must be performed.

For a detailed discussion of each examination, start with the accompanying table. It identifies each of the procedures that are the usual province of this specialist. Suppose your doctor said, "I'll have to cystoscope you to see if your prostate is really enlarged." Find this test and read across its entire line.

Urology

Procedure	Discomfort* (−) to (++++)	Hazard* (−) to (+++)	Hospital (Incl. Short Procedure)	Special Prep.	Physician	Extras*	Informed Consent*	Exam Time* (Hrs.)	Bottom Line* (−) to (++++)	Exam Description (Page)
Physical exam	(+) to (++)	(−)	N	N	Y	N	N	½	(+) to (++)	145
Laboratory tests	(+)	(−)	N	N	N	Y	N	¼	(+)	146
Catheterization	(++)	(+)	N	N	Y	Y	N	¼	(++)	146
Cystoscopy	(++) to (+++)	(+)	N	N	Y	Y	Y	¼	(++) to (+++)	147
Biopsy										
Bladder	(++) to (+++)	(+)	Y	Y	Y	Y	Y	¼	(++) to (+++)	148
Prostate	(++)	(+)	Y/N	Y	Y	Y	Y	¼–8	(+) to (+++)	148
Testicle	(++)	(+)	N	Y	Y	Y	Y	¼	(++)	149
Urodynamic studies	(++)	(−)	N	Y	Y	Y	N	¼	(++)	150
Impotence evaluation	(++) to (+++)	(−) to (+++)	Y/N	Y	Y	Y	Y/N	1–8	(++) to (+++)	150
Infertility (male)	(+) to (++)	(−) to (+)	Y/N	Y	Y	Y	Y	½	(+) to (++)	151
X-ray studies	(++)	(+)	N	Y	Y	Y	Y	1	(+)	151
MRI	(+)	(−)	N	N	N	N	N	1	(+)	151
Nuclear imaging	(+)	(−)	N	N	N	Y	N	1	(+)	152
Ultrasound	(½+)	(−)	N	N	N	Y	N	½	(½+)	152

* See Appendix, Table Details.

A quick synopsis of the pertinent data inherent in this study is listed. (These data are elaborated upon in the Appendix.) The last item on the line is the page number where the study is described in detail.

And finally, after you have read about the particular examination that you are preparing for, reread pages xiv through xvi, General Events Common to All Adult Diagnostic Procedures.

Urologic Evaluation

The familiar term urinary tract, suggesting a single system, is in reality two interrelated systems, and should more accurately be called the genitourinary tract. Particular functions of the body are performed by groups of organs identified by the unique purpose they serve. The designation genitourinary actually combines two groups: those concerned with reproduction—genital —and those concerned with the elimination of bodily wastes through the urine—urinary. The genital system in the female is composed of the ovaries, fallopian tubes, uterus, and vagina. In the male the genital system is composed of the testicles, seminal ducts, prostate gland, and penis. The urinary system is the same for both sexes: kidneys, ureters, bladder, and urethra. (The ureters are the tubes that carry urine, which is made in the kidneys, to the bladder. The urethra is the tube that carries urine from the bladder to the outside world.)

The complexity of this tract is such that three different specialists are concerned with it. First there is the nephrologist (see Chapter 7), who is primarily dedicated to understanding the mechanisms in the production of urine by the kidneys and the nonsurgical corrections that are appropriate for certain types of problems. Next there is the gynecologist (see Chapter 6), who manages the state of affairs in the genital system of women by both medical and surgical means. Lastly, there is the urologist, who is skilled in the surgical correction of both the urinary tract of both sexes and the genital system in men. Diagnostic procedures for urologic evaluation include a physical examination, laboratory tests, catheterization, cystoscopy, biopsy, urodynamic studies, an impotence evaluation, a male infertility evaluation, X-ray studies, magnetic resonance imaging (MRI), nuclear imaging, and ultrasound imaging.

Physical Examination The initial phase of the examination that is performed on both men and women is essentially the same as that which is done by the cardiologist. (See Chapter 2.) But in addition, a pelvic or "internal" examination is performed on all women (see Chapter 6 under Pelvic Organs), and rectal, testicular, and penile evaluations are made on all men.

Rectal Examination You have removed your clothing, and you will lie on your side facing away from the urologist. The doctor will gently but firmly place one hand on your "up-side cheek" and raise it slightly to more easily expose your anus (the opening of your rectum) while gently but firmly inserting a gloved and well-LUBRICATED finger of the other hand into your rectum. That finger will move against the walls of your rectum and you will feel it. The discomfort is a (+) to (+ +), particularly if you add on an embarrassment or indignity quotient. Breathing through your mouth—like panting—may help. You may be asked to "bear down," but that's all you'll have to do. There is no hazard. The elapsed time is one to two minutes, though it may feel longer.

Testicular Examination This is usually performed with you standing. It is a combination of INSPECTION and PALPATION. The palpation is first of each testicle for its size, shape, smoothness, and texture. Then the fingers will go deeper into the scrotum (the bag that houses the testicles), reaching up and to the right and then to the left. You will be asked to turn your head to the side and cough. This maneuver is to test for a certain kind of HERNIA. With the urologist's fingers in this position, and the cough to increase the pressure in your abdomen, if there were any herniation, it would be felt. Give the fingers a (+ +) discomfort. There is no hazard, and the exam requires only a moment for each testicle.

Penile Examination You will be asked to expose your penis, and retract its foreskin, if one exists. Then you are asked to "squeeze and strip" it (applying downward pressure from its base to its tip) with one hand to see if this action will produce any secretions. This is neither uncomfortable nor hazardous, but does rate a good (+) for indignity. It takes only a few seconds to accomplish.

Bottom Line: For men: (+ +) Yuck! For women: (+) This is one time when it is easier being a she.

Laboratory Tests Both urine and blood tests are commonly requested. See Chapter 17.

Catheterization This involves passing a rubber or plastic tube from the opening of your urethra into your bladder. Normally, when you have finished urinating, your bladder will be empty. In some problems there is residual urine remaining after you've finished and thought that the bladder was completely evacuated. It is important to determine whether this is the case. So, after you have been instructed to "empty your bladder" and you believe you have done so, you will be CATHETERIZED to see if there is any residuum. See the section on urine collection in Chapter 17.

Cystoscopy This examination is really an extension of the physical described above. Employing a very specialized instrument designed just for this purpose, the urologist can view the inside of the bladder with exquisite detail. At this time there are two models in common use—the standard and the flexible—and they vary slightly in their technique of insertion.

Standard Cystoscope This is the original model. It is made of metal, is rigid, and is less than a half-inch in diameter. It is best inserted when you are in the lithotomy position—lying on your back with your buttocks at the end of the table, your hips and knees fully bent, and your feet supported in stirrups that extend from upright poles at either side of the end of the table. You will be DRAPED and the area of your urethra will be carefully cleansed. A local anesthetic in the form of a jelly will be applied and will also be used on the outside of the cystoscope. This will numb the urethral opening, but not completely eliminate all feeling. The scope will then be passed into your bladder. Water will be run into your bladder through the instrument. This is done to DISTEND it and thus improve visualization, but from your standpoint it will very quickly make you feel quite uncomfortable because you will have the strong urge (and need) to urinate. Once you have made this condition known, the water addition will end, but you will be exhorted to "try to hold it" until the examination is satisfactorily completed. If any suspicious area is identified, a piece of tissue (a BIOPSY) can be taken through the scope. You probably will not be aware that this is happening. At worst, you may experience an additional "tug" or "pinch." This examination averages about 15 minutes. The bladder is then emptied and the cystoscope is removed. The discomfort is (+ + +). Although this is a routine office procedure, there is a very small possibility that the instrument could poke a hole in the bladder or that the same thing could happen if a biopsy is taken, so give hazard a (+). Most urologists will request an informed consent. There are some aftereffects in the form of urinary burning, possible slight bleeding (particularly if there has been a biopsy), and general discomfort in the area. These could last a day or two. Sometimes you will be given antibiotics to take for several days. Sometimes a medication that may turn your urine orange is given to diminish the pain when urinating. Although not essential, if you can arrange it, taking the next day off is a good idea. Also, observe the rule of BAP—bring a pal to make getting home easier.

Flexible Cystoscope This is the deluxe model. It is of the latest fiber optics technology, which permits the instrument to be made of flexible materials. This results in much greater comfort for you. The flexible scope is easier to insert and does not demand the lithotomy position. But once the scope is in, the rest is the same as described above. Just subtract a (+) from discomfort.

Bottom Line: (+ +) or (+ + +) depending on the model.

Biopsy

Biopsy is a procedure to obtain or collect a sample of fluid, tissue, or cells that are suspect for disease so that it or they may be microscopically studied by a pathologist. See the section Cells and Tissues in Chapter 17.

The problems that you bring to the urologist often make it necessary for a biopsy to be performed. The areas of most frequent concern are the bladder, the prostate, and the testicles. The technique for obtaining a specimen from the bladder is described above under cystoscopy. The other two sites require further detail.

Prostatic Biopsy The most frequent indication for this study is an abnormal finding at the time of physical examination—a "lump" or something "funny" is felt. Recently, some doctors have advocated that the prostate be SCREENED by ultrasound and that this area be biopsied if anything abnormal is discovered. Although the ASPIRATION method is always employed, two different approaches are taken. Their difference is of sufficient magnitude to deserve discussion. One approach is called transrectal. The other, perineal.

Transrectal This method implies that the needle used in the aspiration is placed into the prostate by starting its insertion from inside the rectum. This approach, when possible, is the "kindest" on you, which means that it hurts the least at the time the tissue is actually obtained, and gives you the least amount of difficulty after the procedure is completed. This "kindness" is a consequence of the nature of the nerve supply to the rectum. There are no "pain endings" in this section of the bowel except at its very end. Therefore, once the instrument is inside, as with the insertion of a finger during a rectal examination or the introduction of a tube as for an enema, you will have a sensation of pressure or discomfort, but no true pain. If the needle can be inserted either attached to the doctor's finger or as part of an instrument used to perform ultrasound (see Prostate under Pelvic Section in Chapter 20), the procedure will feel essentially the same as the rectal examination described above, and it will be done in the same way. When the fingertip feels the abnormal change in the prostate or the ultrasound tube "sees" it, the needle will be pushed through the rectal wall and into the prostate. Suction will be applied and prostatic cells will be pulled back into a syringe that has been applied to the needle. This will be felt as a "tugging" and rates only a (+) or (+ +). There is (+) hazard. The procedure is done by the urologist, and takes no longer than 15 minutes. Except for minor discomfort with the next bowel movement or even a slight trace of blood, there are no lingering symptoms.

Perineal In men, the perineum is that area that lies behind the scrotum and in front of the anus. When the transrectal approach cannot be performed, the biopsy is done by entering the skin of the perineum (often but not always with ultrasound guidance), and directing the needle to the prostate. This technique, described by some as a "punch biopsy," is far more painful than the transrectal because the perineal skin does contain pain fibers, and a much larger needle is employed. This procedure usually necessitates general anesthesia. (See Short Procedure Hospitalization in the Introduction.) It also necessitates a discontinuation for several days of certain medications, such as aspirin or steroids, that tend to enhance bleeding. Discomfort is only (+) initially because a general anesthetic is used, but the discomfort will increase and last for several days. Hazard is (+). The procedure will only take 15 minutes, but because of the "general" and the recovery time, allot a full day. Bring your pal to help you get home. Sexual activity is a no-no for the next two days.

Bottom Line: (+) Transrectal; (+ + +) Perineal. Negotiate this one real hard!

Testicular Biopsy When male infertility is suspected, a biopsy of the testicle may be indicated. This can be done as an office procedure. You will be asked to lie on your back with your legs spread apart, probably with your feet up in stirrups. Your scrotum will be bared, draped in sterile towels, and cleansed with an antiseptic agent. The urologist will be dressed in a gown and wear sterile gloves. One of your testicles will be gently grasped to steady it. The doctor will then inject a small amount of local anesthetic into the skin of the scrotum and then deeper into the testicle itself. You will experience a (+) discomfort from the stick, a (+ +) from the sharp burn that will follow, and then joy for the almost instantaneous numbness that results. A small incision will be made through the scrotal wall and a small piece of testicular tissue will be removed. You will be aware only of a slight pulling sensation.

A SUTURE or two may be used to close the incision. The End. Total time—
five minutes. You will be advised to refrain from any real physical activity—
including sex—for one week. There will be mild discomfort through this
period. A second visit to check things and to take the sutures out will be
necessary in about a week.

Bottom Line: (+ +) The thought of it is worse than the deed.

Urodynamic Studies These are procedures to evaluate the act of urinating. They are commonly performed on individuals who are known or are
suspected to have some underlying neurological problem, such as stroke victims and diabetics. The tests are also done in men who may give symptoms of
having an enlarged prostate that is interfering with normal bladder emptying.

You will be asked to arrive with a full bladder. Part 1 is a true relief—you
will be asked to empty that full bladder into a special container that is
equipped to measure and record the rate at which your urine flows. Part 2 is
tougher. You will be asked to lie on your back and be catheterized. (See the
section on urine collection in Chapter 17.) Water or perhaps a gas (carbon
dioxide) will then be run into your bladder in a very controlled manner—
both its rate and its pressure will be carefully monitored. This will result in
your bladder filling, and this is what is being measured by the procedure. How
does it respond to the pressure? Does it accept a normal volume? What is your
tolerance? Can you control the discomfort or does your bladder empty without
your command? Can you then empty it when you *do* command? These are
some of the questions answered.

The whole thing takes about 15 minutes to perform. Score it a (+ +) for
discomfort, for both the catheterization and what comes next. Some find it
embarrassing. There are no delayed problems.

Bottom Line: (+ +) Not a big deal.

Impotence Evaluation Impotence is the term used to describe a condition
in which men are unable to obtain an erection of their penis. This problem
may have either an ORGANIC or an emotional cause. Certain medications can
produce this condition—often those used for depression. Impotence may be
the result of previous surgery—certain types of prostatic surgery have been
known to create this problem. It may be a consequence of longstanding
disease such as diabetes. On the other hand, it may be a consequence of some
emotional trauma, which if resolved will correct the condition. Thus it is
essential to determine which of the two general categories is responsible so
that a reasonable treatment program may be initiated. There are several
procedures that are used.

X-ray There are some who believe that the problem is a result of some change in the blood vessels that supply the penis. Therefore, examination of these vessels can be made. See the section on the heart and arteries in Chapter 18.

Ultrasound Urologists who believe the problem is a result of some fault in the blood supply may elect to explore this possibility using a form of ultrasound known as Doppler. (See Carotid Artery under Neck in Chapter 20, page 279.)

Papaverine Injection Papaverine is a medicinal drug which can produce vascular relaxation. The advocates of this technique believe that the direct injection of this agent into the penis will result in an erection within 15 or 20 minutes if the impotence is of the emotional type. The penis is cleansed and a very thin needle injects it with the drug. The discomfort is (+) to (+ +) and lasts for about one-half hour. There is no hazard and no lingering effects.

Bottom Line: (+ +) It is like adding injury to insult.

Electroencephalography (EEG) It is fair to say that at this time, EEG is considered the most accurate and reliable procedure to establish the correct diagnosis. It is utilized because it is known that men experience erections in their nightly sleep, unless they suffer a true organic impairment. Thus, their sleep is monitored, and the occurrence or absence of erections is recorded. See Chapter 8.

Infertility Evaluation There are two procedures employed to diagnose male infertility. These are the analysis of the sperm (the masculine contribution to reproduction) and the examination of the testicular tissue—the testicles are responsible for the production of sperm.

Sperm Analysis See the Semen section in Chapter 17.

Testicular Biopsy The technique of this procedure has been documented above.

X-ray Studies See the Kidneys, Ureters, Bladder, and Urethra section in the Abdomen and Pelvis category of Chapter 18.

Magnetic Resonance Imaging (MRI) See Chapter 21.

Nuclear Imaging The nuclear medicine procedures that are appropriate—testing the kidneys, the bladder, and the testicles—are described in detail in Chapter 19.

Ultrasound Imaging These procedures are being utilized more and more for urologic diagnosis. The transrectal evaluation of the prostate may eventually prove to be the most sensitive screening study for early problems of this organ. Testicular imaging and Doppler blood flow have been added to examinations of the "old standbys," the kidneys and bladder. See Chapter 20.

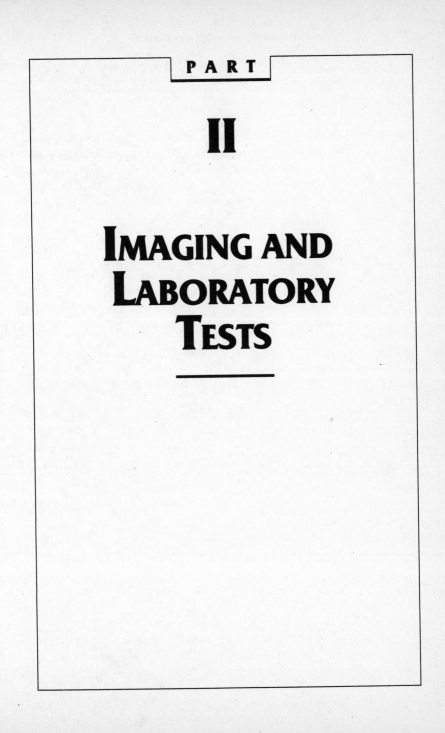

PART

II

IMAGING AND LABORATORY TESTS

CHAPTER

17

Go Get a
Laboratory Test

There is probably only one number that could be larger than the current national debt or Michael Jackson's yearly income, and that is the total tally of laboratory procedures performed in the United States in a year! The figure is essentially nonobtainable, since these tests are initiated at every way station where medicine is practiced: private offices, clinics, public health facilities; national, state, and municipal screening centers of any sort; any place home testing kits are used; independent medical laboratories; and, of course, hospitals. There are doubtlessly countless others that perform diagnostic procedures that would also be covered by that tremendous umbrella called "laboratory." On the road to such a guesstimate some "hard" data can be found. The numbers at two sites in Pennsylvania for the year 1987, for example, are known: hospitals—148,798,426; independent laboratories—43,645,054. So, in one state the quantity of laboratory procedures approaches 200 million (written out for those who, like me, can't remember how many zeroes equal what). As Pennsylvania is but one of fifty states, the total must get into the billions. And this number—for hospitals and independent labs —doesn't touch all the other places where studies are done and not tabulated. In all probability, in any given year, you have been a part of those statistics. Therefore, let's get to know more about "lab tests."

Yes, Virginia, there is a doctor who is in charge of all those tests! That physician, in a hospital, is known as the director of laboratories, and is, by title, a pathologist. One who specializes in the discipline of pathology is a graduate of a medical school, has taken an internship in a hospital for one year, and then has spent an additional four years learning the tools of the trade that permit him or her to be called either an anatomic or clinical pathologist, or both. The anatomical crowd are proficient in evaluating body tissues, commonly by microscopic examination—they are the ones that decide whether the "lump" that was removed is or is not cancer. They are also the ones who do autopsies (examinations of the body after death). They are all the Jack Klugmans of "Quincy" fame. Although some believe it is unfortunate that patients never see anatomic pathologists, it is actually very fortunate, because if you did see them, there would be a good chance that you were on your way to heaven.

The clinical guys and dolls are the ones who oversee all of the multiple procedures that are performed under the common headings of blood tests, urine analysis, and so on. You probably won't get to see these doctors either, because they are only interested in a part of you. The particular "part" (blood or urine, for example) is usually collected by you, your family doctor, a technologist, or the medical specialist you are consulting who requires lab tests as part of the "workup." The part of you is then delivered to the invisible man (or woman) for analysis. So, although you don't get to see him or her, the pathologist is there and performs a most essential role in your health management.

Next, the heart of the matter: What are these tests like from your standpoint? As discussed above, laboratory tests are unlike any other medical experience since you, yourself, are not necessary to the study. It is a "part" of you that can be delivered somewhere that is looked at. Thus, we must identify what part of you goes off for testing and how that part is gotten from you. The technique of collection determines the discomfort, the hazard, the time of involvement, the location, etc. It is essential to understand, in principle, that many, many different determinations can be and are made from the same body part. As an example, there are over 900 different analyses performed on blood alone. But there are only three methods commonly employed to obtain the blood from you that is then given to the analyzer. Thus, only the experience of the specimen collection affects you. (What the results of the tests are and what they mean to you is another matter, but not ours to discuss here. That is between you and your doctor.)

So, let's get to the particulars of each collection. Start with the accompanying tables. They are constructed to identify the general category of thing that is to be tested: blood, urine, feces, sputum, CELLS and TISSUES, fluids, pus, bone marrow, and semen. For example; if your doctor said, "Go get some blood tests done," you would refer to the table and find Blood. On the lines below this heading, you could then find the methods by which your blood can be obtained for those tests. (Most blood tests are initiated by venipuncture.) Scan across the appropriate line—a quick synopsis of the pertinent data, i.e., discomfort, hazard, informed consent, extras, and so on, is listed. (These data are elaborated upon in the Appendix.) The last item on the line is the page number where the detailed description of the procedure is found.

And finally, after you have read about the particular procedure that you are preparing for, reread pages xiv through xvi, General Events Common to All Adult Diagnostic Procedures.

Blood

Everyone knows what blood is. It's that red stuff that comes out of us, mostly when something goes wrong. We get cut; we get bruised; someone bops us on the nose. Everyone knows that it's not a good idea to lose too much blood, so bleeding warrants an emergency visit to the nearest "healer" more often than any other medical complaint. But, after those two headlines—blood is red and we should keep it in us—what more does everyone know?

Blood, indeed, is a very special TISSUE. Although it seems to be only a liquid, more than 40 percent of it is composed of CELLS of many colors: red (those that carry oxygen to all of the tissues of the body); white (those that are involved with bodily defenses against infection); and, no, not blue, but colorless platelets (those that aid in clotting when bleeding does occur). The other 50 percent or so of blood is "juice"—it is plasma. (There is also a liquid portion called serum, but we won't get into all of that here.) The plasma transports the literally hundreds of substances that are dissolved in it— HORMONES, ANTIBODIES, minerals, sugars, vitamins, drugs, proteins (the list is almost endless) to all areas of the body where each is selectively removed and utilized.

Thus, all examinations of the blood can be divided into two major categories: those that are concerned with the blood itself, and those that are concerned with the variety of substances carried in the blood.

Hematology, although actually meaning the scientific study of blood, is also the general name given to all medical examinations of the blood itself.

Examinations of the substances carried in the blood are grouped under three major categories: blood chemistry, blood microbiology, and serology/ immunology.

Blood chemistry measures the amount of particular substances found in

Laboratory Tests

Category/ Procedure	Discomfort* (−) to (+++)	Hazard* (−) to (+++)	Hospital (Incl. Short Procedure)	Special Prep.	Physician	Extras*	Informed Consent*	Exam Time* (Hrs.)	Bottom Line* (−) to (++++)	Exam Description (Page)
Blood										
Venipuncture	(+)	(−)	N	N	N	N	N	¼	(+)	160
Artery puncture	(++)	(+)	N	N	N	N	N	1	(++)	161
Finger stick	(+)	(−)	N	N	N	N	N	¼	(+)	162
Urine										
Spontaneous	(½+)	(−)	N	N	N	N	N	¼	(½+)	163
Catheterized	(+) to (++)	(+)	N	N	N	Y	N	¼	(++)	164
Feces										
Spontaneous	(½+)	(−)	N	N	N	N	N	?	(+)	164
Sputum										
Spontaneous	(½+)	(−)	N	N	N	N	N	¼	(½+)	166
Aerosol	(½+)	(−)	N	N	N	N	N	¼	(½+)	166
Tracheal aspiration	(+)	(−)	N	N	Y	Y	N	½	(++)	166
Bronchoscopy	(+++)	(++)	Y	Y	Y	Y	Y	1	(+++)	166

Category/Procedure	Discomfort* (-) to (++++)	Hazard* (-) to (+++)	Hospital (Incl. Short Procedure)	Special Prep.	Physician	Extras*	Informed Consent*	Exam Time* (Hrs.)	Bottom Line* (-) to (++++)	Exam Description (Page)
Cells & Tissues										
Scraping	(½+)	(-)	N	N	Y	N	N	¼	(+)	167
Aspiration	(+) to (+++)	(+) to (+++)	Y/N	N	Y	Y	Y/N	¼–2	(+) to (+++)	167
Excisional biopsy	(½+) to (+++)	(-) to (+++)	Y/N	Y/N	Y	Y	Y/N	¼–2	(½+) to (+++)	168
Fluids										
Intubation	(++)	(-)	N	Y	N	Y	N	2	(++)	169
Centesis	(++) to (+++)	(++)	Y/N	N	Y	Y	Y	1–2	(++) to (+++)	170
Pus										
Aspiration	(+)	(-)	N	N	Y/N	N	N	¼	(+)	171
Bone marrow										
Aspiration	(+++)	(+)	N	N	Y	Y	Y	½	(+++)	171
Semen										
Spontaneous	(½+)	(-)	N	Y	N	N	N	¼	(½+)	172

* See Appendix, Table Details.

the blood (such as sugar, CHOLESTEROL, digitalis, and alcohol). Blood micro-biology tests for the presence of harmful bacteria in the blood. Serology/immunology attempts to identify the amounts of circulating antibodies and the responses that have been evoked from previous infections or disease states.

Regardless of the tremendous number of different examinations available and the tremendous variety of data they provide, the studies all have one common denominator—they all begin with a sample of your blood. Many different determinations are often possible from a single blood sample. This is sometimes called SMA-12. Almost without exception a technologist will draw the specimen. Depending on what is to be studied, preparation may or may not be necessary. There are certain examinations that require a period of fasting—usually overnight. There are some that demand that certain foods or medications be discontinued for some specific period. Your doctor will give you those instructions. Most tests do not require preparation. Most are initi-ated by venipuncture. Occasionally, an arterial puncture or finger stick is necessary.

How are these done?

Venipuncture   This method involves drawing blood from a vein (a blood vessel that carries blood back to the heart). Veins are thin-walled vessels, often just under the skin, that may appear blue and do not pulsate when you feel them. In some people they are very prominent and snaky—these are the lucky ones if blood has to be taken. In others, the veins are difficult to find. The term "puncture" refers to getting a needle inside the vein and then drawing out some blood by exerting gentle suction (by pulling back the plunger of the syringe that is connected to the needle). The procedure is usually simple. Commonly, the inside of the elbow or the back of the hand is chosen and the part is bared, so wear a loose-sleeved garment that can be pushed up easily. Also, if you know the best arm or a better and easier place from past experience, holler! Some sort of elastic band will be tightly applied above the chosen area to stop the blood flow and make the vein "fatter." This is mildly uncomfortable (½+). The skin will be wiped with an antisep-tic and the person who will draw the blood will then PALPATE the part and choose the vein to be punctured. The person who does the deed is usually not a physician. A technologist, trained in this technique, is most often the one you will meet. The needle will be pushed through your skin and into the vein. If all goes well, and it does in the vast majority of cases, the discomfort will be in the (+) range. If there is a "miss" and more than one attempt is necessary, add another (+). But that's it. Some hypersensitive folks ask for, and should receive, a local anesthetic (either given by injection or applied as a cream or cold spray). Often the anesthetic is more uncomfortable than the puncture itself. But that should be your choice, if you wish to exercise that right. There is no hazard to this procedure. On average, it will be "over and out" in one to two minutes. A Band-Aid may or may not be applied. The part may become black and blue and be tender for a few days.

Bottom Line: (+) No big deal.

Note: Under very special circumstances it may be necessary to obtain venous blood that comes from a particular organ. Such a situation exists in certain studies for HYPERTENSION where it is necessary to sample the renal (from the kidney) vein. Such a sample is far more difficult to obtain than that which is described above. Problems such as these and the techniques of collection are discussed under Veins in the section Heart and Arteries, page 199.

Artery Puncture Arteries are those blood vessels that carry blood from the heart. They are thick-walled and are usually deep under the skin so you can't see them, but they pulsate when you put your finger over them. There are a limited number of studies that require that the blood come from an artery. The commonest of this group is called "blood gases" and serves to measure the amount or percentage of oxygen and carbon dioxide present. The artery chosen for this study is usually in the wrist, near the base of the thumb—it's the one used to take your pulse. Occasionally, the inside of the elbow or even the groin will be chosen. Regardless of the area, the procedure is the same: cleansing of the area with an antiseptic, feeling the vessel, pushing a needle through the skin and into the artery, collecting the blood (which will rush into the syringe that is attached to the needle), withdrawing the needle, and applying pressure over the puncture site. A word about the pressure. Arteries, unlike veins, are under high pressure and once punctured will continue to bleed heavily. Thus, firm pressure directly over the "hole" is necessary until all signs of bleeding have stopped. This usually takes about 5 to 10 minutes. The discomfort of the procedure is similar to or perhaps slightly greater than that for the venipuncture, so give it a (+) to (+ +). There is always a mild hazard of delayed or uncontrolled bleeding when an artery is invaded, so give this one a (+ +). Again, either a physician or technologist does the job. Give the "stick" plus the "hold" about 15 minutes. However, allow another half-hour to hour of hanging around and being watched to make sure there is no delayed bleeding. You will experience some mild discomfort for several days and the area may get black and blue. If, however, there is more than that—if you notice actual bleeding or the site of the puncture appears to be swelling—get yourself to the nearest doctor, *pronto!*

Bottom Line: (+ +) Kind of a big deal.

Finger Stick Not much surprise in this one. A finger is chosen. It is cleansed with an antiseptic swab. The skin is broken with a sharp needle or special instrument called a LANCE (a fancy sharp needle) and a drop or two of blood either wells up or is squeezed out. The technologist who wields the spear will then draw up the blood through a fine glass tube called a pipette and perhaps press a drop onto a glass slide. That's it. You probably won't even get a Band-Aid. The discomfort may be (+)—that little stick can hurt. There is no hazard. Time equals maybe two minutes. The finger will be tender for a day or more. It's not much, but it isn't nothing.

Bottom Line: (+) Compared to the others, almost no "deal" at all.

Urine

Everyone knows what urine is. It's that pale amber to deep yellow fluid that we rid ourselves of several times a day. We probably know that the kidneys make the stuff and the bladder stores it until we "have to go." Any further questions, however, would probably be pushing it. Well, what the heck, let's take it a tad further.

Urine is one of the two major ways the body rids itself of waste products. Your blood moves through your kidneys about twenty times each hour. The kidneys act like an admissions committee for a fancy club—they decide what gets through and what doesn't pass. Their nay vote results in the bad guys getting pulled out of the blood, while the good guys continue to move along. Those that don't make it are a mixed bag of METABOLIC wastes and certain minerals. But sometimes the selection process goes awry. Some club members in good standing are summarily dismissed while obvious villains are not recognized and are let in. So, spot checks may be necessary to ensure that the process is working well. There are nearly 100 different tests that are performed on the urine to ensure you that your kidney "club" is in good working order.

The accuracy of these tests is highly dependent on how the specimen is collected. The collection process varies with the particular test that is to be done. You will be instructed as to how to go about it. Some tests require that the first morning specimen be used since that sample is usually the most concentrated (because it has been collecting in your bladder through the night). Some demand a second specimen. This one is trickier. First you empty your bladder completely. Then you drink several glasses of fluid, wait 30 to 60 minutes (or however long it takes) and collect that sample. This technique may more readily detect sugar and other like substances. Another variation in the collection process occurs when there is a need to analyze all of the urine over a period of time, since its composition varies significantly through the day. This is the 24-hour test and (the name takes all of the suspense out of it) you simply find a big enough container and collect for the total period. It's a good idea to refrigerate the specimen through the collection period. Then there is the clean catch midstream collection, which is designed to decrease the possibility of contamination of the urine by other things that may be around and swept up as you begin to void. This might be material in the urethra (the tube that carries urine from the bladder to the outside world), such as semen, or vaginal products such as menstrual fluid. Begin to urinate into the toilet bowl without collecting the urine. After a couple of seconds— count "one and," "two and," "three and"—and, without stopping the flow—begin to collect your specimen in the container that will go to the lab.

All of the above collection techniques vary slightly one from the other but they have one fundamental similarity—you are delivering the specimen by voluntary urination. So none of the above carry any discomfort or hazard. But there is one type of collection that is not so super. That is the one in which your urine is obtained by having a thin rubber tube (CATHETER) passed up into your bladder. This method is employed when it is essential that the urine not be contaminated because it will be CULTURED (since there is concern of infection), or when you can't "go" on your own, or if there is a possibility that there may still be urine left in your bladder after you think it is empty.

If catheterization is inevitable, here is how it is done: The opening of the urethra must be exposed. In men it is at the tip of the penis. In women it is a small opening just above the opening of the vagina. The area must be thoroughly washed with an antiseptic solution (*wet* and *cold!*). The technologist will then genty insert a well-LUBRICATED catheter into the opening and advance it until it enters the bladder. Average time equals two minutes. Discomfort and hazard each equal (+). Add another (+) or (+ +) for the embarrassment and/or indignity caused by the exposure and manipulation necessitated by the catheter placement.

That's the scoop on urine. All of the tests can be divided into two groups: those using spontaneous collection methods and those requiring catheterized collection.

Spontaneous Collection First morning, second voiding, 24-hour, and clean catch vary only with the instructions of when and how. None cause discomfort or carry any hazard. All you have to do is what you do anyway—just do it their way this time.

Bottom Line: (½ +) Ready, aim, fire.

Catheterized Collection This takes a (+), sometimes a (+ +), for the combination of discomfort and indignity. There is also a (+) for hazard because there is always the possibility—although remote—that the catheter can poke through something. The procedure is usually performed by a qualified technologist, but sometimes a nurse or physician will handle the procedure. It can be done on an outpatient basis. Time of performance is usually only 5 to 15 minutes start to finish. Sometimes there is residual soreness for a day or two when you urinate. There may even be a slight pinkness to your urine for the same couple of days. If there are more symptoms than that, check back with "them that done it to you."

Bottom Line: (+ +) Ugh!

Feces

Feces are known by many names. When being tested in the laboratory, fecal matter is called stool. Normally it is composed of water, digested foodstuffs, bile (a product necessary for the digestion of fats and made in the liver), certain minerals such as calcium and magnesium, and lots and lots of BACTE-RIA. The "good" bacteria may number in excess of fifty different varieties. It only takes one type of "bad guy" to make you very sick. So, a major indication for examination of the stood is the suspicion of infection. Another common concern is whether or not there is any blood being passed. Lastly, the feces are checked for the presence of PARASITES when your complaints and history make this a possibility.

Regardless of the particular study to be done—stool culture for bacteria, a test for occult (not readily recognized) blood, or parasitology—each begins after the specimen is collected and delivered. Collection is the same for all.

There is only one technique of collection. Sometimes there is prepreparation. You may be asked to monitor your diet or medication intake for some short period before the collection. Those details will be provided by the person requesting the study.

The collection itself consists of simply passing some stool into a dry container. *Do not* let it get wet either from urine or from being "fished" out of the toilet bowl. Some laboratories will ask you to take a dab of it with an applicator stick that they provide and place this small sample into a small screw-top tube that they also supply. There is no discomfort and no hazard. The time is what you make it.

Bottom Line: (+) Just try to be a "regular" guy or gal.

Sputum

Sputum is not saliva. Sputum is a mucus-like secretion that is produced in the lungs and bronchi (tubes that carry air to the lungs). It may become infected. It may become bloodstained. It may contain abnormal cells that, if identified, could provide a diagnosis. So, once again, as with all laboratory tests, providing an adequate specimen is the key to success.

Sputum collection is most commonly performed by deep coughing. The "something" that comes up is sputum. You will spit it into a container— usually sterile—that you have been given for the purpose. This might be considered a spontaneous method. Sometimes, however, nothing seems to come up despite how hard you cough. This dilemma can be resolved in several ways. Sometimes a mere tapping on your chest by a trained person will loosen things up so that a specimen can be delivered. If that doesn't work, you might be asked to inhale a steam-like mist (aerosol) that will contain medication that usually enables you to cough up a sample. And, finally, if all else fails, and it is deemed essential that a sputum culture be done, the specimen can be obtained by a physician who will pass a CATHETER down through your nose and into the deeper part of the RESPIRATORY tract, usually to the trachea (windpipe) but sometimes to a bronchus (one of the bronchi). Once the collection tube is in place, some liquid is put in and then "sucked" back out. Since you will not tolerate this maneuver gracefully—you will cough, gag, or fight because you will feel like it is choking you—an anesthetic must be inserted first. It is necessary to deaden the cough REFLEX, which is the body's normal defense against things going down the wrong way. Passing a catheter down for the specimen is called tracheal ASPIRATION. Sometimes a direct collection from a bronchus is obtained by passing down a special instrument —a bronchoscope—during a special examination called bronchoscopy. Usually the bronchoscopy is initiated for a purpose other than just sputum collection. It is commonly done by a physician who is specialized in diseases of the lungs to obtain tissue—a BIOPSY. This procedure is described in greater detail in Chapter 14.

So, the techniques of collection for sputum are spontaneous, aerosol, tracheal aspiration, and bronchoscopy.

Spontaneous Collection This is the usual and routine technique. Cough deeply, spit into a container, over and out. No discomfort or hazard. One minute.

Bottom Line: (½ +) Hardly worth writing about.

Aerosol A short, maybe five-minute, stint of breathing a steam-like mist. (It's like when you were a kid and the folks ran a vaporizer.) The medication in the "steam" may feel a mite irritating and it may make you want to cough. After the session you will be encouraged to cough and bring up the sputum. That's it—perhaps a (½ +) discomfort from the mist, (−) hazard, and a 15-minute experience with a technologist.

Bottom Line: (+) About as exciting as the one above.

Tracheal Aspiration A thin rubber or plastic tube—a CATHETER—will be passed through your nose, down the back of your throat, and into your windpipe (trachea). A small amount of fluid will be injected through the tube, and then "sucked" back. That's the collection. But first local anesthesia is applied so that you can tolerate the placement. It takes 5 to 10 minutes to numb the area. Either a technologist or (more probably) a physician will do it. A spray will be used, which will make your mouth and throat feel very thick. A small amount of anesthetic gel will be put into one of your nostrils so that you won't mind the catheter. And then the deed is done. It is about a (+) discomfort. There is no true hazard. It will take a good half-hour. A big reminder: *Remember* not to eat or drink anything for about two hours after the procedure! If a catheter could get down, so could anything else—so hold off until the good old cough REFLEX is back on the job.

Bottom Line: (+ +) A mild pain in the neck.

Bronchoscopy This is really a big-time study and is rarely initiated for sputum collection alone. But if your doctor tells you that is what he or she has in mind, turn to pages 130–32, where this technique is described in detail.

Cells and Tissues

CELLS and TISSUES are commonly examined to determine whether or not they are abnormal. This examination is performed by the pathologist, and this type of study is called cytology. There are several different techniques that are performed to obtain the appropriate specimen, all falling under the general term of BIOPSY. The collection is usually performed by the medical specialist that initiates the examination. To offer an example: The Pap test is a cytologic evaluation of the cells on the surface of the uterus and its canal. The cells are obtained by a general physician or gynecologist by a technique called SCRAPING. Another common type of collection is ASPIRATION. Still another method is EXCISIONAL biopsy. Biopsy techniques are also described in detail on pages 226–27.

Techniques of collection for cells and tissues include scraping, aspiration, and excisional biopsy.

Scraping The part that is to be studied is bared. A wooden stick that looks something like a long Q-tip, except its end is slightly flared and V shaped, is used for collection. The collector is usually a physician and commonly one who specializes in the area from which the scraping is made. He or she will rub the stick gently but firmly over the part until some cells are scraped off. The stick will then be rubbed again over a glass slide, making what is called a smear (or perhaps the stick will be placed into a tube which is then capped). The specimen will be sent to the laboratory where it will be examined by the pathologist. The entire procedure, from your standpoint, takes only minutes. It rarely reaches a (+) discomfort level, and there is no hazard. There may be some minimal irritation about the area for several days. Just check occasionally to see that there is no infection.

Bottom Line: (+) Consider it just another minor scrape.

Aspiration *Aspiration,* when used nonmedically, identifies a strong desire to achieve something high or great. The physician who performs aspiration has a high desire, and it is to achieve a great specimen from you by a suction technique. The procedure requires that the skin over the part be cleansed by an antiseptic solution and draped with sterile towels. Usually a local anesthetic will be injected just under the skin. This is felt as a small "prick" (½ +) and then a sharp burn (+). Then a needle is inserted. The needle is attached to a syringe. When the needle is correctly positioned, the plunger in the syringe will be pulled back, creating suction, thereby pulling fluid or cells (or both) from the part into the syringe. Most of the time, this is felt as pressure and mild pulling but not real pain. The specimen is thus collected. It will be packaged correctly by making "smears" or whatever is appropriate, and then sent to the laboratory for pathologic analysis. The discomfort and hazard depend on just where the area of concern is. If it is a soft little bump just under the skin the procedure can be done in the doctor's office and take just a minute and a half. If it is something in your lung that was seen on an X-ray, then it could require your being hospitalized with the examination being performed under CT guidance (see detailed description, page 226, in Chapter 18 under Biopsy Guidance in the Miscellaneous section). In the former example, the discomfort is ($\frac{1}{2}$+) and the hazard (−). In the latter, it is (++) or even (+++) for each, and it will be necessary for you to give informed consent. Usually, when your physician says you need just an "aspiration" it suggests the easy kind; but if the recommendation is for an "Aspiration biopsy," get set for the "big number."

Bottom Line: ($\frac{1}{2}$+) to (+++) I hope yours is the easy one.

Excisional Biopsy   When there is no other way to get a specimen—it can't be scraped off, it can't be sucked out—then it must be gotten by cutting it out. As with the other described techniques, the magnitude of the procedure depends on where the deed needs to be done. If the problem is a small "crust" on the side of your nose, a five-minute office visit to a dermatologist will suffice. If, on the other hand, your SCREENING mammogram identifies "something" deep in one of your breasts, the excisional biopsy becomes a hospital surgical adventure. So, one description does not fit all. There is an obvious commonality—each will be done with either local or general anesthesia. But you should know the specifics about the one you are being asked to undergo. To resolve this problem there is an appropriate description of biopsy in each chapter where a biopsy is part of the testing being suggested by that particular medical specialist.

Bottom Line: ($\frac{1}{2}$+) to (+++) This group is really too variable for a one-liner.

Fluids

Fluids are nonsolid substances—liquids. Many different types are found normally throughout the body. Under certain conditions, such as infection or tumor, both the volume of a fluid and its composition can be altered. Additionally, these same (and many other) abnormal states may attack certain structures which do not normally produce fluid—the linings of the lungs (pleura) and of the abdomen (peritoneum) for example—but now respond by fluid formation.

Either the increase in volume—often noted as swelling of the part—or the altered functions that result from the presence of fluid where none should be or for the changed nature of the fluid, necessitates "getting some" to find out why these events are occurring.

"Getting some" is then dependent on where the "some" is. Two general techniques exist that permit this collection: INTUBATION or passing a tube into a hollow organ, and CENTESIS, which means to pierce or puncture.

Intubation   When the desired fluid is within a hollow ORGAN such as the stomach or the duodenum (the first portion of the small intestine), it can be collected by passing a tube from either your nose or mouth down to the part and then "sucking out" a sample.

For this one there is a "prep." Nothing by mouth (yes, that includes water) for at least eight hours. Then to wherever the collection will be made. (Often it is at a laboratory; often this procedure is done by the gastroenterologist.) It is necesssary to pass a thin rubber or plastic tube through the back of your nose and down into your stomach. A LUBRICANT containing a local anesthetic will be put into one of your nostrils first. (If you know that one side is better than the other—*tell!*) The person who is placing the tube (usually a technician) will ask you to swallow as the CATHETER is being pushed in. The tube, almost always, slides right down and into your stomach. There may be a momentary "gagging" sensation. The maneuver takes about one to two minutes and rates a (+) for discomfort. (−) is the hazard mark. This step is known as Intubation and is Part 1.

Part 2 is the actual collection. A syringe will be attached to the end of the tube—the part that sticks out of your nose—and gentle suction will be applied. This will yield a liquid specimen (often colorless) which will then be put into a tube and capped. This collection will be repeated every 15 minutes for an hour. Except for a mild tugging sensation that you may experience as the fluid is being pulled up there is no discomfort.

At the end of the first hour you will be given an injection into the muscle of your arm—a sting and a mild ache—of something that normally stimulates the stomach to produce acid. Another hour of collections will then follow. It will be no different than the first—just the intermittent mild tugging. But there is boredom! You must keep "hanging around" with that "thing" also hanging around the outside of your nose, for over two hours. Therefore, bring a book, some knitting, a crossword puzzle, or a pal. When the tube is finally removed, you are finished, and may leave. A long tale for a (+ +) discomfort and a (−) hazard. Except for a mild irritation that may linger for a few days at the back of your throat there should be no other problem.

Bottom Line: (+ +) A drag, but the coffee that follows never tasted better.

Centesis Fluids that cannot be reached by intubation require the insertion of some type of needle into the part of concern. This approach is known as *centesis*. Usually the name of the part that will be entered precedes the word "centesis"; for example, if there is a need to see the fluid that lines the surfaces of the lungs, the chest or thorax will be tapped and the study is called a thoracentesis. The same would apply to the study of the fluid around the heart—a pericardiocentesis; within a joint—an arthrocentesis; and so on. (There is another term for this technique often used by the in-crowd, and that is "tap." The identical name is used outside of medicine for essentially the same purpose—to obtain fluid. A beer keg is tapped, as is a maple tree. For kegs and trees an appropriate bore or drilling instrument is inserted and the "good stuff" is caught in a mug or bucket. In medicine the tools are a needle, tubing, and a bottle.)

It should be noted here that spinal fluid collections are usually referred to as "taps" rather than spinalcentesis. The detailed description of this particular technique is under Myelography in the Spine section of Chapter 18, pages 204–6. The general technique for the other centeses follows.

You will be positioned appropriate to the "best shot" for the part to be "tapped." If it's your knee you would be lying down on your back; if it is your chest you might be lying on your side; if it is your abdomen you might be sitting up. The "target area" is bared, carefully cleansed with an antiseptic agent, and draped with sterile towels. The performer of the deed is usually a physician and usually one specializing in that part of the body from which the fluid is to be drawn. A local anesthetic will be injected under the skin overlying the part. This is done with a fine, short needle, so expect a mild prick and a momentary "burning." When the part is numb a longer and thicker needle will be inserted deeply enough to reach the CAVITY containing the fluid. The needle is connected either to a syringe or tubing that in turn is connected to a collection bottle—often of the vacuum type, so that the fluid is "sucked out." Once the specimen is obtained the needle is withdrawn, pressure is applied over the puncture site for a minute or two, and a small dressing—often no more than a Band-Aid—is applied. The discomfort varies with the part but rarely exceeds (+ +). The hazard score is also (+ +). The time, too, is dependent on the "where," but an hour is a safe average. Most of the time you can go home with only the warning to watch the dressing to be sure it isn't leaking. Sometimes, however, the study requires that you remain in the hospital overnight so that you can be more closely observed. The procedure, regardless of where, usually requires an informed consent.

Bottom Line: (+ +) to (+ + +) It hurts more than a "tap."

Miscellaneous

There are always a couple of pieces that don't quite fit. (Remember when you were a kid and took the clock apart? When you put it back together, oh so carefully, there were always a couple of parts still on the bed. That's miscellaneous!) We will consider them here: pus, bone marrow, and semen.

Pus Pus is a thick fluid, usually yellowish white, often foul-smelling, and where it's found almost always hurts. It has a calling card that says, "I'm here so that means you have an infection." This material is a consequence of the body's protective mechanism against infection and usually found in it are some of the "germs" (BACTERIA, viruses, fungi, rickettsia, and even PARASITES) that caused the event. It is often important that the causative agent be known so that it may be treated with the antibiotic or other medicines that are known to be most effective against it. A specimen of the pus is therefore obtained, CULTURED, and then studied microscopically by our friendly pathologist. This scientific discipline is known as microbiology.

A small amount of pus is obtained either by rubbing an applicator (like a Q-tip) over the sore area or even by drawing it up through a needle. Either way is mildly uncomfortable and warrants a (+). If the collection is from a difficult location,—the back of your throat, for example—the collection can produce additional discomfort. There is no hazard. The sample may be obtained by either a technologist or a physician. The time averages about five minutes, and there should be no significant aftereffects.

Bottom Line: (+) Why does everyone hate pus?

Bone Marrow Marrow is a highly specialized TISSUE that is responsible for the manufacture of blood cells and is found in the hollow part of most bones. (When you crack open a chicken drumstick the brown stuff on the inside is marrow.) When you have a problem with your blood—perhaps there's not enough, or perhaps too much, or perhaps the cells "look funny"—analysis of the marrow may be indicated.

Collection of a sample is called bone marrow ASPIRATION. (It really is a bone marrow BIOPSY. Aspiration has been described earlier—see page 167.)

Bone marrow is taken from either the back of your pelvic bone—not the base of your spine, but on either side of that bone—or from your breastbone. The procedure is similar for both. The part is exposed, cleansed with an antiseptic, and draped. A physician—commonly a hematologist (a specialist in diseases of the blood)—will do the job. The skin overlying the bone will be numbed with a local anesthetic (a fine needle prick, a slight instantaneous burn) and then a larger and thicker needle will be inserted and pushed through the bone and into its CAVITY. You will certainly feel the pressure (+ +). Sometimes you can even feel the penetration of the needle through the outside shell of the bone. This is a (+ + +) pain, but it only lasts for a few seconds. There is a (+) hazard that the needle could go all the way through the bone and hit something on the other side. Although this is quite rare, you will probably be asked for an informed consent. The procedure takes about one-half hour. You may be asked to hang around for another half an hour to make sure there is no bleeding and that you are O.K. Except for the soreness that will linger for a week or more, you shouldn't have any problems.

Bottom Line: (+ + +) For this one, take a pal along. You'll appreciate the company going home.

Semen   Semen is the medical name given to the fluid that is ejected from the penis as a consequence of stimulation of that part either by sexual intercourse, masturbation, or emotional stimulation (as in nocturnal emissions, or "wet dreams"). This fluid is usually milky in color, rather thick, and somewhat sticky. It contains the sperm (highly specialized cells produced by the male body that are essential for reproduction) plus some other material. When there is a problem of infertility (the inability to conceive a child) the analysis of the sperm is immediately included in the search for cause. (Perhaps as many as one-third of all such problems are due to the male partner.) This analysis is usually initiated by a medical specialist in fertility—commonly a gynecologist—or by a urologist.

First the "prep": There should be no sexual activity that results in ejaculation for five to seven days before the actual collection. This direction may vary slightly depending on who is ordering the test, but all will invoke some "cold shower days." Next, the collection itself: This, too, can vary. A specimen may be obtained by masturbation into a sterile container. It may be achieved by intercourse using a special condom supplied by your doctor. (The commercially obtained propyhylactics contain powders or lubricants that may affect the specimen.) Regardless of how, the sample must be delivered and analyzed within two hours of its collection and it must not be refrigerated or tampered with in any way. And, lastly, the score: discomfort and hazard are (−).

Bottom Line: (−) Except for the emotional pain that undoubtedly exists as a consequence of the reason for which this study is being done, it is tempting to suggest that all examinations should be this tough.

18

Go Get an X-ray

Hazard: Ionizing Radiation Is Detrimental to Health!

This is a one-paragraph-fits-all disclaimer that applies to all X-ray examinations: X-ray procedures subject the recipient to ionizing radiation. The amount varies with the examination. The effects are cumulative. The potential for harm is greater in the young than in the old, and is greatest in the fetus. Thus, each study must be weighed carefully and the risks-to-benefit ratio established by those most knowledgeable to make this decision —your referring physician and the radiologist. Except for the pregnant patient, and even in this example there are exceptions, the hazards are more theoretical than real. The benefits from an indicated examination far outweigh the risks. But, if you do have fear, discuss it with your professional advisors. If you are or even might be pregnant, let this fact be known. Keep records of all your previous X-ray examinations and review them with the radiologist prior to each new study. Concern is warranted. Panic is not.

In 1985 (according to figures from the American College of Radiology) the command "Go get an X-ray" was honored some 265,000,000 times in the United States alone. That figure includes only the numbers obtained from hospitals or private offices where the studies were performed by a radiologist. How many more examinations were performed in outpatient centers or in private doctor's offices by physicians other than radiologists cannot even be guesstimated. However, despite the impossibility of providing absolute numbers there is agreement by those who concern themselves with these data, the counters at both the federal and the state governmental agencies responsible for health-care delivery, that X-ray examinations, year in and year out, are with laboratory tests the most commonly performed diagnostic procedures in medicine. Thus, there is hardly a soul in the United States who has not already had an X-ray. But, having had a "picture taken" at some time in the past does not necessarily prepare you for the "now" experience, which could be totally different. There are obvious similarities from one study to the next, but there are also considerable differences possible. Thus, each specific examination will be described in detail.

First an overview of those things that are similar to all X-rays.

The Equipment Up until some ten years ago radiological procedures were performed by machines that were all quite similar in their design and appearance. Then the world was enriched by the addition of the CT (Computerized Tomographic) or CAT (Computerized Axial Tomographic) scanner. This is an X-ray machine, but its design and appearance are sufficiently different from the older conventional apparatus that it has been dignified by its own name. Thus it is commonplace, now, to refer to one's examination as being performed by "X-ray" or by "CT," and the decision of which to employ for a given diagnostic problem (on occasion both are necessary) is made after consultation between your doctor and the radiologist.

Procedural Terminology As noted above, the terminology now used to identify a radiological (X-ray) procedure is to refer to the ones using standard equipment as "conventional," and those employing CT scanners as "CT." "Conventional" is further divided into "Conventional-Routine" and "Conventional-Special."

Conventional-Routine Examinations that are categorized as routine rarely require the presence of a radiologist (a medical specialist in X-ray), and they rarely cause discomfort, impose hazard, require hospitalization, need informed consent, or produce any delayed or lingering problems.

Conventional-Special These examinations almost always require a radiologist in attendance, and frequently cause discomfort, and may impose hazard and delayed or lingering problems. Some may also require both hospitalization and informed consent.

The Equipment-Room Configuration Despite the fact that all of the examinations to be described are produced by X-rays, physical variations in the equipment, and thereby the room, are required between one study and the next. Lest these differences in physical appearances cause you concern, a few lines about each. Three general equipment-room configurations exist:

Standard The conventional room consists of an X-ray tube which looks like a small box, usually mounted on rails on the ceiling but occasionally on a pole or a stand, and a table which may or may not move. The table will contain a drawer-like part underneath its top that will permit an X-ray cassette (which holds the film) to be stored within it.

Fluoroscopic FLUOROSCOPY is a form of X-ray image production whereby the examined part is seen on a special screen rather than on film. It permits visualization of the part in motion, like the heart beating or toes wiggling. It is what is used to examine your luggage at airports, and—for those old enough to remember—how they once fitted kids' shoes. Fluoroscopy is the province of the radiologist. The equipment in the fluroscopic room is far more bulky than that found in the standard suite and the space is usually larger. The tube is housed in a large cylinder or tower that can be moved over the X-ray table and is positioned above you. The radiologist guides the tower to the area of examination. When the tube is activated, images are created that are viewed on a monitor (like a small TV screen) and depict the part as it is at that instant and over the time of viewing. Thus, if the stomach is looked at, it will be seen to be moving, and this motion can be evaluated. This differs from the X-ray picture, which displays only a static image. (If you ask, the monitor that displays all the action can be positioned so that you, too, can see what is happening. It's better than instant replay!)

A note on the sartorial splendor of both the radiologist and technologist who are in the room with you. They wear special aprons and gloves—made of lead—for their protection. Did I hear you say, "What about my protection?" You are protected in that you receive the absolute minimum exposure consistent with a diagnostic study. You'll absorb some radiation, of course, just as you do when lying in the sun, but here it is controlled, and where possible lead shields will be used. The professionals who examine you are subject to exposure many, many, times each day. Don't begrudge them the eighteen-pound apron they wear.

CT (or CAT) The CT suite is completely different. The machine looks like a large freestanding wall with a large hole cut out of its middle. A long slender table mounted on tracks, called the *gantry*, stands in front of the wall and at the same height as the midportion of the hole. You lie on the table and the table is then moved into the aperture so that the part of you that is to be examined is within the "bagel." At one end of the room a technologist sits behind a large window and operates the computer that controls the study.

The Picture Experience Examinations done by the conventional techniques often vary significantly, so the experience for each can be different. Therefore, each such experience will be detailed here with the description of each study. However, the experience when having an examination by CT varies only in whether you lie face up or face down and whether or not you're given an injection. It would therefore be redundant to repeat the same words with each CT procedure described. However, a one-time waltz through the CT experience is appropriate, since it is completely different from all other X-ray surveys. But then, and forever after, whenever reference is made to CT, it will not repeat these details.

The CT difference is that only a relatively small body area is examined at one time and this area is SECTIONED (sliced like a loaf of bread) by a series of exposures, each of which images only a very fine part. All of the slices are then displayed after a great deal of heavy-duty computer manipulation and offer information obtainable in no other way.

You are asked to lie on the table on either your back or stomach. The table is moved into the machine to a depth appropriate to the body part to be examined. Each exposure requires several seconds and it is probable that each will be accompanied by a detectable whirring sound. The table will move slightly (about one-quarter to one-half inch) between each exposure, bringing the next area to be sectioned into position. You will be instructed when to hold your breath and when to breathe by the technologist, whose voice will sound close to your ear since there is a sound system built into the machine. This system also permits you to speak and express any concerns, difficulties, or questions that you may have to the technologist who is watching you through the large windowed wall at the end of the room.

There is no real discomfort or hazard unless the nature of the study requires injection of an X-ray "dye." ("Dye" is discussed in detail in the Appendix under Extras.) This injection is mildly uncomfortable and does carry a potential hazard to those who may be sensitive to iodine, from which these "dyes" are made. So if no "dye" is required, the studies are rated (−) for both discomfort and hazard. When "dye" is necessary, the score is (½ +) for each.

On occasion, being moved into the machine evokes ACUTE anxiety (an overwhelming sense of apprehension and fear). It may be triggered by a

CLAUSTROPHOBIC reaction. If you experience this reaction or can anticipate its occurrence based on earlier similar experiences, *holler!* Medication can be given that will control the fear.

Picture Taker   The image that is the end product of an X-ray examination is created, for the most part, by a specially trained individual known as an X-ray technologist. This person is specifically, carefully, and thoroughly grounded in the methodology inherent in achieving the goal for each of the products sought. This person is not a physician. However, when the product has been obtained it is then given to another trained specialist who will interpret it so that it has medical meaning.

Picture Reader   The trained specialist who will interpret the images is a physician. This person, after graduating from both college and medical school, has spent an additional four or five years becoming versed in the specialty of radiology. When that study has been satisfactorily mastered, as attested by successful passage of examinations known as boards, a degree is awarded proclaiming the person to be a certified radiologist.

For the particulars of each examination, start with the accompanying table. It is constructed so as to divide the body into six general sections (plus a miscellaneous group for whatever stuff is left over). Within each major area are listed the parts that are found there. For example, if your doctor said: "Go get a CT of your brain," you would refer to the table and find head—the general body area in which the brain is found. You would find brain and read across its entire line. A quick synopsis of the pertinent data inherent in this study—discomfort, hazard, informed consent, extras, etc., is listed. (These data are elaborated upon in the Appendix.) The last item on the line is the page number where the study is described in detail.

And finally, after you have read about the particular examination that you are preparing for, reread pages xiv through xvi, General Events Common to All Adult Diagnostic Procedures.

Head

Many consider the head as that body part where we really live. It is, after all, where we store our brain and many of the ORGANS that initiate our senses— our eyes, ears, and nose, for example. These "inhabitants" are so well known that they require no particular introduction as to the "wheres, whats, and hows" that are necessary when discussing lesser-known organs. But celebrity status does not carry any more immunity to danger than exists for the more lowly. Thus, the tenants of the head are subject to the same types of ills as the rest of the body: the brain, for example, is the site of headache, losses of sensory and/or motor functions, infections, and injury; the skull, consisting of the cranium, the facial bones, and the jaw, can be injured and is subject to infections and abnormal development or function; and the salivary glands are subject to abnormalities that cause changes in saliva production or discharge.

But not everything above the neck lends itself to X-ray examination. What can be examined in this way is described below. Some of the individual structures can be examined together with others. Some of the procedures of study are identical to each other. When either is the case, the descriptions of the techniques are lumped together. All three types of X-ray—conventional-routine, conventional-special, and CT—are explored for each body part when applicable.

Brain

Conventional-Special These studies are reserved for problems that suggest the possibility of tumor, vascular abnormalities such as a stroke, infections, or other complaints that cannot be readily dismissed and which might be recognized if the blood vessels within the brain could be seen and analyzed. This is accomplished by ANGIOGRAPHY. The details of this procedure are included in the general discussion of all vascular examinations, since they are all performed in essentially the same manner. Refer to pages 194–200.

CT For the brain, CT has been a diagnostic prayer and dream come true. When you consider that until its advent there was neither a simple nor a NONINVASIVE technique to investigate one of the top three most common complaints in medicine—the headache—it becomes clear why radiologists hailed its coming in the same ranking order as fire, the wheel, and pizza.

To begin the procedure you must remove all removables from your head and neck, including hair fasteners or adornments, glasses, earrings, and dentures. You lie on your back on the gantry. The rest is identical to all other CT experiences. See pages 177–78 for the details. The total time is approximately one half hour. There is neither discomfort nor hazard. No lingering complaints.

Bottom Line: (½ +) Easy.

For certain problems, such as the possibility that there has been bleeding into the brain or that there may be some abnormality of the vessels, a second

X-ray

Body Part/ Procedure	Discomfort* (−) to (++++)	Hazard* (−) to (+++)	Hospital (Incl. Short Procedure)	Special Prep.	Physician	Extras*	Informed Consent*	Exam Time* (Hrs.)	Bottom Line* (−) to (++++)	Exam Description (Page)
Head										
Brain	(½+) to (++++)	(−) to (+++)	Y/N	Y/N	Y/N	Y/N	Y/N	¼–2	(½+) to (++++)	179
Skull										
Cranium	(½+)	(−)	N	N	N	N	N	½	(+)	187
Facial bones										
Orbits	(½+)	(−)	N	N	N	N	N	½	(+)	187
Nasal bones	(½+)	(−)	N	N	N	N	N	¼	(+)	187
Sinuses	(½+)	(−)	N	N	N	N	N	½	(+)	187
Jaw	(½+)	(−)	N	N	N	N	N	½	(+)	187
Salivary glands	(+)	(+)	N	N	Y	Y	N	¾	(+)	187
Neck										
Larynx	(−) to (+)	(−)	N	N	Y/N	Y/N	?	¾	(+) to (++)	188
Pharynx	(+)	(−)	N	N	Y	Y	N	¾	(+)	189
Chest										
Breasts										
Mammogram	(++)	(−)	N	N	Y/N	N	N	½	(++)	190
Ductagram	(+)	(+)	N	N	Y	Y	N	1	(+)	191
Mass localization	(++)	(+)	N	N	Y	N	N	1	(++) to (+++)	192

Body Part/ Procedure	Discomfort* (−) to (++++)	Hazard* (−) to (+++)	Hospital (Incl. Short Procedure)	Special Prep.	Physician	Extras*	Informed Consent*	Exam Time* (Hrs.)	Bottom Line* (−) to (++++)	Exam Description (Page)
Cage										
Ribs	(½+)	(−)	N	N	N	N	N	½	(½+)	192
Sternum	(½+)	(−)	N	N	N	N	N	½	(½+)	192
Clavicle	(½+)	(−)	N	N	N	N	N	½	(½+)	192
Scapula	(½+)	(−)	N	N	N	N	N	½	(½+)	192
Sternoclavicular joint	(½+)	(−)	N	N	N	N	N	½	(½+)	192
Acromioclavicular joint	(½+)	(−)	N	N	N	N	N	½	(½+)	192
Heart										
Routine	(−)	(−)	N	N	N	N	N	¼	(½+)	194
Heart and arteries										
Coronary	(+++)	(+++)	Y	Y	Y	Y	Y	2	(++++)	194
Brachial/ subclavian	(+++)	(+++)	Y	Y	Y	Y	Y	1	(++++)	194
Aorta—thoracic	(+++)	(+++)	Y	Y	Y	Y	Y	1	(++++)	194
Carotid/vertebral	(+++)	(+++)	Y	Y	Y	Y	Y	2	(++++)	194
Cerebral	(+++)	(+++)	Y	Y	Y	Y	Y	2	(++++)	194
Pulmonary	(+++)	(+++)	Y	Y	Y	Y	Y	1	(++++)	194

X-ray—cont'd

Body Part/Procedure	Discomfort* (−) to (++++)	Hazard* (−) to (+++)	Hospital (Incl. Short Procedure)	Special Prep.	Physician	Extras*	Informed Consent*	Exam Time* (Hrs.)	Bottom Line* (−) to (++++)	Exam Description (Page)
Aorta—										
abdominal	(+++)	(+++)	Y	Y	Y	Y	Y	1	(++++)	194
Celiac	(+++)	(+++)	Y	Y	Y	Y	Y	2	(+++++)	194
Superior/inferior										
mesenteric	(+++)	(+++)	Y	Y	Y	Y	Y	2	(++++)	194
Renal	(+++)	(+++)	Y	Y	Y	Y	Y	1	(+++)	194
Iliac-femoral	(+++)	(+++)	Y	Y	Y	Y	Y	1	(+++)	194
Veins										
Brachial/sub-clavian	(++)	(+)	N	N	Y	Y	N	½	(++)	199
Superior vena cava	(++)	(++)	N	N	Y	Y	?	½	(++)	199
Inferior vena cava	(++)	(++)	N	N	Y	Y	?	½	(++)	199
Renal	(++)	(++)	N	N	Y	Y	Y	1	(++++)	199
Iliac	(++)	(++)	N	N	Y	Y	?	¾	(+++)	199
Femoral	(++)	(+)	N	N	Y	Y	N	½	(+++)	199
Lungs, bronchi	(++)	(−)	N	Y	Y	Y	N	¾	(+++)	200
Esophagus	(+)	(−)	N	Y	Y	Y	?	¼	(+)	201

Body Part/Procedure	Discomfort* (–) to (++++)	Hazard* (–) to (+++)	Hospital (Incl. Short Procedure)	Special Prep.	Physician	Extras*	Informed Consent*	Exam Time* (Hrs.)	Bottom Line* (–) to (++++)	Exam Description (Page)
Upper Extremity										
Shoulder	(½+)	(–)	N	N	N	N	N	¼	(½+)	202
Humerus	(½+)	(–)	N	N	N	N	N	¼	(½+)	202
Elbow	(½+)	(–)	N	N	N	N	N	¼	(½+)	202
Radius/ulna	(½+)	(–)	N	N	N	N	N	¼	(½+)	202
Wrist	(½+)	(–)	N	N	N	N	N	¼	(½+)	202
Carpal/metacarpal	(½+)	(–)	N	N	N	N	N	¼	(½+)	202
Phalanges	(½+)	(–)	N	N	N	N	N	¼	(½+)	202
Joints arthrogram	(++)	(+)	?	N	Y	Y	?	½	(++)	203
Lower Extremity										
Hip	(½+)	(–)	N	N	N	N	N	¼	(½+)	202
Femur	(½+)	(–)	N	N	N	N	N	¼	(½+)	202
Knee	(½+)	(–)	N	N	N	N	N	¼	(½+)	202
Tibia/fibula	(½+)	(–)	N	N	N	N	N	¼	(½+)	202
Ankle	(½+)	(–)	N	N	N	N	N	¼	(½+)	202
Tarsal/metatarsal	(½+)	(–)	N	N	N	N	N	¼	(½+)	202
Phalanges	(½+)	(–)	N	N	N	N	N	¼	(½+)	202
Joints arthrogram	(++)	(+)	?	N	Y	Y	?	½	(++)	203

X-ray—cont'd

Body Part/ Procedure	Discomfort* (–) to (++++)	Hazard* (–) to (+++)	Hospital (Incl. Short Procedure)	Special Prep.	Physician	Extras*	Informed Consent*	Exam Time* (Hrs.)	Bottom Line* (–) to (++++)	Exam Description (Page)
Spine and Bony Pelvis										
Cervical	(½+)	(–)	N	N	N	N	N	½	(+)	204
Dorsal	(½+)	(–)	N	N	N	N	N	½	(+)	204
Lumbar	(½+)	(–)	N	N	N	N	N	½	(+)	204
Sacrum	(½+)	(–)	N	N	N	N	N	½	(+)	204
Coccyx	(½+)	(–)	N	N	N	N	N	½	(+)	204
Pelvis	(½+)	(–)	N	N	N	N	N	½	(+)	204
Myelogram ("dye")	(+++)	(++)	Y	N	Y	Y	Y	1	(+++)	204
CT	(½+)	(–)	N	N	N	N	N	½	(½+)	206
Abdomen/Pelvis										
Abdominal survey	(½+)	(–)	N	N	N	N	N	¼	(½+)	207
Gastrointestinal										
Stomach/ duodenum	(+)	(–)	N	Y	Y	Y	N	¼	(+)	207
Jejunum/ileum	(+)	(–)	N	Y	Y	Y	N	2	(+)	207
Colon	(+++)	(++)	N	Y	Y	Y	N	1	(+++)	209
Gall bladder	(+)	(–)	N	Y	N	Y	N	½	(+)	210

Body Part/ Procedure	Discomfort* (−) to (++++)	Hazard* (−) to (+++)	Hospital (Incl. Short Procedure)	Special Prep.	Physician	Extras*	Informed Consent*	Exam Time* (Hrs.)	Bottom Line* (−) to (++++)	Exam Description (Page)
Pancreas										
ERCP	(+++)	(+++)	Y	Y	Y	Y	Y	1	(+++)	212
CT	(½+)	(−)	N	N	N	N	N	½	(½+)	212
Liver										
Transhepatic cholangiography	(++)	(+++)	Y	Y	Y	Y	Y	1	(++)	214
CT	(½+)	(−)	N	Y	N	Y	N	½	(½+)	214
Spleen	(½+)	(−)	N	N	N	N	N	½	(½+)	215
Genitourinary										
Uterus/tubes										
Hysterosalpingography	(++)	(+)	N	Y	Y	Y	N	¾	(+++)	215
CT	(½+)	(−)	N	N	N	N	N	½	(½+)	217
Ovaries	(½+)	(−)	N	N	N	N	N	½	(½+)	215
Prostate	(½+)	(+)	N	N	Y	Y	Y	¼	(½+)	217
Kidneys/ureters										
IVU	(+)	(+)	N	Y	Y	Y	Y	1	(+)	218
Retrograde pyelogram	(+++)	(+++)	Y	Y	Y	Y	Y	1	(+++)	219

X-ray—cont'd

Body Part/ Procedure	Discomfort* (−) to (++++)	Hazard* (−) to (+++)	Hospital (Incl. Short Procedure)	Special Prep.	Physician	Extras*	Informed Consent*	Exam Time* (Hrs.)	Bottom Line* (−) to (++++)	Exam Description (Page)
Bladder										
Retrograde cystogram	(++)	(+)	N	N	Y	Y	N	½	(++)	221
Chain cystogram	(++)	(+)	N	N	Y	Y	N	½	(++)	221
Voiding cystogram	(++)	(+)	N	N	Y	Y	N	½	(++)	221
Urethra	(++)	(+)	N	N	Y	Y	N	½	(++)	222
Adrenal glands	(½+)	(−)	N	N	N	N	N	½	(½+)	222
Lymph glands	(++)	(+)	N	N	Y	Y	Y	4–24	(++)	223
Miscellaneous										
Surveys	(+)	(−)	N	N	N	N	N	½	(+)	225
Biopsy guidance	(++) to (++++)	(++) to (+++)	Y	Y	Y	Y	Y	1	(++) to (+++)	226
Postoperative	(+)	(−)	N	N	Y	Y	N	½	(+)	227
Recheck	(++)	(−)	N	N	Y	Y	N	1	(++)	227

* See Appendix, Table Details.

similar series of exposures will be made. For this series there is an "add-on." This one requires the injection of "dye" (see the Appendix, Table Details) into a vein. This injection will be given by the radiologist, after explanation and approval. This second part will also take about a half hour. Except for the discomfort of the injection (½ +), there is no pain. There is no hazard, except for those few who are iodine-sensitive, for whom the hazard is (+).

Bottom Line: (+) Still pretty easy.

Skull   Cranium, Facial Bones, and Jaw

Conventional-Routine   The skull is best understood by considering it to be composed of three major parts, with each part being composed of more than one bone. These parts are the cranium, which is the box that houses the brain; the facial bones, which make up the orbits that house the eyes, the nasal bones, which make up the nose, and other structures, such as the sinuses; and the jaw. All of the major parts as well as the particular parts unique to each are studied in the same way and can be considered together.

If you are wearing anything that can cast a shadow on the picture, such as earrings or glasses or necklaces, you will have to remove it. You will either be seated or asked to lie down on the X-ray table. Your head will be positioned by turning it from side to side, up or down, or front or back, and the pictures will be taken. That's it. There is no anticipated pain. There is no hazard. The whole thing takes about half an hour. No afterblues.

Bottom Line: (½ +) Piece of cake.

CT   You will lie either on your back or stomach depending on the part to be studied. Discomfort index is (−). Hazard index, (−). The examination time is about one-half to three-quarters of an hour.

Bottom Line: (½ +) Ho-hum.

Salivary Glands

Conventional-Special   The salivary GLANDS are specialized structures that produce saliva (spit) which they then deliver into the mouth through tiny tubes called ducts. The glands are located inside each cheek, under the base of the tongue, and at the angles of the jaw. They can only be seen if they are OPACIFIED. This is accomplished by the radiologist inserting a fine plastic tube into the orifice (the mouth or opening) of the duct and carefully injecting a very small amount of "dye." Sometimes the opening is hard to find. In that case you will be given a slice of lemon to get the spit flowing. The radiologist can then see where the saliva is entering the mouth and thus locate the opening. Sometimes the orifice is too tight to admit the tubing. A fine metal blunt-tipped PROBE is inserted to stretch it a mite. Once the tube is positioned —usually a matter of minutes regardless of the maneuvers required—and after the "dye" has been injected, the technologist will take several films of the area. The tube is then removed, and it's over. There may be mild discomfort associated with the tube placement—(+). There is a (+) hazard whenever ducts are entered. Figure about half an hour for the whole job. The site of injection could be mildly sore for a day or so.

Bottom Line: (+) Not as bad as it reads!

Neck

Although the neck is the bridge that connects the head to the rest of us and therefore is heavily trafficked with all the connecting links between the two parts, there are only a few structures that lend themselves to X-ray investigation—the larynx (the voice box and/or Adam's apple) and the pharynx (often referred to as the throat). The larynx is studied whenever there is some unexplained problem with speaking; the pharynx when there is some difficulty in swallowing.

Larynx

Conventional-Routine The larynx is located in the front of the neck and lives inside the cartilaginous box called the Adam's apple. It can be examined conventionally using laminographic techniques. LAMINOGRAPHY is a technique of examination requiring specialized X-ray equipment. The particular machine differs from standard types in that the X-ray tube moves during the exposure—often traveling in an arc over the part of interest. You lie on your back with your head bent back to bring the front of your neck forward. The tube is above you and swings from a point behind your head to one above your upper chest with each exposure. Don't be frightened; the tube won't hit you. There is neither discomfort nor hazard. It takes about one-half hour.

Bottom Line: (½ +) Boring!

Conventional-Special There is another method to image the larynx, preferred by many throat specialists (laryngologists) because it provides superior detail over the conventional-routine technique. This method requires that a CONTRAST MATERIAL ("DYE") be placed into the larynx before the pictures are taken. This placement is not difficult but does require that the area be anesthetized first to prevent you from coughing. The technique of preparation and "dye" placement is detailed in Bronchoscopy, Chapter 14, pages 130–32. The whole thing takes about 5 to 10 minutes. You will then be placed behind a FLUOROSCOPE and the necessary X-rays will be taken.

Discomfort rates a (+ +) and hazard a (−). Allot an hour. You'll feel the aftereffect of numbness of the throat for perhaps one to two hours, so you may have *nothing by mouth* until it is completely gone!

Bottom Line: (+ +) Not too bad.

Pharynx "Throat" is really a general name for the front portion of the neck. It contains the pharynx, which is a tube-like extension of the mouth. Food or liquids that you swallow move into the pharynx. When the swallowing function is working properly these materials will be moved further along the DIGESTIVE TRACT and into the esophagus. However, problems in the pharynx could result in misdirection of that which has been ingested (swallowed). This material might end up in your lungs (down the wrong tube) or it might be propelled backwards and end up coming out of your nose. Thus, the pharynx must be looked at on occasion. The study is called a swallowing function.

Conventional-Special Swallowing (deglutition) function is studied by observing and recording the swallowing act. You will be positioned behind a fluoroscopic screen (usually in the standing position) and given a glass to hold. This glass contains a liquid called barium. Barium is used in almost all examinations of the digestive tract. It is almost always flavored and, although somewhat chalky, is easily tolerated. The radiologist, who is on the other side of the fluoroscopic screen, will ask you to take a mouthful and hold it there until you are directed to swallow. When so instructed, swallow the whole thing in one mighty gulp. Pictures will be taken as you do this and will permit review and study of the act. The pictures will either be individual shots—so-called spot films made through the fluoroscope—or rapid sequential exposures like those taken by a movie camera. Except that each of these machines makes a different sound, it shouldn't matter to you how the picture-taking is done. (In some fluoroscopic rooms the monitor can be positioned so that you can watch what is happening. Ask. It's fascinating.)

Discomfort rates a (+) only because of the barium. There is no hazard. Allot a half-hour.

Bottom Line: (+) It's as difficult as swallowing.

Chest

Just about everyone knows where the chest is. It's that part of our body we like, in moments of deepest sincerity, to get something off of. But not everyone knows how many things comprise it. Starting from the outside, there are the breasts. Then come the bony parts; the ribs, the breastbone, and a part of the spine called the cage. Finally, there is the inside, which is composed of well-known residents, the heart and lungs, and lesser-known dwellers, the tube that carries food from your mouth to your stomach (the esophagus), the tubes that carry air from your nose to your lungs (the trachea and bronchi), and some major blood vessels (the aorta and superior vena cava).

All of these good things are, unfortunately, subject to bad things. The examinations used to discover and root out evils such as infections, tumors, and injuries are many and varied. Let's look at them all.

Breasts   *Mammography* is the name for this study. It must be done on dedicated (specially designed to be used for no other purpose) equipment. Experience has shown that the least radiation exposure and the best images of the breasts are obtained when the machines employed for this examination are made especially for this duty. These units are also designed to permit uniform pressure to be applied to your breast at the time of the exposure. This pressure, called compression, is also an essential element for an appropriate study today.

Conventional-Routine   No special preparation is absolutely necessary, but the discomfort experienced by many may be significantly reduced if all caffeine is eliminated from the diet for two weeks prior to the examination. Caffeine and certain medications have been shown to cause fluid retention. This can make your breasts more sensitive, particularly when compression is applied. So, if there is no urgency for the examination—if it's not being done for "cause," but is simply a routine SCREENING study—and if your breasts tend to be sore or tender to the touch, particularly around the time of your period, discuss a short dietary purge of caffeine and similar "baddies" with your doctor. Although not mandatory, examination at midcycle may be the preferred time for menstruating women.

You will be asked to remove all clothing from the waist up and will be given a gown that opens in the front. The technologist will perform the study, which will consist of a minimum of two views of each of your breasts. These are obtained with you either standing or sitting and with your breast carefully placed on a small shelflike surface that extends out from the vertical pole that also supports the X-ray tube. Your breast will be positioned so that it is as flat and smooth as possible and then you will be gently but firmly pushed forward so that the edge of the shelf presses into your chest just below your breast. Then the compression device will be brought down onto the breast and as much pressure applied as you will permit. So psych yourself up before it starts: tell yourself that you will accept some discomfort, yes, even some pain, so that the most detailed pictures possible can be obtained. The technologist will be guided by your directions. The whole compression application time is less than a minute. As soon as the exposure has been made the device will be released.

If the study was simply for screening (you have no complaints; you are just of the age that it should be done) then you might not see a radiologist. If, however, you are there for "cause" (you have a complaint—a lump, a discharge from the nipple, a change in the skin) then you will be seen and examined by one. The physical examination by the doctor, except for any embarrassment that it might evoke, should not cause discomfort and takes only a few minutes. That does it. The discomfort rating is a function of your breasts' sensitivity to pressure and how much pressure you will allow. It should be at least a (+ +). Score (−) for hazard. Allow an hour. Although there are usually no aftereffects, you may notice some breast discoloration. This is a consequence of the compression and will gradually disappear. Infrequently, there is a nipple discharge for several days. Ignore this too, unless it persists beyond the accepted time.

Bottom Line: (+ +) It won't be fun—but do it!

Conventional-Special There are two examinations that are performed: ductography and mass localization.

Ductography Ducts are tubes that carry fluid. There are many ducts in your breasts and they all converge and end at your nipples. When there is a nipple discharge from only one breast and it occurs without pressure, it may be due to a problem within a duct. Discharge from both breasts or discharge only under pressure, regardless of its color, is rarely significant. The ducts can be examined in greater detail than that which is obtainable on the routine mammogram by putting "dye" into them. This addition is performed by the radiologist. It is a relatively simple procedure in which the nipple is cleansed and a very fine tube is gently inserted into it. A very small amount of "dye" is then injected and pictures are obtained. No compression is applied, so you are spared that discomfort. The tube insertion rates about a (+). There is also a (+) hazard rating only because of the very remote possibility that the nipple might be injured. Allot about an hour. Expect some discharge—but you already had it.

Bottom Line: (+) Easier than the conventional screening study.

Mass Localization This examination is done when something of concern has been found on your earlier X-rays but that "something" can't be felt. The concern is sufficient to warrant a BIOPSY. But if the LESION (area of "badness") can't be felt then the surgeon will be unable to find it. Help is provided. Just before the biopsy is to be performed you will be sent to X-ray. The radiologist will reexamine the original films and find the site in question. Small metallic markers—often BBs—will be applied to the skin of your breast overlying the lesion. The breast will then be X-rayed again (without compression). The lesion thus will be aligned to a particular marker, and its depth within your breast can be measured. Your skin will be cleansed and the radiologist will insert a special needle down into your breast along the path decided upon from the marker picture. Sometimes a local anesthetic will be injected under your skin before the localizing needle is inserted. However, there is little or no additional discomfort from the big needle than from the one used for the anesthetic, so the "local" is often skipped. But it is your choice! If you would prefer anesthesia, ask! A second film will be made with the needle in place. If its point is at the lesion, the job is done. If not, needle replacement and recheck for correct position will be continued until the mission has been accomplished. The needle or a fine wire that can be inserted down through it to the area of concern is taped in place on your breast and covered by a special dressing. You will then be taken back to the operating room where the biopsy will be performed. The localization time varies depending on the number of realignments that are needed. Average time is 30 minutes. Discomfort (+ +). Hazard (−). Although the whole thing sounds like some medieval torture to obtain a confession, it really isn't too, too terrible.

Bottom Line: (+ +) Good luck with the biopsy!

Chest Cage (Bony Thorax)

The chest cage (bony thorax) is composed of the ribs, the breastbone (sternum), the collar bone (clavicle), the shoulder bone (scapula), breastbone joint (sternoclavicular joint), and the collarbone joint (acromioclavicular joint). All of these structures are imaged in a similar manner and can be considered together.

Conventional-Routine No preparation is necessary except taking off everything from your waist up and putting on a gown. You will be positioned in the standing, sitting, or lying down position—depending on the particular part of interest. The X-ray beam is centered to that part, and the film is behind it. Two or three views are obtained by simply turning you appropriately. There is no discomfort. There is no hazard. A quarter- to a half-hour is maximum.

Bottom Line: (½ +) They should all be this easy.

The conventional-routine study of the acromioclavicular joint is slightly different. It is performed when there is concern that there could be a separation of the collarbone from the shoulder bone. This concern is almost always a result of injury. There is no preparation except stripping from the waist up and putting on a gown. Then you stand in front of the film holder with your arms at your sides. An exposure is made. You are then given something heavy, commonly a sandbag, to hold in each hand and another exposure is made. (The sandbags act to pull the arms and shoulders down. If there is a true separation the arm comes down but the shoulder doesn't.) That's it. No discomfort. No hazard. This takes about half an hour.

Bottom Line: (½ +) "Nuthin' to it!"

Heart   The heart, whose office address is the chest, is the best-known member of the work gang called the circulatory system. Big Red is the leader who oversees the operation of supplying the entire body with blood. The heart is a master pump whose tireless energy drives the Elixir of Life, the blood, to every cell in the body. The conduits that carry the payload are a miraculous network of pipes—the blood vessels. The vessels are of two types: arteries and veins. The arteries receive the blood that leaves the heart after being oxygenated (receiving the oxygen that we have breathed into our lungs). The arteries get the oxygen to all of their customers. Because the flow is away from the heart, a strong push is required to move it and this is the blood pressure. As the arteries must withstand this constant thrust, their walls are thick and muscular. The veins, on the other hand, return the blood to the heart after the oxygen has been removed, so the cycle can begin again. Since this part of the cycle is is a low-pressure system, veins are thin-walled.

Because of these differences, the examination of the component parts varies. The commonest and simplest examination is used to see the heart's size. This is also the study that is done to see the overall appearance of the lungs. This procedure is referred to as the "routine chest." When more detailed information about the heart and/or blood vessels is required, the examination becomes far more complex and difficult. The heart and arteries are studied in a similar manner and can be considered together. The veins are examined somewhat differently. However, the same type of vessel, regardless of where it is in the body or what organ it supplies, will be examined in the same way.

Conventional-Routine The "routine chest" is usually performed while you are standing. You face the holder of the X-ray film and press your chest against it. You head is mildly stretched up and your chin rests in a holder. You will be asked to place your hands on your hips and then to roll your shoulders forward. The X-ray tube is behind you. You will then hear those immortal words that have been spoken since Roentgen Antiquity, "Take in a deep breath. Hold it. You can breathe." There may be a need for X-rays taken in other positions, which could include sideways (lateral view), partially turned (oblique view), lying flat on your back (supine view), or even on your side (decubitus view). There may be need to use laminographic equipment. That's where you lie flat on your back and the X-ray tube moves in an arc over your chest while the exposure is being made. But regardless of your position or the style of hardware used, that's the ballgame. No hits (discomfort), no runs (hazard), no errors (radiologist). The whole procedure takes five to fifteen minutes.

Bottom Line: (½ +) Why can't they all be this way?

CT All of the structures of the chest are seen beautifully by this method. Sometimes contrast material will be injected when the blood vessels need to be seen in better detail. Other than this mild discomfort (½ +) with the mild hazard always invoked by contrast (½ +), it's the same old CT routine, with you positioned on your back. In and out in a half-hour.

Bottom Line: (+) Tough to stay awake.

Heart and Arteries ANGIOGRAPHY is the name applied to all definitive examinations of the heart and blood vessels. Arteriography is the term that relates to studies of the arteries alone. Examination of the heart chambers— ventriculography—can also be included in this section because it is performed the same way. Regardless of the particular artery or system of arteries that is being evaluated, the conventional-special method is identical: an artery must be entered with a special needle; contrast material—"DYE" (see the Appendix, Table Details)—must be injected so that the vessels can be seen; pictures must be taken; the hole in the artery caused by the needle must be closed. Each of these components—the arterial puncture, the "dye" injection, the picture taking, and the hole closure—must be understood.

• Arterial puncture: In ARTERIOGRAPHY the puncture is everything! Entering an artery is both difficult and hazardous. It is difficult because arteries, unlike most veins that are used for injection (which lie just under the skin and can be seen and felt), are deeply positioned in the body so they cannot be seen and must be found by touch alone. It is hazardous because once the arterial wall is violated, bleeding can be massive and life-threatening. But the specially trained radiologist is capable of surmounting both obstacles. Here is how the injection is made:

First the puncture site is chosen. This decision is based on how best to get the contrast material into the artery that supplies the area that requires study. There are four common sites of entry: the groin area; the region of the armpit; the hollow of the elbow; the neck. The groin is selected most frequently.

Next the site is prepared. This is done by cleansing the region with an antiseptic agent. Sometimes it might even require removal of hair by shaving. The area is then draped with sterile towels. A local anesthetic is injected under your skin and into the deeper structures surrounding the artery. You will feel minimal burning and pain (+) for several seconds in the region— then, numbness.

Finally the puncture itself. A radiologist dressed in a sterile gown, wearing sterile gloves and assisted by a similarly garbed physician, nurse, or technologist, will do the deed. The artery will be entered by inserting a special needle through your skin (occasionally a small INCISION is made just through the numbed skin to facilitate the insertion) and into the vessel. The needle is special because it has an internal wire running through it, called a stylette, that prevents blood from escaping from the needle. When the radiologist believes the needle is correctly positioned within the artery the stylette will be removed. If the position is correct there will be a sudden spurt of blood out of the back end of the needle. It's like striking oil, only this minigeyser is red. Don't panic! It means that the puncture has been made correctly. The radiologist will immediately insert another very fine wire, called a guide, back through the needle. This will stop the bleeding. The guide wire will be advanced under FLUOROSCOPIC guidance to the area that requires study. The needle will then be removed, leaving only the wire. A thin flexible tube called a CATHETER will be slid over the wire and it, too, will be advanced to the proper position. The wire will then be withdrawn, leaving only the catheter in place. The end of the catheter is equipped with a valve that prevents blood from escaping. These maneuvers may take minutes to hours. They require extreme skill, care, and remarkable patience on the part of the radiologist, and extreme understanding and cooperation from you. During all this you experience little or no discomfort. You will be aware of some pressure and mild tugging where they are working. But what will probably bother you the most is just the tedium of lying reasonably still on the X-ray table. If it is "your thing," you can relieve the boredom by watching what they are doing. This can be accomplished by having the monitor that shows what is going on positioned so that you can see, too. When these steps are completed the "dye" can be injected.

• "Dye" injection: (See the Appendix, Table Details.) It is now the moment of truth. All of the above has been performed in preparation for the delivery of the contrast material to the artery. This is accomplished by the injection. It must be noted that the injection in this situation is unlike any other injection you may have previously experienced. The volume of "dye" given is large and it must be delivered to the part rapidly lest it become diluted. Thus the instillation is most often made by a mechanical injector—a device that can propel the "dye" at high velocity to the part. The sensation experienced when a large volume of contrast material is expelled at high pressure is highly variable from one patient to the next. Some report severe pain (+ + + +) in the location at which the "dye" enters the artery, while others state that the sensation experienced is only uncomfortable (+ +). Many complain of a generalized feeling of heat. This, too, varies in intensity from one patient to the next. Other unpleasantness, though less common, is also possible: headache, chest pain, dizziness, and/or a change in heartbeat. Blessedly, almost without exception, these sensations—even the most severe —last only for seconds. You will be warned that the "dye" is coming. The irony is that you will also be asked to remain absolutely still at the instant that the sensation is worst because that is when the pictures are being taken.

One last word on the injection, or more accurately, on the contrast materials. There has been a remarkable breakthrough in the composition of opaque agents. They can now be made such that most of the reactions described above will not be experienced. But, at this writing, the cost of these new products is prohibitive for routine use. Hopefully, by the time you read this section, injection miseries will be a thing of the past.

• Picture taking: Because of the nature of blood flow in the arteries, the imaging techniques are unique in these studies. Pictures are being made of blood that has been contrast-enhanced. Because the rate of flow in arteries is so rapid, the pictures must be obtained in rapid sequence before the "dye" runs off. This is accomplished by a mechanical device known as a film changer. It automatically exchanges an exposed film for a new one, permitting almost continuous filming. All that this means to you is that this phase of the procedure will be noisy. Each change is accompanied by a mild bang and perhaps a mild vibration because all of this is occurring right under you. Another possibility is that actual X-ray movies will be taken. Again, all this means is that there will be a different sound—a whirring noise. It is more the rule than the exception that the picture taking will be done in several sequences. These may be associated with changes in position of the catheter to "see" other vessels or even changes in your position to "see" the same vessels in a different view. Each sequence, unfortunately, necessitates another injection of contrast. So, all of the above is repeated.

• Hole closure: When the arterial puncture "dye" injection and picture taking have been completed, it is time to quit. That means getting the catheter out of your artery so you can leave. This is a very critical time. The catheter is withdrawn slowly and gently, causing you no discomfort (or at worst a mild pulling sensation). But the instant the catheter is out of your artery you will feel heavy pressure being applied to the puncture site. This pressure serves to seal the hole made by the catheter and to prevent bleeding until this closure is achieved. It will be done either by the doctor placing both hands over the area and leaning down with heavy force or by a mechanical device that will do the same thing. Whichever method is used, you will really feel it—and it will hurt (+ +). This pressure will stay on for some 10 to 15 minutes and will then be gradually released. If there is any evidence of bleeding, pressure will be reapplied. The pressure is the "finger in the dike." Remember, it was an artery that was punctured and bleeding can be profuse and even life-threatening if the hole is not properly sealed. So, although it hurts and you are mighty weary after all that has been done, hang in there for another few minutes.

Those are the nuts and bolts of arteriography. They apply to all such studies. There will be some variation between one region and the next, as some arteries can be isolated more easily than others and some arteries supply ORGANS that are more complicated than others. Some locations, such as the heart itself, may be more sensitive to the "dye" injection or to the presence of a catheter wiggling and bumping about. This in turn might evoke changes in function such as alterations of heart rhythm or blood pressure, which in turn might necessitate immediate treatment measures to correct. Therefore, in certain studies where the risks are known to be great, the radiologist may be supported by other medical specialists who will monitor you and initiate any remedial measures that may be demanded. Indeed, in studies of the coronary arteries and the chambers of the heart, the probability of side effects requiring immediate management is so high that it has become more the rule than the exception that the entire procedure be performed by a cardiologist specially trained in angiography.

Now for personal details: Nothing by mouth for at least eight hours before the examination. In preparing you, monitors—small sensory devices that look like disks about the size of a dime—may be placed on your chest and connected to a machine that prints out tracings of your heart function. Medication may be given with the intent of relaxing you about an hour before. An IV LINE (a needle connected to a bottle containing fluid that will be inserted into a vein in your arm) will be started—(½ +) discomfort. This is to permit the rapid administration of medication if it should be required. The rest of it you know.

In the majority of situations hospitalization will be necessary. (At one time this was an absolute rule but it seems to be bending slightly, and there are some who will perform these studies as an "in and out" (see Short Procedure Hospitalization on pages xvi–xviii). For our discussion, let's stay with the conservative folks who are going to keep you "in." The specifics of this confinement vary. You may be asked to enter the night before, or on the morning of the study. Be prepared to stay the night following the procedure. This is done mostly to ensure rapid and appropriate attention if bleeding should occur. This complication is not frequent, but is always a real possibility, particularly if you become active too soon after the procedure is completed. During your stay, both nurses and doctors will check the puncture site regularly. They will check your blood pressure as well, to be certain that there is no evidence of "silent" bleeding.

You will be asked to "take it easy" for several days, meaning that you should not act in any way that could put strain on the puncture area. It might be a good idea to take the rest of the week off—your employer probably owes you sick days anyhow. The puncture region will be sore for about a week. It may also be discolored—black and blue—for several weeks. It may be "hard" under the skin surrounding the point of the "stick." This is due to a HEMATOMA that developed because of some bleeding at the time of the study. This, too, requires weeks before it totally disappears. You will also be instructed to pay close attention to the area and if anything seems to be changing except for the better, "get thee to thy doctor," pronto! Arteriography is a (+ + + +) discomfort and a (+ + +) hazard all the way. The hospital will want your signature on its informed consent form!

Bottom Line: (+ + + +) You will put this one in your scrapbook.

Whereas arteriography can be used on all arteries, only the very largest can be studied by CT. But this may be enough to diagnose your problem. If that is the case, great, because this technique does not require that the artery be violated at all. You are placed on your back on the table and moved into the gantry. A needle will already have been positioned in a vein in your arm. The radiologist willl inject "dye" rapidly and picture taking will begin. CT won't provide nearly as much detail here as the angiographic procedure described above. The study will take 30 to 60 minutes. Except for the discomfort of the injection $(1/2+)$, that is it. The "dye" makes the hazard rating $(+)$. There are no aftereffects.

Bottom Line: $(+)$ Another easy one.

Veins As discussed above, veins are the vessels that return blood to the heart. Because they are not under pressure, their walls are thin and when they are violated bleeding is slow, and almost without exception, readily controllable. For these reasons examination of veins—venography—is significantly easier and far less hazardous than the examination of their vascular cousins—arteries. Venography is a conventional-special procedure that also requires an injection.

Many veins are found just under the skin, so that entering one with a needle is usually relatively simple. The particular veins that are to be studied will govern the injection site. Most of the time it will be possible to use your hand, the hollow of your elbow, or your foot. Sometimes it is necessary to enter a larger vein in your groin, shoulder, or neck. On occasion, however, it is necessary to study a vein that is deeply situated in the abdomen or chest, such as the major veins returning blood to the heart—the superior and inferior venae cavae—or the vein that drains the kidneys. When this is the case the vessel must be reached by a catheter. This is a technique similar to that used in arteriography, but again, since it is a vein that is entered and not an artery, the procedure is both simpler and far less hazardous.

As with the arteriogram, once the vessel has been entered "dye" must be added to make the veins visible on the X-ray. All of the problems and risks inherent when contrast agents are used must be clearly understood. (See the Appendix, Table Details.) Usually a far smaller volume of "dye," as compared to that used in an arterial study, is employed. Usually the contrast is injected by hand rather than machine-injected. Both of these variations considerably reduce the degree of discomfort.

For some studies an eight-hour fast will be necessary. For most, no preparation is needed except removing clothing and other "removables" from the area of examination and donning a gown. Unless you are unusually tense, no medication will be given. You will be asked to lie on your back on an X-ray table that is equipped to perform fluoroscopy or DSA (Digital Subtraction Angiography, which is a form of computer magic that, in some specialized situations, permits vascular examinations to be performed utilizing smaller quantities of "dye"; from your standpoint nothing will be detectably different). The site selected for the puncture will be cleansed with an antiseptic solution. If the injection site is superficial (close to the skin), a piece of rubber tubing or sometimes a blood pressure cuff will be be wrapped around either your arm or leg—depending on the site of entrance—and tightened. This acts to obstruct the flow of blood in the chosen vein, making it "fatter" and thus easier to puncture. The radiologist will insert the needle and when satisfied that it is in correct position will secure it with adhesive tape. The rubber tubing will be released. The "dye" injection is then made and the pictures are taken. If the site of injection is deep and requires the placement of a catheter, the procedure is more involved, and is similar to that which is performed for arteriography (see arterial puncture above), except that it is less hazardous. The "dye" will be hand-injected, and pictures will be made. The catheter will be withdrawn, and the puncture sites will be sealed by direct hand pressure. Unlike the arterial puncture, closure is accomplished in just a few minutes, and the pressure is less.

Discomfort rates a **(+)** to **(+ + +)** depending on which vessels are being studied. Hazard is only for the "dye" and equals **(+)**. The time of study averages an hour. It would be nice to have a pal there to help you home because the study is fatiguing. You might want to take the rest of the day off, but you'll have no real aftereffects except the black and blue marker at the injection site, which will last for at least a week. The same spot could also be a tad sore for a few days.

Bottom Line: **(+ +)** or **(+ + +)** Like an encounter with a less-than-favorite relative—it could be painful but, as a rule, it is only a minor trauma.

Lungs, Trachea, and Bronchi The lungs are paired organs residing in the chest, one to the right of the heart and the other to the left of it. Together with the tubes called the trachea and the bronchi, they comprise the RESPIRATORY SYSTEM. This system is responsible for respiration, or the act of breathing, which as we all know is essential to life. In order for each cell in the body to live, it must have a substance called oxygen, a gas found in the air. This gas must be brought to suitable depots, loaded aboard a carrier, and shipped out to each client. The shipping is done via the trachea and bronchial tree, the depots are the lungs, the carriers are the red cells in the blood, the clients are all the cells of the body.

Like other body parts, the lungs, trachea, and bronchi are subject to the threats and attacks of infection, tumor, developmental abnormalities, injury, and so on. In most situations, or at least to start an investigation, the routine chest examination described earlier in the chapter on page 190 will suffice. However, in many problems more extensive studies of the trachea, bronchi, and lungs are required.

Sometimes it is necessary to see the breathing tubes (the bronchi) in more detail than is obtainable in the routine chest X-ray. This can be accomplished by a conventional-special procedure which involves putting something into the tubes to make them "stand out" from the rest of the lung. That something is "dye." How to get it in and how to make you keep it there is what makes this examination special. The exam is accomplished by passing a thin rubber tube (a catheter) about 20 inches long through your nose (after an anesthetic gel has been placed into a nostril), down the back of your throat, through your voice box (larynx), into your central breathing tube (trachea), and then into the breathing tube (or tubes) of either lung (or both lungs). (See page 130 for a discussion of the suppression of the cough reflex). The contrast material is then instilled into the catheter and it runs down and fills the tubes. This is performed by the radiologist under fluoroscopic control, and appropriate pictures are taken. The study is called a bronchogram.

You will have a "thick throat" for about an hour until the anesthetic wears off. You may not eat or drink anything until all of its action is gone. This procedure ranks a (+ +) for discomfort and a (−) for hazard, and takes one-half to three-quarters of an hour.

Bottom Line: (+ +) So-so tough.

Esophagus The swallowing tube or esophagus is a part of the DIGESTIVE TRACT. This tract is a long, continuous tube extending from the mouth to the anus. In different parts of the body it takes different diameters and shapes according to the digestive function performed at that particular way station. It also takes different names in the journey. Let's start at the top—the mouth. Behind it, the pipeline through the neck is called the pharynx. When it reaches the chest it is known as the esophagus. (We will pick up the trail again when we reach the abdomen. But for those of you who can't rest until you know "who done it," it will be called stomach, small intestine, and large intestine.)

Conventional-Special The esophagus can be seen on X-ray only if something is put into it. That something is barium. (Barium is explained more fully in the Appendix, Table Details). You must arrive for the X-ray in the morning, having had nothing by mouth (yes, that includes water and coffee!) for at least eight hours preceding. If the examination is limited to the esophagus, you will have to disrobe only from the waist up. You will be placed behind the fluoroscopic screen, probably in the standing position, with a glass of barium in your hand. On the other side of the screen will be your friendly radiologist. He or she will instruct you when to swallow and when to change positions. While you are doing your thing, and undoubtedly making disparaging remarks about the "drink," the radiologist will be watching the barium moving through your esophagus and taking appropriate pictures. (In some fluoroscopic rooms the monitor is so positioned that you, too, can watch. Ask. It's fascinating.) The table that had been behind you while you were standing will probably be lowered, and you will be placed on it, so that additional views can be obtained. Your only discomfort will be drinking "that stuff"—(½ +). There is no hazard. If only the esophagus is being examined you should be in and out in about 15 minutes. Usually, other parts of the tube, such as the stomach and small intestine, will be looked at too. If so, add another half-hour.

Bottom Line: (+) Strawberry-flavored barium isn't bad.

Upper and Lower Extremities

All of the examinations of both the upper and lower extremities, with the exception of certain special studies of the joints, are performed in a similar manner and can therefore be described together. All of the special techniques for visualizing the joints are also similar, so they, too, can all be described together.

Arms and Legs

Conventional-Routine The entire arm is more correctly identified as the upper extremity, consisting of the bones of the shoulder (scapula), upper arm (humerus), elbow, forearm (radius and ulna), wrist, hand (carpal and metacarpal bones), and fingers (phalanges). The entire leg is more correctly identified as the lower extremity, consisting of the bones of the hip, the thigh (femur), knee, leg (tibia and fibula), ankle, heel (calcaneus), foot (tarsal and metatarsal bones), and toes (phalanges). With the exception of examinations of the joints, the X-ray beam is centered on the part of interest. Two or three different views are taken—for instance, the part may be held out straight, then rotated, then positioned sideways—anything that will permit a comprehensive viewing of it. There is mild discomfort (½ +). There is no hazard. Budget a quarter- to half-hour.

Bottom Line: (½ +) Really a snap!

Joints

Conventional-Special When the conventional-routine X-rays are normal but pain or limitation of motion exists, particularly after there has been an injury, it may be necessary to reexamine the part in a more detailed manner. A special procedure known as arthrography permits the structures that compose the joint—the cartilage, the tendons, and the other soft TISSUES—to be evaluated. Here is how the deed is done:

You lie on the X-ray table. The joint of concern is bared, cleansed with an antiseptic solution, and surrounded with sterile towels. A trained physician, either an orthopedist, who may have ordered the study, or the radiologist, will take over. Wearing both a gown and sterile gloves, he or she will inject a local anesthetic into your skin. You will feel a prick, a few seconds of mild burning (+), and then numbness. A longer needle will then be inserted into the joint. Small amounts of air, or "DYE," or perhaps both, will be injected. This will produce mild to moderate discomfort (+ +)—that's all. Someone will then manipulate or move your arm or your leg to get all of the joint surfaces covered with the CONTRAST MATERIAL that was added. This consists of bending and straightening the joint several times. Again, mild discomfort. The radiologist will then view the joint through the FLUOROSCOPE and appropriate pictures will be taken.

Discomfort is moderate—(+ +); hazard is minimal—(+). It will be over and you'll be out in a half-hour. Afterwards, you will probably have soreness, swelling, and perhaps even some funny sounds—kind of like squeaks —when you bend or straighten the part. These problems may last for several days. Try to rest the joint as much as possible until it feels okay. Don't worry unless the condition lasts more than a week.

Bottom Line: (+ +) You will know you were there!

Note: In the near future, all or at least some of the above may become obsolete. MRI (see Chapter 21) may replace arthrography as the method of choice in the evaluation of joint PATHOLOGY.

Spine and Bony Pelvis

Time out for a short anatomy lesson: The spine is composed of a line of bony boxes placed one below the other and extending from the base of the skull to the tip of the coccyx (tailbone). Each box (vertebra) is separated from the next by a padlike structure (intervertebral disk) that acts as a shock absorber. At its back surface each box has a thin band of bone that makes the unit look something like a huge diamond engagement ring—the diamond is the box up front, the bony ring is the band behind. This configuration creates a hole (where the finger would go if it were a ring) that is completely surrounded by bone. When the boxes are aligned so are the holes, such that they form a long bony tube. This tube is the spinal canal and it functions to protect the spinal cord, which is the name given to all of the nerves that leave the brain and extend downward to the base of the spine. Individual nerves leave the canal at specific levels to go to the body part that each supplies. Attached to the lower spinal segments, the sacrum and coccyx, are another group of bones that form a large, cup-shaped ring called the bony pelvis. Although the bony pelvis is not really the spine, the close relationship of the parts makes it logical to include it in any general discussion of the spine.

Many problems of the back that are due to aging, certain forms of arthritis, injuries, infections, and even tumors that either have originated there or spread from another site can be seen on routine examination. However, there are problems such as "slipped disks," other types of arthritis, and different types of tumors, to mention the most common, that produce symptoms because they affect the nerves in the canal. These particular changes cannot be seen on the routine examination. Fortunately, there is a special study that permits detection in most cases; it is called *myelography.*

The entire spine, including the neck (cervical region), the upper back (dorsal or thoracic region), the lower back (lumbar region), the tailbone (sacrum and/or coccyx), and the pelvis (ilium, ischium, pubis) can be considered as a group.

Conventional-Routine There is no preparation, except for disrobing (taking off your clothes) and then robing (putting on their gown). You are positioned appropriate to the part of your spine being examined—most often lying, but perhaps sitting, or, occasionally, standing. The X-ray tube is in front of you, the film behind. The number of exposures varies with the part and the problem, but is usually between two and five. There is no discomfort. There is no hazard. There is one-quarter to one-half hour of your time.

Bottom Line: ($\frac{1}{2}$ +) Boring!

Conventional-Special The special examination of this region, called myelography (*myelo* = spinal cord, *graph* = picture), is really a study of the spinal canal and is essentially the same for all parts of the spine. It requires that a "dye" be placed in the spinal canal so that the spinal cord and the other structures within the canal can be seen and evaluated. This is accomplished by the physician performing a spinal tap, and when that has been obtained, "DYE" is then instilled.

After you have removed all of your clothing except your socks and shoes, you are positioned on the X-ray table in one of two usual ways—either on your stomach (with pillows placed underneath your stomach), or on your side with your knees bent up and your head bent down. Either position acts to arch your back and widen the spaces between the vertebrae. Your lower back is then bared, cleansed with an antiseptic (always wet and always cold), and surrounded by sterile towels. A physician—a radiologist, an orthopedist, or a neurosurgeon—highly trained in this technique will then place a needle into your spinal canal. He or she will do this by first "freezing" your skin by injecting a local anesthetic just under the surface through a very small needle. You will feel a prick, a second of burning (+), and then numbness. A larger needle will then be inserted. It will pass through the space between adjacent vertebrae and into the canal. This step may be accomplished with little discomfort, but more often than not you will experience real pain that cannot be avoided. The pain may be at the spot where the needle is, or it may travel (radiate) down either or both of your legs. The degree of discomfort can vary anywhere from a loud *"Ouch!"* (+ +) to *"My God,* knock it off!" (+ + +). Additional anesthetic solution will be given to you, and this should end the misery. At this point, you will no longer feel your legs. The physician will then attach a syringe to the needle and apply suction. If the needle is correctly positioned, spinal fluid will be ASPIRATED. "Dye" will then be instilled.

Those were the coming attractions. The feature show now begins and is always performed by a radiologist. You will be positioned on your stomach and the X-ray table will be energized to move from the level horizontal position and to incline any degree toward the vertical, in either direction, so that you may be head up and feet down or head down and feet up. There is a shoulder support at the top end of the table and a footboard at its bottom end to keep you from sliding off. These maneuvers are performed under FLUORO-SCOPIC guidance all with the purpose of moving the CONTRAST MATERIAL to all parts of concern in the canal. Exposures are made by the radiologist. (If seeing what the radiologist sees is your thing, ask that the monitor be moved so that you can watch, too.) When the examination is over the "dye" is removed through the same needle by which it was injected—the needle having been left in your back. (Some dyes do not have to be removed because they are absorbed into the blood, so this last step may not be necessary.) This examination can be very painful, so be prepared—(+ +) to (+ + +). It is also moderately hazardous (+ +). It is best to remain in the hospital over-night, although the current rage of "in and out" may prevail where you are examined. (See Short Procedure Hospitalization, pages xvi–xvii). If this is the case, make sure your pal is with you to get you home! A big-time headache for the rest of the day and a mild back pain for the rest of the week is a possibility. Figure a good hour in the X-ray room.

Bottom Line: (+ + +) Big-time study!

CT This is a superior method of examining the spine. It is particularly good for the same problems that myelography seeks to uncover, and in many, if not most, situations it has replaced the more invasive procedure. However, in some institutions CT may be done immediately following myelography. Those who espouse this suspenders and belt approach assert that the combination is superior to either alone. But the majority of authorities go with CT first since it is so innocuous and easy. If this approach does not answer the question, then there may be no alternative but to "stick the back."

Study time is about 30 minutes for each spine section. Add the appropriate increment for any additional parts. There is neither discomfort nor hazard.

Bottom Line: (½ +) Hard to stay awake.

Note: Coming up fast on the outside is the horse that may someday replace all of the above—magnetic resonance imaging (MRI). See Chapter 21.

Abdomen and Pelvis

There are seventeen specific organs whose address is Abdomen and Pelvis— the Belly. Each one is a star in its own right. Some choose to perform almost independently, doing mostly one-person command performances, such as the liver and spleen. Most, however, choose to pool their individual talents, forming stock companies called ORGAN systems or tracts, to achieve masterpiece performances. Their achievements are well known and applauded. Examples are "digestion," starring Stomach and Colon with a lesser cast of Duodenum, Jejunum, and Ileum, and "reproduction," featuring such female luminaries as Ovaries and Uterus, while the male leads are played by Prostate and Testicles.

Considering the stature of these superstars it is best to view them independently. Let's look at the abdomen, gastrointestinal tract, gall bladder, pancreas, liver, spleen, genitourinary tract, adrenal glands, and lymphatic system.

Abdomen Before any detailed examination of any of the specific parts is initiated it is common practice to obtain one overview of the entire abdomen. Therefore, the first picture that begins almost all of the other examinations will be an abdominal survey (sometimes called a "flat plate").

There is one general exception to this rule. When your doctor is concerned that your complaints could be the result of an ACUTE PROCESS such as an obstruction or a PERFORATION of your bowel, or suspects that a stone (calculus) is passing, an "acute abdominal survey" might be performed.

Conventional-Routine for a Routine Survey No preparation except trading your clothes from the waist down for a gown that opens in the back. Then you get onto the X-ray table on your back, for a single film. There is no discomfort and there is no hazard. The technologist will do it all in about two minutes.

Bottom Line: (½ +) Hardly worth mentioning.

Conventional-Routine for an Acute Survey No preparation except trading your clothes from neck to knees for a gown. Films of your abdomen will be exposed with you lying flat on your back, on your side, and standing. A single view of your chest will also be made. None of this causes discomfort (−), and there is no hazard (−). It takes only 15 minutes, but it will seem longer because you are hurting.

Bottom Line: (+) Easy—but with the pain, you won't agree.

Gastrointestinal Tract In order for the body to perform particular functions—in this case, digestion—a group of structures, commonly referred to as organs, are linked together. The term gastrointestinal (GI) refers to that portion of the DIGESTIVE SYSTEM (or tract) that is found in the abdomen. A general description of the tract can be found in Chapter 5.

Stomach and Small Intestine This study is commonly referred to as an upper GI because it includes only the stomach and small intestine. (The lower GI refers to the large bowel or colon.)

Conventional-Special Preparation is essential. The stomach must be completely empty. This is accomplished by your adherence to the rule of "Nothing by mouth after bedtime of the night preceding the study." This examination is scheduled in the morning so that your fast will be better tolerated.

The examination will be performed by both a radiologist and a technologist in a FLUOROSCOPIC room. The radiologist will start by giving you some medication by injection either in a vein or under the skin. The needle is thin, the prick is instantaneous and minimal —a (½ +) discomfort. The medication, glucagon, markedly diminishes the movements of your stomach and bowel (peristaltic activity), thus permitting a more detailed and superior look at what is happening to the liquid you will be asked to drink. Its effect lasts for only 10 to 15 minutes. (A note of warning: Glucagon may cause mild nausea and/or dizziness in some people. If it does affect you this way, the feeling will last only about 15 minutes.)

Next, you will be given a small cup containing some granular material and be asked to throw the granules into the back of your mouth and swallow them. (These granules are like Alka-Seltzer. They produce gas—effervescence—that acts to distend the stomach and to improve the detail of the coming pictures. Try not to burp.)

You will be given a glass of flavored barium (see the Appendix, Table Details), and asked to stand with your back to the X-ray table, which has been placed in a vertical position. The fluoroscopic screen will be positioned in front of you. The radiologist, who is on the other side of the screen, will request that you take small individual swallows of the barium, on command, as he or she watches the filling of your stomach. (Ask that the wall-mounted monitor be turned so that you can see the action, too, if you'd like.) You will be instructed to assume different positions—back to the table, face to the table, sideways, whatever. Additionally, the table will be made to move, with you on it, so that it may be in any position from straight upright to horizontal. All of these maneuvers are performed to coat and thus outline the inner surfaces of your stomach and intestine with both the barium and gas. (This technique is referred to as "double contrast," as opposed to older methods in which barium was used alone—"single contrast." Double contrast is now considered by most authorities to be the superior method of examination.) While all of these gymnastics are going on, the radiologist will be making exposures—taking pictures. You may be asked to hold your breath while this is being done and you may hear some machine-like noises. Nothing more. At the end, the doctor may leave and the technologist will take a few more pictures.

If only the stomach and duodenum (the portion of the small intestine adjoining the stomach) are being studied you will be finished. If your doctor has asked for the entire small intestinal tract (the duodenum, jejunum, and ileum)—"a detailed small bowel study"—then the examination goes on. You will be taken from the X-ray suite back to the dressing or waiting area and returned to the suite every 15 to 30 minutes for a film. When the barium has completely filled the entire small intestine you will be finished. Along the way the radiologist may reappear and take another look with the fluoroscope.

Some special views may be taken. Not to worry. Discomfort equals (+). Hazard is (−). A stomach and duodenum study averages about one-half hour. If the entire small bowel is to be analyzed, the time is less predictable, varying from one to three hours. And then you may eat.

Bottom Line: (+) Easy as swallowing a glass of barium (yuck).

Large Intestine Preparation for an examination of your large intestine, known as a barium enema or sometimes as a double contrast barium enema, is big time. It is essential that the bowel be completely empty. Things that are being looked for may not be much larger than a pinhead in size. Any residual debris retained in the bowel can mask and confuse the findings. Therefore, the better the prep, the better the study.

The recommendations to accomplish this end often vary from one radiologist to the next. But they are sufficiently similar that a general idea can be identified: lots of laxatives, lots of fluids, and no solid food. An example of one popular protocol is as follows: you must completely stop eating solid food two days before the scheduled study. Only clear juices, clear soups like chicken broth or bouillon, and gelatin are permitted. (Milk is excluded.) You take citrate of magnesia (a laxative) at 4:00 and 8:00 pm of the second day. And two enemas are necessary on the morning of the study. This will be one time in your life when the common expression "feeling all washed out" will be literally correct!

The conventional-special examination is performed in a fluoroscopic room. Once you're in a gown, having removed all of your clothing, you will be asked to lie on the X-ray table and a single film will be made (see page 207).

Before the barium enema is started, the radiologist must examine your rectum to ensure that an enema tip (that short firm piece at the end of the tubing attached to the enema bag) can be inserted into you safely. You will be positioned on your side with your top leg bent forward. Your back will then be exposed and the doctor will insert a gloved and LUBRICATED finger into your rectum. It will be (+) uncomfortable. If no CONTRAINDICATION is discovered, the tip will be inserted. (It should be noted that the tip used here is not the same as the one on bags sold for home use. It is designed to include a built-in balloon. Once inserted, the balloon can be inflated. The inflated balloon acts as a "safety valve" for those who are concerned that they will be unable to retain the enema. The decision of whether or not to inflate is yours. Add a (+) discomfort point if the decision is Yes.)

Another decision must be faced: "To glucagon or not to glucagon?" Glucagon is a medicine that can overcome or at least diminish the discomfort experienced when the bowel is distended by an enema. This feeling is inter-preted as "fullness," and it may cause patients sufficient distresss to require termination of the enema because they fear loss of control. Glucagon acts to paralyze the bowel's nerve endings that cause this sensation. It is given in the arm, either by injection into a vein or under the skin. The drug's action is very short-lived; it is over in about 15 minutes. In some people glucagon may induce both a mild dizziness and nausea which can last for 5 to 10 minutes. Additionally, its use tends to make the study longer. Thus, you must decide whether or not it will be used. (My own vote is usually "Yes," use it, because it tends to diminish overall discomfort.)

There's nothing left now but to do it. The radiologist will bring the fluoroscopic screen over you and instruct the technologist to begin the enema. The liquid used is a barium solution. You will be instructed to relax. *Breathe slowly and deeply through your mouth.* When you breathe this way it is impos-sible to tense your abdominal muscles. Meanwhile, in back of the fluoroscope, things are happening. The amount of fluid you are getting is being scrupu-lously monitored so that you won't receive a drop more than is necessary. You may hear a slight whirring motor noise and perhaps see a faint flash of light as the pictures are being taken. Just about the time that you think you can't take any more the radiologist will happily announce that the enema part is over. The enema bag, which acts to siphon off much of the fluid, will be lowered to the floor. A moment of relief! That ends Part 1 of two.

Part 2: Air will now be put into you. (The air is an important component of the examination. It mixes with the barium that is left and produces a double contrast. This significantly improves the detection sensitivity for rec-ognizing any abnormality.) The addition of the air will cause the same or perhaps even greater discomfort than the barium. But it takes much less time! Again, remember the deep breathing. Lot of pictures will be made in lots of different positions. And then it's over!

You'll experience a (+ + +) discomfort and a (+) hazard. Time aver-ages one hour. Bring a pal to help you get home. You will feel beat from the combination of the days of preparation and the procedure itself. Plan to take the rest of the day off. You may feel abdominal discomfort for some hours because of the air.

Bottom Line: (+ + +) One word says it all—tough!

Gall Bladder The gall bladder is the organ that is concerned with fat digestion. It has been described in Chapter 5.

Conventional-Routine Preparation is required. Special medication must be taken the night before the study. This material will be in capsule or tablet form and the usual dose is four to six. The medicine is to be taken in the late evening and will not cause you any distress. You will be requested to take nothing by mouth, except the capsules, from after your dinner until after the examination the next morning. You might also be asked to go on a fat-free diet for several days preceding the study and to take an enema on the morning of the examination.

Once you're in the X-ray room the rest is a song. You will be put into different positions—standing, lying, sideways. Films will be made by the technologist. The whole process takes 15 minutes on a slow day. You'll experience no discomfort and be subject to no hazard. No lingering memories.

Occasionally after the first set of films you may be given something to drink which will have a creamy taste and is a little slippery. It is a high concentration of fat and its purpose is to see how the gall bladder responds to this stimulus. Does it contract as it is supposed to? It takes about 15 minutes for the fatty meal to do its thing. Then back you go for a repeat of what you just had done. Add 30 minutes for the double-feature. All else is identical.

Bottom Line: (+) A laugher.

Note: Prior to the advent of ultrasound the above description of a gall bladder examination represented the rule. Now, it is probably the exception. Most routine studies are initiated by ultrasound techniques. (See Chapter 20.)

Pancreas Your pancreas is located just below and slightly behind your stomach. This organ has two major functions and belongs both to the digestive system and to the ENDOCRINE SYSTEM. Its endocrine system role can be found in Chapter 4. Its digestive role is discussed in Chapter 5. The pancreas is particularly prone to tumor formation and infection.

Conventional-Special The pancreas cannot be seen on conventional-routine X-rays. The entire pancreas cannot be seen even with conventional-special X-ray techniques, but certain of its parts can. It is possible to see both its blood supply and ductal structures. Visualizing either or both permits the skilled viewer to make accurate assumptions about the condition of the entire organ.

Blood Supply The techniques for visualizing the arteries to any body part are very similar. See page 17.

Ductal Structures Ducts are tubes. They exist for the purpose of transporting a product found or manufactured within one part of your body to another part where it is needed. The ENZYMES made in the pancreas must be delivered to a special location in the small intestine (the duodenum). This is accomplished by a tube within the pancreas called the pancreatic duct. If these ducts can be seen and are normal, it can be inferred that the surrounding parts of the pancreas are also normal. If, however, the ducts exhibit abnormality—that's big-time trouble.

The ducts to be studied must first be OPACIFIED by the instillation of "DYE." This is accomplished by a procedure known as ERCP—Endoscopic Retrograde Cholangiopancreatography. "Cholangiopancreatography" refers to the location of the body parts that will be X-rayed—the duct of the pancreas and the major bile duct coming into the pancreas from the liver.

The endoscope is passed through your mouth, down your esophagus, through your stomach, and into your duodenum, where an opening of the duct that has come from the pancreas is found. A thinner tube is then passed down through the original scope and into the opening of the duct, and the "dye" is injected.

To accomplish this difficult passage the navigator of the tube is a specialist in diseases of the digestive tract—a gastroenterologist. To obtain the pictures once the "dye" is placed into the duct requires an X-ray specialist—a radiologist. The two physicians work together on this mission. You, the recipient of this attention, must accept the following conditions: nothing to eat or drink for at least eight hours before the study; mild SEDATION that will enable you to tolerate the discomfort; local anesthesia of your throat that will last for about one-half hour; the rigors of the tube being in you for one-half to three-quarters of an hour; the possibility of having to remain in the hospital overnight; the probability of a mild sore throat for several days; the very small but real risk that something serious could happen as a result of the examination. (In any procedure in which an instrument is inserted there is always the risk that there could be a PERFORATION of the part.) Figure an hour for the study, a (+ + +) discomfort, a (+ + +) hazard, a couple of days to feel right. BAP—Bring a Pal.

Bottom Line: (+ + +) Real tough!

CT CT is to the pancreas what peanut butter is to jelly and gin is to tonic—made for each other. The previous sections have given you some ideas of the extreme difficulty of evaluating this organ by conventional X-ray. Those procedures are not only extremely difficult on you, often requiring hospitalization, but also do not show the entire organ. Thus, the diagnostic decision is inferential rather than direct. CT, on the other hand, shows the entire pancreas! And it is so very easy.

It begins with your drinking a barium-like fluid. Then on your back on the table and into the gantry, 15 to 20 minutes; no discomfort; no hazard; no aftershocks.

Bottom Line: (½+) To paraphrase that singing commercial—"I love CT!"

Note: There are often multiple alternatives for the examination of a particular part. The pancreas is a prime example of this surfeit of riches. In addition to those techniques described above is the examination employing ultrasound. (See Chapter 20.) The decision of which to use is the province of the medical specialists faced with your problem. However, you do have the absolute right of being informed of the various alternatives, understanding your options, and feeling satisfied. Get into the act!

Liver Your liver is the largest SOLID ORGAN in your body and is perhaps the most complex. It lives in the upper right corner of your abdomen, tucked up under your lowest ribs, and is separated from the bottom of your right lung by a muscle sheet called the diaphragm. The liver is a veritable conglomerate of industries and organizations. It is a merger of Du Pont and Dow Chemical when the host of chemical products that it manufactures are added up. It is the Red Cross for the body's white cells, both accepting and storing donations it receives from other organs and then returning them—like a transfusion— back to the body when they are needed. It is a major "detox" center and dump site for a host of circulating toxins—alcohol being but one. This is one organ that we truly cannot live without.

Conventional-Special The entire liver cannot be seen even with conventional-special X-ray techniques, but certain of its parts can. It is possible to see both its blood supply and ductal structures. Visualizing either or both permits the skilled viewer to make accurate assumptions about the condition of the entire liver.

Blood Supply The techniques for visualizing the arteries to any body part are very similar. See page 17.

Ductal Structures Ducts are tubes. They exist for the purpose of transporting a product found or manufactured within one part of your body to another part where it is needed. One of the group of products that the liver manufactures is bile, a fluid that contains ENZYMES necessary in the digestion of fats. Bile must be transported to a special location in the small intestine (the duodenum). This is accomplished by tubes within the liver called hepatic ducts. If there is any interference with this delivery, a very serious condition known as jaundice develops. (It's often called "yellow jaundice" because the blockage of bile results in discoloration of the skin.) The cause for this problem must be identified and one of the measures taken is to look at the ducts.

The ducts to be studied must first be opacified by the instillation of "dye." This is accomplished by a procedure known as transhepatic cholangiography. (*Trans* is a word for direction, meaning "across"; *hepatic* is another name for the liver; *cholangiography* is the term for the parts that will be X-rayed, the bile ducts.)

You'll be required to maintain a fast for over eight hours. Once in the X-ray department, you will be asked to remove everything and "gown up." You may (by your choice) be given a mild sedative by injection (½ +). Then into a room where you will be placed on your back on the X-ray table. Your upper right abdomen will be exposed. The radiologist will then cleanse the part with antiseptic solutions and drape the area with sterile towels. He or she will then find a spot between two of your lower ribs and anesthetize the area with a local agent. (You'll feel a needle prick and experience a momentary burning sensation—(+) discomfort.) When the area is good and numb the doctor will insert a long, very fine needle into your liver. These maneuvers are done under the fluoroscope. (If you want to see what is going on, ask. The radiologist usually can adjust the monitor so you can watch too.) You will feel the pressure but no real pain. Simultaneous with the needle insertion is the injection of a small amount of "dye." The purpose of these manipulations is to blindly find a duct in the liver bed and fill it with "dye." This search may be successful with a single pass of the needle, but odds favor several. You will be affected more by the time it takes than by the doctor's activity. Once a duct has been found and entered it is appropriately filled by injecting additional CONTRAST MATERIAL, and X-rays are taken. After all the films have been checked and found technically satisfactory the needle is withdrawn and you are finished. Total study time averages about an hour. The discomfort index is (+ +). This study carries a (+ + +) hazard rating. The movements of the needle through the liver always risk the possibility—however small—of causing serious bleeding or bile spillage. If either or both of these complications should occur it might require surgery for correction at the worst, or a day or so in the hospital for observation at the least.

Bottom Line: (+ +) Sometimes easy, sometimes tough.

CT This is a good way to go for information about the liver. No discomfort. No hazard. One-half hour.

Bottom Line: (½ +) A joke.

Sometimes the whole thing is repeated, giving you "dye" (see the Appendix, Table Details) by vein for a second series. If this is the case then change discomfort to (½ +), hazard to (+), and add another half an hour.

Bottom Line: (+) Still a joke, just not quite as funny.

Spleen   The spleen is another solid organ, but it's not nearly as complex in its functions as the liver. It concerns itself with matters of the blood—both the red cells (which it manufactures throughout your life, and removes from the circulation when they become damaged), and the white cells (the spleen serves as a major producer of lymphocytes). It lives tucked under your ribs in your upper left abdomen—to the left of and slightly behind your stomach. The spleen is an organ that we can generally live without.

Conventional-Special   The only special studies of the spleen that are still performed in this age of CT, ultrasound, and nuclear medicine are those to visualize its blood supply—both arterial and venous. As has been said in previous sections, all studies of vascular structures regardless of where they are or what they supply are similar and are described on page 17.

CT   A most splendid and civilized approach. On your back on the table; 15 minutes to half an hour. No discomfort, hazard, or aftereffects.
Bottom Line: ($\frac{1}{2}$ +) A big yawn.

Genitourinary Tract   The familiar term urinary tract suggests a single system. There are in reality two interrelated systems which should more accurately be called the GENITOURINARY tract. The composition of the genitourinary tract has been described in Chapter 16.

For our purposes the genital and urinary systems are discussed separately, and the appropriate examinations, for either the entire system or its component structures, are detailed.

Uterus, Fallopian Tubes, Ovaries

Conventional-Special   The uterus and the fallopian tubes are HOLLOW ORGANS. A hollow organ is one in which there is a central CAVITY (in contrast to a solid organ, which has no such cavity). The heart, stomach, and colon are other examples of the hollow group. The liver, spleen, and pancreas exemplify the solid. With the hollow organs, introduction of an appropriate contrast material will often permit diagnostic judgments to be made. The trick is to get the contrast material in. For the uterus and tubes this is quite a trick and it is known as hysterosalpingography. (*Hystero* means "uterus," *salpingo* refers to tubes.)

The examination is best performed in the first two weeks of the menstrual cycle. What comes next is indistinguishable from the initial steps in a routine "internal" examination (see pages 57–58). It may even be done by your own gynecologist, but more frequently it will be the radiologist and a female technologist who will do the deed. The only other difference up until this point is that you will be on an X-ray table rather than the typical gyn couch.

Now the new part: after the SPECULUM has been positioned and the inside of your vagina cleansed, the opening of your uterus (cervix) is found and grasped by another instrument. Although you will be warned before it is done, it is a (+ +) jolt. Blessedly, the pain is only for the second that the actual pinch is made. Now, a third instrument is inserted. This one is a hollow tube (cannula) whose end will be passed into your cervix. This should cause no discomfort. When all this has been accomplished, and it usually takes only 5 to 10 minutes, you will be gently pulled back so that you can straighten your legs. (Yes, the instruments are still in.)

Another radiologist will fluoroscope you. (If you are interested in seeing what the doctors will be watching, ask!) Radiologist one, whom you already know from the preceding events, will then inject "dye" into the hollow tube that was positioned earlier. The "dye" will enter your uterus and flow from it into your fallopian tubes. If the tubes are open, as they should be, some of the "dye" will flow out and enter your abdomen. (Not to worry; the "dye" will be quickly absorbed and will cause no ill effects.) Radiologist two (the fluoroscopist) will observe the filling and take appropriate pictures. You will be told that an exposure is about to be made, and asked to hold your breath. You'll experience a slight sound and vibration—nothing more. If your tubes are patent (open) the addition of "dye" will not increase your discomfort. If, however, there is some tubal abnormality that impedes the flow, the injection can be painful. It may be similar to a menstrual cramp, or it may be sharp if a narrowed or blocked area is suddenly forced open. Sometimes patients experience pain between their shoulderblades. Usually discomfort is no more than (+ +).

When the pictures have been taken and are deemed satisfactory, you will again be placed in the knees-up posture and all of the instruments will be removed. The technologist will wipe away any traces of the lubricant that might remain, and provide you with a pad.

The procedure, start to finish, takes about three-quarters of an hour. Evaluation of the discomfort index is somewhat difficult in this case. The first part of the study is no different than a routine pelvic examination, which has both a true discomfort and an added indignity component as givens. The second part—the instrumentation—adds additional pain. A (+ +) or (+ + +) is the best judgment for discomfort. A (+) is a fair value for the hazard. Bring a pal both for moral support and to help you get home. Expect drainage on the pad for two or three days. It might even be blood-tinged. Don't be alarmed unless true bleeding occurs, fever develops, or you have continuing abdominal pain. For any of the above, consult your gynecologist.

Bottom Line: (+ + +) Unfortunately, your memories of this one will not be fond.

CT It is possible to "see" the general size and position of the ovaries and uterus by this method of study, but not the inside of the uterus, and usually not the tubes. No preparation is required. No "dye" is used. The routine is: on your back on the table. Into the gantry to the level of your pelvis, 5 to 10 minutes of SECTIONING, out of the gantry, and out the door. No discomfort, no hazard, no aftereffects.

Bottom Line: (½+) A four-leaf-clover day if this will pinpoint the problem.

Note: Ultrasound techniques are being used more and more for certain gynecological problems. Review the discussion of uterine and ovarian examination in Chapter 20 as well.

Prostate Gland Of the structures that compose the genital system in the male—the penis, testicles, seminal ducts, and prostate—only the prostate GLAND lends itself to routine evaluation by X-ray studies, and even these are limited. Conventional techniques offer only indirect data. If the prostate is enlarged it may produce indentation of the floor of the bladder, but this is a coincidental finding when the bladder is being studied. It is not an examination of the prostate as such. Only CT offers a direct evaluation.

CT In some cases the prostate examination is done with no preparation. However, it is more usual to fill the bladder with "dye," which acts to improve the detail of the prostate, because it lies just below and slightly behind the bladder. The "dye" (see the Appendix, Table Details) is given by injection into a vein in your arm, and it takes about 15 minutes for it to fill your bladder. Then it's ho-hum. On your back on the table and into the gantry. You'll hear "whiz-bang" sounds and feel the slight table movements for about 10 minutes of imaging. Then you're finished. Discomfort rates (½+) for the "stick." Hazard equals a (+) for the "dye." No aftereffects.

Bottom line: (½+) Let's hear it again for CT!

Kidneys, Ureters, Bladder, Urethra

Conventional-Routine A film of the abdomen (see page 207) is capable of providing some information about the general size and position of your kidneys and perhaps some indication of the size of your bladder; in addition it may highlight abnormal shadows that could be stones somewhere in the tract. But that's about all. If this very limited look is all that is deemed necessary, it takes about five minutes and is associated with neither pain nor discomfort.

Bottom Line: (½ +) Hardly worth mentioning.

Conventional-special techniques are really the routine for examination of the urinary tract. Four different studies are performed, as described in the following.

Intravenous Urography (IVU), also known as KUB (kidneys, ureters, bladder) This is the examination that is requested for most problems that may be of a urinary tract nature. Its performance requires that a rather large volume of "dye" be injected. (A full discussion of iodine can be found in the Appendix, Table Details.)

Preparation is preferred but can be skipped if the study is of an EMERGENT nature. This "prep" includes a laxative in the afternoon of the day preceding the study, a light or liquid dinner that night, and then nothing by mouth until the examination is completed the following morning.

Once you arrive at the place of the examination, you will be asked to strip from the waist down and wear a gown, so bring along your own socks, slippers, or even robe if that will give you comfort. Then it's on with the show.

You will lie on your back on the X-ray table. A preliminary film will be made of your abdomen by the technologist. The radiologist will then appear and talk to you about the "dye." He or she will select a vein (if you know from sad experience that one arm is better than the other, speak up!), insert a needle, and inject the "dye." This may be done in one continuous "push," or the "dye" may be diluted in a bottle of fluid and allowed to "drip" in slowly. In either case you may experience a sensation in your arm above the site of injection, and this may be followed by a general feeling of warmth throughout your body. Some people develop a "funny" taste in their mouth. All of these experiences are momentary and do not constitute a "reaction." The technologist will make exposures on a timed sequential basis. Often the first few pictures will be made by laminographic techniques. (LAMINOGRAPHY is described on page 188.) Often a compression device (in this case, a wide belt—exactly the same as a blood pressure cuff, only large enough to encircle your abdomen) will be placed about the level of your belly button to put pressure on your abdomen just below each kidney. Doctors do this to slow down the flow of urine from your kidneys; this causes a better concentration of "dye," and thus a better "look." It may produce mild discomfort (½ +). The compression device is used only for the first 10 to 15 minutes of the study, after which it is removed. When the radiologist, who reviews each picture immediately after it has been taken, is satisfied that all of the obtainable information has been gotten, you will be placed in the standing position. Another film will be made. After that one, you may go to the bathroom and empty your bladder. Then, one last picture, and you are free. The elapsed time from entering the room to parole averages 45 to 60 minutes. Anticipate (+) discomfort and consider hazard to be (+) for the "dye." There should be no aftereffects. Best to bring a pal.

Bottom Line: (+) Lots of words for "No big deal."

Retrograde Pyelogram "Retrograde" is a term used to describe direction, and means "against the normal flow"; *pyelo* is another name for the hollow portion of the kidneys. Thus a pyelogram is a picture of the hollow portion, or collecting portion, of a kidney—where urine that is made in the solid portion of the organ collects and then flows down each ureter or tube to the bladder. In this procedure "dye" is not injected by vein, but is instilled directly into either the kidney itself or the tube that is connected to the kidney. Getting the "dye" into your kidney requires the participation of three different medical specialists: an ANESTHESIOLOGIST, a urologic surgeon, and a radiologist. What a lineup! The game plan is divided into three parts.

Part 1: You must come into the hospital as a patient, either the night before or the morning of the examination. (Review Short Procedure Hospitalization on pages xvi–xviii.) It is essential that you have nothing to eat or drink for at least eight hours before. You will be dressed in a hospital gown and will be taken to the operating suite according to a prearranged schedule. There you will be met by the anesthesiologist who will explain, and, with your informed consent, perform a spinal tap. (See page 204.) When the needle is correctly positioned, an anesthetic solution will be injected and you will lose all sensation from the waist down. Except for the oddness of this new condition, it is not unpleasant. You are now ready for Part 2: the urologist.

Part 2: The urologist will reposition you so that your pubic area will be exposed, permitting him or her to find the opening of your urethra. (In men the opening is at the tip of the penis; in women just in front of the opening of the vagina.) This entire area will be cleansed with an antiseptic solution (you won't feel anything because of the "spinal" you just got) and draped with sterile towels. The urologist will insert an instrument into your urethra and gently advance it until it enters the bladder. This instrument is one of many similar optical devices that permit direct inspection of different body cavities. For the bladder, the instrument is a thin flexible tube called a cystoscope. It has a hollow center that not only permits fluids to be put into the bladder but also provides a means of emptying it of urine. Special instruments can be inserted through the scope, thereby allowing certain surgical procedures to be performed. And, lastly, a very fine flexible tube (CATHETER) can be threaded through the cystoscope into the bladder and then up into a ureter which opens into the bladder. This catheter can be gently pushed all the way up to the kidney. The cystoscope will then be removed, leaving the catheter in position with the outside end taped to your thighs. (Under special circumstances both kidneys may be examined at the same time.) This entire procedure is performed in some 15 to 20 minutes. Because of the anesthesia you will experience no true discomfort, although you may be aware of some sensations of mild pressure or tugging. So much for Part 2.

Part 3: On to the radiologist. You may remain in the operating suite, or you may be transported to the X-ray department. In either case you will be placed on an X-ray table and the radiologist will determine the position of the catheters that are in you by using a fluoroscope. If any adjustments in their position are made you might be aware of mild tugging sensations. Syringes containing "dye" will be attached to the ends of the catheters and the contrast material will be injected under fluoroscopic guidance. You won't feel this. Pictures will be made, and checked. When all are satisfied that they have captured the real you, the catheters will be pulled out—again a minor tug. Mission accomplished!

You'll experience (+ +) or (+ + +) discomfort—mostly due to the spinal tap; a (+ +) hazard due to the spinal and catheter insertion. Schedule about two hours for the actual procedure and another three to four hours before the anesthesia wears off and you feel everything belongs to you again. You might experience a headache for some hours and a backache for several days. There is an element of embarrassment during the urological portion of the procedure. There may be some increase in the frequency of your urination and perhaps some pinkness in your urine for a day or so. Whether or not you can go home the same day is a decision made after the study is over. Have a pal in attendance.

Bottom Line: (+ + +) A real drag.

Cystogram Cysto refers to the bladder. Most of the time the bladder can be seen well enough for evaluation when an IVU (described above) is performed. Sometimes, however, that study is not good enough. Your problems may be such that a more detailed study of the bladder alone is necessary. When that is the case, three different techniques, each for a different set of symptoms, are available.

• Retrograde: The examination begins with the catheterization of your bladder. (Review this technique on pages 163–164.) With the catheter in position a solution containing "dye" will be run into your bladder. You will begin to experience the sensation you know as "having to go." When this fullness becomes really uncomfortable the technologist will turn off the flow. Your bladder is now full. The catheter is removed. The technologist will take X-rays in several views. These maneuvers are neither stressful nor unpleasant. You can then go to the bathroom. You return for one more film, and then you're done. The study takes about 30 minutes. Discomfort rates a (+), hazard (+). There may be some slight increase in the number of times you will go to the bathroom in the next day, and some pinkish hue to your urine for the same period.

Bottom Line: (+ +) A big ugh!

• Chain: In some women where there is concern that the bladder has "dropped" (a condition known as cystocele) and needs surgical correction, another study of the bladder, called the chain cystogram, may be indicated. It is in many respects identical to the retrograde cystogram just described, but besides "dye" being put into the bladder, a fine chain is also inserted through the catheter. This causes you no additional discomfort or embarrassment. The catheter is then removed, leaving the chain lying on the floor of the bladder and extending down through the urethra to the outside. When X-rays are taken with you in the standing position the angle formed between the bladder floor and the urethra can be determined by measuring the angle formed by the chain. If the angle is abnormal, appropriate surgical correction is considered. From your standpoint this procedure is identical to the retrograde.

Bottom Line: (+ +) A big ugh, with a chain!

• Voiding: "Voiding" is another word for urinating. For certain problems, particularly in children, it is most helpful to get pictures of the parts while the patient is actually voiding. In this study, your bladder is filled by the retrograde method described above. You are then asked to urinate right there on the table. (Men are given urinals, women a stack of towels.) While this is occurring the Peeping Tom of medicine, the radiologist, is watching through the fluoroscope and taking pictures. The voiding is the most difficult part of the whole thing. Most of us consider this to be a private act and "choke up" when asked to perform. But after a bit of prompting, it gets done. Discomfort and hazard are the same as described above.

Bottom Line: (+ +) Who thinks these things up?

Retrograde Urethra "Retrograde" describes a direction which is opposite to the usual movement of a fluid. The urethra is the tube that extends from your bladder to the outside world. In women it is about half an inch long. It is much longer in men, running the length of the penis. None of the examinations described above are designed to satisfactorily visualize this final segment of the urinary tract, except perhaps a carefully performed voiding cystogram. Thus, when symptoms suggest that the urethra may be the source of your problem, it must be studied by techniques that optimize its visualization.

"Dye" must be instilled from the end of your urethra so that it runs backwards to its origin, which is at the bottom of your bladder. The filling is not difficult, but keeping the urethra filled long enough for picture taking is. Without a special "gadget," anything put into it will either run backwards and into your bladder or will spill out the front end. So—"the gadget please." A special tube (catheter) has been developed that has a balloon at one end and another along its length that can be moved. Neither balloon is inflated initially. Your urethra is cleansed with an antiseptic solution, and the catheter is slid in to the correct depth—in this case into your bladder. The end balloon is then inflated and the catheter pulled back gently. When the balloon gets to the mouth of your bladder it acts like a plug in the bathtub. The second balloon is then inflated and slipped up to the mouth of your urethra, acting as another plug. Now, sufficient "dye" is injected to fill the urethra—which isn't very much. X-rays are then taken—two or three pictures. The balloons are then deflated and the catheter slipped out. Elapsed time is about 15 minutes. Physical discomfort is only (+), but add one more (+) for embarrassment. There may be residual discomfort in the area for a day or two, but it's usually only an awareness of a difference, no more.

Bottom Line: (+ +) Another one where the bark is worse than the bite.

CT Except for the urethra, the entire urinary tract—the kidneys, ureters, and bladder—can all be seen after "dye" has been given by vein. (See the discussion in the IVU description on page 218.) You will be on your back on the table. The table will be moved into the gantry. Sequenced exposures will be made. From 15 to 30 minutes should do it. Expect a (½ +) for the discomfort of the "stick," (+) for the hazard. Bring a friend just in case the "dye" and you don't agree. There should be no aftereffects.

Bottom Line: (+) A CT ho-hum.

Adrenal Glands If a recognition poll of body parts were taken the adrenal glands might well finish last. Yet these small (about one inch long and triangularly shaped) bodies that live on top of each of our kidneys are critical to our well-being. Among the products that they manufacture and regulate are steroids and adrenalin, HORMONES that undoubtedly are better known than the glands themselves. So we offer here a salute to that anonymous pair that serves us so gallantly.

A more complete description of their bodily role can be found in Chapter 4.

Conventional-Special The blood supply to these glands can offer important information. As stated earlier, the techniques that are used to visualize the blood supply to any part are similar, and are discussed together on page 17.

CT Can do! On your back on the table and into the gantry. A quarter-hour will do it nicely. Neither discomfort nor hazard. Nothing to remember after.

Bottom Line: (½ +) Boring.

Lymph Glands Everyone knows about swollen glands, especially when they occur in the neck. "They have something to do with infection, or something." But that's about all that most of us have to say about them. Actually, those glands, swollen or not, are part of an entire system—the LYMPHATIC SYSTEM—which consists of a network of fine vessels and nodes that circulate a fluid called *lymph* throughout the body. Nodes are small specialized clumps of TISSUE that serve as collection stations along the vessel network. They are also capable of making some types of white blood cells that the body requires to combat infection. Nodes are the "glands" that you can feel when they become enlarged, either because of infection or other causes such as the presence of a MALIGNANCY (a lymphoma that originates within the lymph nodes or develops in them as a consequence of tumor spread —metastasis). In many medical workups it is most essential to know the state of these nodes. In many places, such as your neck, armpit, and groin, they can be felt. But in many other places they are too deep to be PALPATED and other means to determine their condition are sought.

Conventional-Special This study is called lymphangiography. As in other X-ray procedures in which the desired part cannot be seen without contrast material, so, too, with the lymphatics. Since the lymphatic system is very similar to the CIRCULATORY SYSTEM why not do the same thing that is done when it is necessary to "see" a vein or an artery—stick a needle into it and inject "dye"? The logic is faultless and that's what's done, but it isn't quite the same. Blood vessels can usually be felt and since they carry a red fluid can also be seen. Lymph vessels have the thickness of a single hair and carry a colorless fluid. They can neither be felt nor seen.

Question: What to do?

Answer: (1) Make them visible. (2) Make them fatter. (3) Get a needle into one and inject "dye." This 1-2-3 procedure takes about one, two, or even three hours to accomplish. Here's how it is done:

Almost without exception the site of injection is in the feet. (If another location is selected, for instance, the hands, the technique that is used is very similar to the one described here for the feet, and need not be specifically detailed.) You will lie on your back on an X-ray table after removing your shoes and socks or stockings. The radiologist will prepare each foot by cleansing it with an antiseptic solution and then surround each with a sterile towel. A very small amount of a special blue stain containing a local anesthetic will be injected into the skin on the top of each foot between several of your toes. You will feel a slight prick with each "stick." No worse. You will be able to see a blue blob at each injection site—almost like a small blue tattoo. Following this, there is a wait of 10 to 20 minutes. A look down now will show that extending from each blob are one or more fine snaky blue lines. These snakes are lymph vessels that have picked up the injected stain. End of Step 1—now they can be seen! Begin Step 2 —making the vessels fatter.

The radiologist will choose one of the blue snakes to attack. A local anesthetic will be injected into your skin over the vessel and a small INCISION will be made in your skin to the depth of the vessel. You will feel mild pressure but no pain. The vessel will be isolated and a clamp will be put around it to temporarily block the movement of its fluid. This will cause the part below the blockage to distend. Step 2 accomplished.

Next—the injection of "dye." A very fine needle is inserted into the vessel and "tied" into it with a piece of black silk thread. The clamp is removed, restoring flow. The needle is connected to tubing that is connected to a syringe containing the "dye" (see the Appendix, Table Details). Because of the fineness of the vessel, only minute amounts of "dye" can be injected at a time or the lymphatic will rupture. Thus, the syringe is placed into a special pump mechanism that will control the rate of injection. It takes almost an hour to put in enough contrast. Since the same procedure is also done on your other foot that side will be started as soon as the first foot injection begins. When all is accomplished the needles will be removed and the incisions closed by "stitches." Dressings will be applied. One or two X-rays will be taken over your abdomen and perhaps your chest. That's it for Day One.

Oops, almost forgot to tell you that the major X-ray imaging occurs on Day Two. So, back again the next day for pictures. These will consist of exposures made in different positions over your abdomen. They should take about 15 minutes to obtain. The radiologist will look at your feet to make sure that they are O.K., and then re-dress them. Unless there is a special circumstance that requires additional views on Day Three, that's it!

The actual "doing" is only a (+) discomfort because everything is performed under local anesthesia. But there is the tedium of lying on your back while all that stuff is going on down below—maybe two to four hours in duration. For some it rates a (+ +). The hazard rates a soft (+). Allow four to six hours on Day One, and another hour on Day Two. Bring something to read to pass the time. Bring a pal to assist you home because you will be weary and your feet will begin to ache when the anesthesia wears off. Bring slippers because your shoes may be too tight now that your feet are bandaged. The dressings should be changed every day to avoid infection. You can probably do that yourself. Plan a visit back to either your doctor or the radiologist in about a week to get the stitches out. Lest you tend to forget the experience, the small blue blobs between your toes will help you remember because the stain persists for months.

Bottom Line: (+ +) You hereby become a valued member of the Blue Foot Club—a most elite group.

CT Lymph node enlargement, in many locations, can be detected by this technique and no special preparations are necessary. If the area of concern is one which lends itself to this approach—super! It is a 15-minute procedure with you on your back and the part of interest centered in the gantry. No discomfort, no hazard, no returns.

Bottom Line: (½ +) Joy.

Miscellaneous

It is inevitable that even after the most careful of deliberations, some things are left over because they just don't quite fit the greater scheme. But they are too important to be left on the table. What to do? Simply again thank that unsung genius who solved the problem for us all by inventing the category miscellaneous! When it comes to X-rays, this category includes surveys, biopsy control, and postoperative and recheck tests.

Surveys A survey is a comprehensive overview of a particular condition or problem. Physicians know that particular diseases are likely to attack certain locations in the body more than others. So examinations for a known or suspected condition are tailored to X-ray only those higher-probability sites. For example, when there is advanced kidney disease, there may be associated changes in one or more bones. Certain bones, such as the vertebrae, are affected more commonly than others. The recognition of these changes is important to the overall management of the patient. Therefore, in this example an examination of the most commonly affected bones, a metabolic survey, is performed.

The name of the survey—metabolic, metastatic, or rheumatoid—denotes the problem being explored and each has its own routine pattern of examination. However, they are all otherwise similar and thus can be considered together.

Conventional-Routine No preparation is necessary. You will have to get undressed and put on a gown—so bring your own stuff if that will make you more comfortable. Once in the X-ray room you will be positioned according to the parts to be studied. None will cause you discomfort and none are hazardous. Schedule about half an hour. There will be no take-home misery.

Bottom Line: (½ +) A piece of cake.

Biopsy Guidance A BIOPSY is the removal of sufficient TISSUE suspected to be abnormal so that it may be identified and an appropriate treatment plan initiated. There was a time not too long ago when most of these procedures were surgical adventures, often major, which almost without exception required hospitalization, general anesthesia, and a period of recovery. If the tissue findings were such that the entire abnormal tissue had to be removed —for example, if it was found to be cancerous—then another, more extensive surgical intervention would follow. With the advent of CT and ultrasound (see Chapter 20), intrepid radiologists got into the act. They realized that with this new way of seeing the body, many problem areas requiring biopsy could be reached and the deed could be done by simpler techniques, thereby making an open surgical encounter unnecessary. This is what is done:

Let's assume that an atypical "shadow" was discovered on a conventional-routine X-ray of your chest and a biopsy to determine its nature is required. Your chest is now reexamined by CT and the LESION reidentified. If the problem is nearer the front of your chest you will lie on your back; if closer to your back then your position will be on your stomach. Markers—often in the form of barium paste—are applied to the skin overlying the abnormality. The part is then reimaged with the CT scanner and the marker closest to the "badness" chosen. The skin is then prepared by antiseptic cleansing and draping with sterile towels. A local anesthetic is injected under the skin marker—you'll feel a slight prick and a slight burn. Additional anesthesia is injected at deeper levels until the entire area is numb. A longer needle is then inserted with the intention of placing its tip in the tissue requiring biopsy. The part is again imaged with the needle in place to check its position. This is repeated, with adjustments in positioning, until the placement is precise. Suction is then applied to the other end of the needle by a glass syringe sufficient to draw up some cells from the area of abnormality. These acts of needle placement and suction are felt, in most cases, only as sensations of pressure and tugging (+). Occasionally it is painful, but that is the exception, not the rule. The content of what has been sucked up is then placed onto slides and into a "fixing" solution, and sent to a PATHOLOGIST for an answer. The needle is withdrawn and a dressing is applied. The part is reexamined for the last time to see whether the procedure has caused any undesirable new problems, such as excessive bleeding. If everything is cool, that's it.

All biopsies that are done under CT, ultrasound, or FLUOROSCOPIC guidance are performed by a radiologist and helpers. The time is highly variable, but allow two hours. It will probably be less. Although the discomfort is only (+)—maybe (+ +)—the hazard is (+ + +). There is always the real possibility of complication. However, the decision to attempt the procedure by a PERCUTANEOUS technique rather than by open surgery was reached because all concerned physicians involved in the case concluded that the "bottom line" risks were less this way. If all goes as anticipated—and it does in about 90 percent of all cases—you should have no significant aftereffects. The area attacked may be sore and black and blue for a couple of days. If the tissue report is good and no further management is demanded, you should be able to resume all normal activities. Always bring a pal.

Bottom Line: (+ +) Good luck.

Postoperative and Rechecks This is a catchall category for any examination that is required after a surgical procedure to evaluate the immediate results or after an X-ray examination whose findings were such that later "looks" are required to see what—if anything—has happened. It is impossible to detail this entire group because it is so varied and individualized. However, there are two conventional-special procedures that are done with sufficient frequency that their story should be told:

T-tube Cholangiogram A T-tube is a thin rubber tube shaped like a T. *Cholang* relates to the biliary system (see page 49). *Gram* means a picture. A small group of people who have their gall bladders removed also have some problem in the ducts that connect to the gall bladder. In these instances, the surgeon may elect to insert a rubber tube into one of these ducts—a T-tube —at the time of surgery, to be certain that the duct is clear. The part of the tube that is inserted is the short crossbar of the T. The long limb extends out of the incision and onto the skin. This procedure provides a way to "see" the inside of the duct and ascertain that it is free of disease. "DYE" is injected into the external end of the tube. X-rays are taken when the CONTRAST has reached the duct. If everything is normal the tube is withdrawn.

All of the above is done while you are under anesthesia, so you are unaware of these events. However, if the films identify a problem which the surgeon does not feel he or she can correct at this surgery, for any number of reasons, the T-tube is left in. You leave the hospital with the outside of the tube in a small plastic bag taped to your abdomen. At some prearranged time you return for another look.

No breakfast the morning of the study is the only "prep." You will be asked to lie on a fluoroscopic table on your back. The radiologist will free the tube from its bag and attach a syringe containing "dye" to its end. The contrast material will then be injected into the tube under fluoroscopic guidance. Films will be made. You will be instructed to hold your breath when it is appropriate. You will hear the whirring of the machine and see the flash of the X-ray exposure. But that's usually all. There is rarely any discomfort. There is no hazard. There are no anticipated delayed miseries. The job takes about half an hour. If the findings are normal—hurrah! They will remove the damn tube. If there is still concern the tube stays in and you will be back another day for the same study. Sorry.

Bottom Line: (+) Anyone for a coming-out party?

Barium Enema Through a Colostomy Opening This one is pretty obvious. You have had surgery and are left with a colostomy (an artificial anus; the new end of the colon is created by bringing it up to the skin on the front surface of the abdomen). It may be necessary to periodically examine your colon to ensure that there is no recurrence of the problem that initiated the original surgery or to monitor healing which may permit your bowel to be rejoined and the colostomy closed.

The study is not unlike the barium enema you experienced way back before you were operated on (see page 209) except now the enema tube is inserted into the stoma (mouth) of the colostomy. This tube will have a special balloon at its tip that can be inflated once it is in place so that it will prevent the barium from spilling out. The preparation is essentially the same as for a colon examination (see page 209). You should monitor your diet for several days, take laxatives as directed, and bring a buddy along. Once the enema tip is in and the radiologist is ready, the show begins. You may receive glucagon. Spot films will be made during the filling of your colon. Overhead views will be made after. What can I tell you that you don't already know about this one? It probably isn't as uncomfortable as the original, but it still is a chore.

Bottom Line: (+ +) Hope that this is the last one!

19

Go Get a Nuclear Study

> **Hazard: Ionizing Radiation Is Detrimental to Health!**
>
> This is a one-paragraph-fits-all disclaimer that applies to all nuclear medicine examinations: Nuclear medicine procedures subject the recipient to ionizing radiation. The amount varies with the examination. The effects are cumulative. The potential for harm is greater in the young than in the old, and is greatest in the fetus. Thus, each study must be weighed carefully and the risk-to-benefit ratio established by those most knowledgeable to make this decision—the referring physician and the nuclear medicine physician. Except for the pregnant patient the hazards are more theoretical than real. The benefits far outweigh the risks. If you do have fear, discuss it with your professional advisors. If you are or even might be pregnant, let this fact be known. Keep records of all your examinations and review them with the nuclear physician prior to each new study. Concern is warranted. Panic is not.

Since the atomic explosions at Hiroshima and Nagasaki and more recently the accidents at Three Mile Island and Chernobyl, the word "nuclear" evokes a knee-jerk response in many that equals *bad!* or *evil!* or *awesome!* or *immoral!* And, indeed, I share this response, when the word "nuclear" precedes certain other words, such as "bomb" and "missile." But when it precedes "medicine," I think it is very, very *good*.

To understand the basis of nuclear medicine requires a smattering of basic physics. I will try to explain in the next few paragraphs that which has filled lifetimes of scientists who have helped to clarify some of the mysteries of our physical world.

Here goes . . .

All things found in nature are composed of combinations of fundamental building blocks called elements. Each element has a unique configuration, which is its atomic structure. (The atom is the smallest particle of an element that can exist alone.) An atom is composed of a nucleus (the nucleus is the central portion of the atom and comprises almost all of its weight) and electrons (an electron is an elementary particle that is negatively charged) which orbit around the nucleus.

The nucleus of the atom is our main interest. It is composed of two fundamental particles: the proton (a proton is an elementary particle of matter that possesses a positive charge and a mass greater than that of an electron) and the neutron (a neutron is an elementary particle of matter that possesses no charge but has a mass almost equal to that of a proton). It is the particular number of protons and neutrons in their combination that distinguishes one element from another. Thus the atom that is oxygen will always contain the same number of protons in its nucleus, and almost always the same number of neutrons. When the neutron number varies, either naturally or as a result of processes designed by man, that atom, although still oxygen, is now a special ISOTOPE (one of two or more atoms having the same proton number, but different numbers of neutrons) of oxygen and is likely to be radioactive. Why?

This why can be satisfied by beginning with the broad generalization that the desired combination of protons and neutrons in any atom results in a balance between them. When this exists the atom is *stable* or at "ground level." When the neutron number is altered from ground level that combination may no longer be in balance—and if it is not balanced, that atom, although the same element, is *unstable*. It is a radioactive isotope of the stable atom. Since the desired natural order of things is stability, this unstable atom will rearrange its combination to become stable by releasing energy. This energy release is called radioactivity. The release occurs in the form known as alpha particles, beta particles, or gamma rays. For the sake of simplicity—and sanity, since the first two have no further role in our saga—the definition of alpha and beta will be ignored. For our purposes gamma radiation can be considered as identical to the photons of energy that we call X-rays.

To understand what nuclear medicine is all about let's choose the thyroid GLAND as an example. This ORGAN's function is to extract the element iodine, which is found in normal diets, and convert it into HORMONES that are then released back into the general circulation. Let us assume that after hearing your complaints your doctor decides it is appropriate to investigate the function and condition of your thyroid. Knowing that your thyroid will extract any ingested iodine and knowing that there are radioisotopes of iodine that are safe for human consumption, the nuclear physician gives you such an isotope. Your thyroid "takes up" the isotope, being unable to distinguish the unstable from the stable. Because the iodine now in your thyroid is radioactive and will release gamma rays, the function of the gland can be measured and a detailed picture of its structure can be obtained. Images thus created originate from energy sources inside your body and reflect the function and configuration of the part which incorporated the isotope. This is in contrast to X-rays, where the energy is passed through your body from the outside and is neither dependent upon, nor necessarily a reflection of, function.

To understand who directs the nuclear medicine show, meet the nuclear medicine physician. He or she is a person who has quite a bit of training. First, he or she graduates from both college and medical school, and spends three additional years either studying the vast array of diseases that are included under the umbrella of internal medicine or tilling the fields called radiology. When these efforts are successful, as attested by passage of examinations known as boards, the physician is awarded a degree proclaiming that he or she is a certified internist or radiologist. The physician then undergoes a second period of study that will last one or two more years and is devoted only to those problems that can be either diagnosed or treated with radioisotopes. Again, there are examinations, and a second certification, proclaiming the doctor is a nuclear medicine physician, is awarded.

We will concern ourselves only with procedures that are of a diagnostic nature. Diagnostic examinations performed by nuclear medicine techniques are of two general types—imaging and laboratory. *Imaging* is the technique whereby a picture is obtained similar to an X-ray. In *laboratory* procedures, a measurement is obtained that can then be compared to values known to represent normal function.

Imaging

Nuclear medicine studies differ from all other imaging modalities in one fundamental characteristic. The energy that is responsible for the creation of a picture using X-rays, ultrasound, or magnetic resonance originates from a source outside of your body, is passed through your body, and is captured as it exits from your body to produce the image. The image created in nuclear medicine is derived from an energy source that is first placed into your body; then as it passes through and leaves the body, it, too, is captured to produce the picture. This energy source is a radioactive ISOTOPE. Thus, all procedures require the administration of a radioactive isotope (henceforth identified solely as an isotope, radiosotope, TRACER, or nuclide). This is done by injection, swallowing, instillation, or inhalation. A word about each follows.

Administering the Isotope

• *Injection:* For all routine and ordinary procedures the injection is made into a vein—the biggest and most easily accessible one you have. (This procedure, venipuncture, has been described earlier. See Chapter 17.) That which is injected is a RADIOPHARMACEUTICAL. (A PHARMACEUTICAL is a drug used in medicine. A radiopharmaceutical is such a drug to which an isotope has been attached.) The drug will then carry the isotope to the part of your body that is to be imaged.

• *Swallowing:* Some isotopes can be put into capsules or in a liquid that can be taken by mouth. With those, it's down the hatch.

• *Instillation:* There are certain examinations that require the isotope to be put directly into the part of interest. The bladder is often such an example. Tubes, also known as CATHETERS, are carefully passed to the area of interest and the material is put in. The degree of discomfort and hazard will depend on the location of the part requiring the instillation. In most cases neither will exceed (+). Usually the procedure is accomplished in minutes.

• *Inhalation:* Certain isotopes are in the form of a gas. They are administered through a tube that is connected to a special mask that is placed over your nose and mouth. You are asked to take in a deep breath. The gas is drawn into your lungs. It sounds dreadful but except for the mask it is no different from taking in a breath of air. The gas has neither odor nor taste. The mask may cause you momentary concern but once it is explained and fitted to your face, and once you realize that it does not impair your normal breathing, the fear will be gone. You will remain completely awake throughout the entire event. So—a possible (+) for discomfort and a (−) for hazard.

The nuclide is now inside you. Its precise location is not a matter of chance. It has been put into a specific place if the introduction is by instillation or inhalation. If the administration is by injection or swallowing it is taken to the desired body site by being attached to something else that "knows where to go." (The something else is a pharmaceutical agent. For example, an aspirin "knows where to go" when you have a headache.) The isotope is in place. All systems are "Go." Now what happens?

The Equipment You will be taken to a room that contains special machines. There are those known as scanners that can capture the isotope's energy and convert it into an image. There are others, known as probes, that measure the amount of isotopic accumulation in a particular body part. Scanners are usually referred to as *gamma cameras.* They, as well as probes, come in different models.

• *Stationary gamma camera:* This machine is composed of three parts. There is a base and a vertical column that is perhaps seven or eight feet tall. An arm comes off the column and supports a large object resembling a bass drum —the camera. The "drum" will vary in size depending on the diameter of its crystal. Some crystals are 15 inches across. Others may reach 30 inches in diameter. The whole thing looks something like a lamppost. The camera on its arm can be raised or lowered and the camera itself can be rotated and angled. Its face is smooth and flat. An attempt is made in each examination to position the camera as close to the part of interest as possible. You may lie flat on your back or stomach. Sometimes your position will be sitting or even standing. The decision is based on the closest "fit" of the scanning head to the part of concern. Once this is established there is no further movement of the camera. In those situations in which the part of interest—it could be your whole body—is larger than the "field of view" of the camera, the process is repeated until all of the area is covered and the desired information is obtained.

• *Rotating gamma camera:* This machine is also known as a SPECT scanner. (SPECT is an acronym: S = single, P = photon, E = emission, C = computed, T = tomography.) This term explains that the energy source used to create the images is obtained by the emission of single photons, in this case gamma rays, and that the picture is derived employing computerized tomographic (CT) technology (see Chapter 18). The SPECT scanner differs from the stationary gamma camera in its ability to move while the image data is being collected. The large camera head—some models have two cameras suspended at right angles to each other—is mounted on an arm attached to the inside of a large open metal ring. The arm can move in a circle inside the ring. You are placed on a special table that is mounted on rails and called the *gantry.* The table is made to move into the open ring to a position that places the body part of concern at the level of the camera. The scanner can then make a 360-degree rotation, or any lesser arc, around the body part. Unlike the CT gantry which moves the patient into the enclosed machine, making some people anxious, this table is completely open. Additionally, unlike the arrangement in CT, there is always a technologist in the room with you during the examination, and this, too, helps to allay fear. The scanner does not touch you. However, examinations performed on this machine may be long—20 to 40 minutes—and demand total immobility. Thus, discomfort (+) or (+ +) may develop from the necessity of lying still.

• *PET scanner:* PET is an acronym for positron emission tomography. (Positrons are one group of subatomic particles possessing a positive charge; they are found in the nucleus of an atom. Certain elements, when in the radioactive or unstable state, emit positrons. So, this instrument is employed to create images from isotopes that release positrons and to format the images in a tomographic presentation.)

For those who have experienced CAT or MRI imaging the PET is very similar. The machine appears as a freestanding wall with a hole in its center. There is a table that is positioned at right angles to the hole. You lie on the table on your back. The table is moved so that your head enters the opening. Very precise measurements are made to ascertain that the position is correct. Once this has been established, no further movements are necessary (unlike CT, in which the table moves between exposures). Except for the time each study takes and the claustrophobia (fear of being in a confined space) that some people occasionally experience, there is no anticipated discomfort. An additional soothing plus is that the technologist remains in the room with you.

As of this writing, PET is used almost exclusively for examinations of the brain, and is considered to be more of a research than a clinical tool. However, it is highly probable that over time its use will be expanded to permit study of other body areas, and it will become more commonplace.

• *Probe:* This instrument, like a scanner, is capable of detecting gamma rays, but it is not capable of converting the energy into pictures. It records the amount of energy it "sees." Thus, it is used to measure the quantity of ionizing radiation emanating from a specific location. This data is then compared to normal expectations, and conclusions about function—normal, increased, decreased—are obtained. Probes can come in different sizes, but all are metallic and have a tube-like contour. The probe may be hand-held or attached to some type of suppport. When in use it is pointed at the site of interest. It rarely touches the part and therefore does not produce any discomfort.

Laboratory Procedures

Laboratory procedures identify that group of diagnostic studies that are performed to either measure or analyze some body fluid or TISSUE. These may be done on the body itself (in vivo), or on specimens taken from the body (in vitro). For example: How many red cells are in the blood? Is the thyroid gland functioning normally? Is there albumin (a type of protein) in the urine? (It doesn't belong there.) Most, but not all, of these determinations are made on specimens taken from your body, blood and urine being the most common. The procedure might be looking through a microscope. It might be placing a specialized detector over the body part of concern. It might be performing a complicated set of chemical manipulations. The technique chosen for the particular job is the one which will provide the greatest accuracy in the shortest time with the least inconvenience and discomfort to you.

Enter radioisotopes! ISOTOPES are useful and valuable not only in creating images but also in assessing certain bodily functions. These materials may be used, in certain situations, to "tag" onto bodily substances such as blood or urine, and then the signal that they emit can be "heard" by appropriate instruments and thus be measured. From these data normal and abnormal values can be established.

These are the nuts and bolts of the nuclear medicine experience. If a laboratory study is called for, the body part or body TISSUE or fluid of concern is analyzed by an appropriate technique. If an image is made—a scan—then the appropriate isotope for the body part of concern is administered in one of several ways and the picture is obtained by one of several types of imaging devices. In general, the procedures are all very similar from your standpoint. It hardly matters to you whether you are receiving technetium-99m or indium-111. Who really cares whether the scanning instrument is a conventional gamma camera, a SPECT, or a PET? What is of vital concern to you are: the possibility of discomfort, and how bad it might be; the fear that something will be done that could be embarrassing or dehumanizing; the degree of inconvenience to your schedule imposed by the time required; the hazards of a particular study; and lastly, the anxiety that there could be aftereffects, both immediate from the examination itself and/or delayed because of the dread radioactivity.

The news is good! Almost without exception (the few exceptions that "prove the rule" are carefully described) nuclear procedures can honestly claim little discomfort, no embarrassment, little inconvenience, little hazard, and no aftereffects!

For the particulars of each examination, start with the accompanying table. It divides the body into five general sections (plus a miscellaneous group for those procedures that do not easily fit into a single body area, such as infection). Within each major area are listed the specific body parts that are found there and, in some cases, different specific procedures that can be done on that particular part. Your doctor will identify the desired test by its specific name. For example, if your doctor said, "Go get a nuclear scan and uptake of your thyroid," you would refer to the table and find neck, the general category in which the thyroid gland is found. Next you would find both scan and RAI uptake under thyroid and read across the entire line of each. A quick synopsis of the pertinent data inherent in each study is listed. (These data are elaborated upon in the Appendix.) The last item on the line is the page number where the study is described in detail.

And finally, after you have read about the particular examination that you are preparing for, reread pages xiv through xvi, General Events Common to All Adult Diagnostic Procedures.

Head

Of all the structures found in the head, only the brain itself and several of the brain's component parts—the ventricular system (a group of CAVITIES that manufacture and circulate cerebrospinal fluid, a necessary fluid for both the brain and spinal cord) and the blood supply to different areas—lend themselves to nuclear investigation.

Brain Prior to the easy availability of CT (circa 1974) and magnetic resonance imaging or MRI (circa 1986) there was no NONINVASIVE technique to image the brain except for ISOTOPES. The "brain scan" was one of the hottest tickets in the nuclear medicine repertory. But, in truth, although it was far superior to the skull X-ray (which was the only possible alternative and all there was before isotope scanning), the information offered by the brain scan was limited. Thus, with the emergence of the magic of CT the hot ticket became yesterday's news. Well, no more! Thanks to the brilliance of the radiopharmacologist (one who is skilled in the science of both radioisotopes and drugs and is concerned with the research and development of new agents

Nuclear Medicine

Body Part/ Procedure	Discomfort* (−) to (++++)	Hazard* (−) to (+++)	Hospital (Incl. Short Procedure)	Special Prep.	Physi-cian	Extras*	Informed Consent*	Exam Time* (Hrs.)	Bottom Line* (−) to (++++)	Exam Description (Page)
Head										
Brain scan	(½+)	(−)	N	N	N	Y	N	3	(+)	237
Ventricular system	(+++)	(++)	Y	N	Y	Y	Y	24	(+++)	242
Regional cere-bral blood flow	(+)	(−)	N	N	N	Y	N	1	(+)	243
Neck										
Thyroid										
RAI uptake	(½+)	(−)	N	Y	Y	Y	N	24	(+)	245
RAI scan	(½+)	(−)	N	Y	N	Y	N	24	(+)	245
Tc-99m scan	(½+)	(−)	N	N	N	Y	N	½	(½+)	246
Hormone assay	(+)	(−)	N	N	N	Y/N	N	¼–¾	(+)	246
Parathyroids	(++)	(−)	N	N	Y	Y	N	1	(++)	246
Chest										
Chest cage	(+)	(−)	N	N	N	Y	N	4	(+)	247

Body Part/ Procedure	Discomfort* (-) to (++++)	Hazard* (-) to (+++)	Hospital (Incl. Short Procedure)	Special Prep.	Physician	Extras*	Informed Consent*	Exam Time* (Hrs.)	Bottom Line* (-) to (++++)	Exam Description (Page)
Heart										
Infarct	(½+)	(-)	N	N	N	Y	N	½	(+)	249
Stress	(++) to (+++)	(++)	N	Y	Y	Y	Y	4	(++) to (+++)	249
Wall motion	(++)	(-)	N	N	N	Y	N	2	(++)	250
Ejection fraction	(-)	(-)	N	N	N	Y	N	—	(-)	251
Blood vessels										
Circulatory integrity	(½+)	(-)	N	N	Y	Y	N	¼	(½+)	252
Venous infection	(+)	(-)	N	N	Y/N	Y	N	1–120	(+)	252
Blood										
Blood volume	(+)	(-)	N	N	N	Y	N	½	(+)	254
RIA	(+)	(-)	N	N	N	N	N	¼	(+)	255
Lungs										
Ventilation	(+)	(-)	N	N	N	Y	N	½	(+)	257
Perfusion	(½+)	(-)	N	N	N	N	N	½	(+)	257
Skeletal System										
Bone scan	(+)	(-)	N	N	N	Y	N	4	(+)	258
Bone density	(½+)	(-)	N	N	N	N	N	½	(½+)	258

Nuclear Medicine—cont'd

Body Part/ Procedure	Discomfort* (−) to (++++)	Hazard* (−) to (+++)	Hospital (Incl. Short Procedure)	Special Prep.	Physician	Extras*	Informed Consent*	Exam Time* (Hrs.)	Bottom Line* (+) to (++++)	Exam Description (Page)
Abdomen and Pelvis										
Gastrointestinal										
Stomach:										
Reflux	(+)	(−)	N	Y	N	Y	N	½	(+)	260
Emptying time	(+)	(−)	N	Y	N	Y	N	3	(+)	261
Small/large bowel:										
Schilling test	(½+)	(−)	N	N	Y	Y	N	24	(+)	262
Acute GI bleeding	(++)	(−)	N	N	N	Y	N	1–24	(++)	261
Gall bladder	(+)	(−)	N	Y	N	Y	N	1–4	(+)	263
Liver	(½+)	(−)	N	N	N	Y	N	½	(½+)	264
Spleen	(½+)	(−)	N	N	N	Y	N	½	(½+)	264

Body Part/ Procedure	Discomfort* (−) to (++++)	Hazard* (−) to (+++)	Hospital (Incl. Short Procedure)	Special Prep.	Physician	Extras*	Informed Consent*	Exam Time* (Hrs.)	Bottom Line* (−) to (++++)	Exam Description (Page)
Genitourinary										
Testicles	(½+)	(−)	N	N	N	Y	N	½	(+)	264
Kidneys	(½+)	(−)	N	N	N	Y	N	¾	(+)	265
Ureteric reflux	(++)	(+)	N	Y	Y	Y	N	½	(++)	266
Bladder emptying	(++)	(+)	N	Y	Y/N	Y	N	½	(++)	267
Lymph glands	(++)	(−)	N	N	Y	Y	N	4	(+++)	268
Miscellaneous										
Infections	(½+/+)	(−)	N	N	N	Y	N	24–72	(+)	269
Monoclonal antibodies	(½+)	(−)	N	N	Y	Y	N	?	(+)	270

* See Appendix, Table Details.

that can be used for diagnosis and treatment) and the engineers who design scanning equipment, the brain scan is back! Isotopes are now available that result in images that provide data not obtainable by any other diagnostic study. New equipment is available that permits utilization of certain of these isotopes—the PET and the SPECT scanners (see pages 234–35). Both the newer nuclides and the scanners have been tremendously helpful and are responsible for the recent and ongoing explosion of brain research. Areas of the brain can be "mapped," pinpointing what functions are performed where. Patterns are being discovered that permit the diagnosis of certain types of dementia (mental deterioration) such as Alzheimer's disease. The diagnosis of stroke (the rupture or obstruction of an artery in the brain) can be validated by images days sooner than with modalities such as CT. And that may be only the beginning. So, it is most appropriate to welcome the brain scan back and describe it.

The vast majority of all brain scans will be done by a gamma camera that has tomographic capabilities—the SPECT. Under very special circumstances the study will be obtained on a PET imager. The examination is essentially the same for each—only the equipment behaves differently. The study is divided into two parts: immediate and delayed.

Immediate: You are positioned on the scannning couch lying on your back. The couch is moved to a position that places the camera just above your head. The technologist (or, on occasion, the physician) will inject the isotope into a vein in your arm—(½ +) discomfort. The scanner will "see" the isotope as it is carried to your head and rapid sequential images are obtained. You will feel nothing. You will be asked only to keep your head still. Total elapsed time is three minutes. That's it for Part 1.

Delayed: One to two hours later additional images will be made. No additional isotope is needed. You are again positioned under the camera. Allot about half an hour. There is mild discomfort (½ +), no hazard, and no aftereffects.

Bottom Line: (+) Boring!

Ventricular System The system is composed of a specialized group of interconnected and communicating cavities (ventricles) within the brain that also communicate with the cavity of the spinal canal. These structures manufacture cerebrospinal fluid—the fluid that bathes the brain and cord. Any obstruction to the free flow of this fluid results in serious consequences to the normal function of the central NERVOUS SYSTEM (the brain and spinal cord). If such a problem is suspected, images of the ventricular system should be obtained.

This is a big-time examination. Fortunately CT and MRI have significantly reduced the need for this procedure. But it is occasionally still the study of choice. (The decision of whether or not to go this route should be made by either a neurologist or neurosurgeon—a specialist in diseases of the nervous system—rather than by your family physician or even the nuclear medicine specialist.) So, if it is warranted, here is how it is done: Since it requires that an isotope be placed in your spinal canal so that it will mix with the spinal fluid, a spinal tap must be performed. (This procedure is described in detail on page 204.) This is a $(+ + +)$ discomfort and a $(+ +)$ hazard.

When the needle is correctly positioned, the isotope will be injected. The needle will then be removed and you can get up. Actual imaging does not begin for one to two hours following the isotope instillation. It takes that long for it to move with the spinal fluid from the lower portion of your back up into your brain. Multiple pictures will be made with a gamma camera positioned against your head. The instrument will barely touch you so there is no discomfort. The necessary scans can be acquired in about 15 minutes. Images are again obtained two to four hours later and the next day. Therefore, you will remain in the hospital overnight.

You may experience delayed headaches for several days and some soreness where the needle was inserted, so you might try to take some sick time.

Bottom Line: $(+ + +)$ Whenever they tap your spine, it is a big-time event.

Regional Cerebral Blood Flow   Doctors now know that the blood supply to the brain (the cerebral blood flow) and to particular areas or regions of it is altered in certain vascular, neurologic, and psychiatric disorders. Identifying these regional changes in CIRCULATION is extremely helpful in the diagnosis of these problems. Techniques for detecting these changes have been developed utilizing an isotope known as xenon-133. This material is a gas that can be inhaled. The gas will travel to your lungs where it will enter the circulation. Thus the TRACER will be carried to the brain in the blood that supplies that ORGAN. Its distribution in the brain reflects the state of the blood supply to the particular area. This distribution can be evaluated by obtaining pictures or by obtaining measurements.

If imaging is used, you will be positioned under a gamma camera. Prior to either picture taking or measurements, however, the xenon must get to your brain. This is accomplished by your inhaling it. Sounds easy—yes? No. No, because if there is any xenon left over after you inhale, it would naturally be expelled on your breathing out. Since this gas must not enter the room air where others could inhale it, it must be captured and stored. Thus, you will be asked to breathe in a "closed system." (The details of xenon inhalation are described on page 257. The only difference is that in this study, the camera would be positioned to image your head.)

Immediately following the inhalation, imaging is begun. It is really no different from other scans of the brain. It probably is shorter in time although the inhalation procedure may be repeated several times. The whole thing requires about one hour. Expect neither discomfort nor hazard. When it's over, it's over—no side effects.

Bottom Line: (+) The mask may be a drag—the rest is plain dull.

Much of the same information regarding regional blood flow can be obtained without pictures. A different device is necessary. This one looks something like what could be found in a beauty parlor. It consists of many (32 is now the usual) thin metal cylinders—PROBES—which are detectors. They are meticulously positioned on each side of your head. You inhale the xenon as described above. Each detector records the activity it receives from the xenon as it moves through its particular region, for about 10 minutes. The information from each of the detectors is fed into a computer and the amount of blood flowing to each brain region is calculated. None of these maneuvers produces discomfort. There is no hazard. You can go home when all is over—after about an hour—and forget about the procedure because there will be no complaints to remind you of what happened.

Bottom Line: (+) Secod verse same as the first.

Neck

The particular structures found in the neck that lend themselves to investigation by nuclear techniques are the thyroid and parathyroid glands.

Thyroid Gland The thyroid is a GLAND located in the front of the neck. The hormones that it produces regulate your body's METABOLISM. Sometimes the thyroid's production is too bountiful, a condition that is called hyperthyroidism; sometimes the yield is too sparse, a condition known as hypothyroidism. In a condition sometimes called goiter, the thyroid becomes enlarged. Sometimes the thyroid makes lumps or bumps of abnormal cells, a condition called nodule formation. Information on your gland's function and images portraying its size and composition are essential when your symptoms suggest some problem. (See the listing of symptoms suggesting thyroid disesase on page 30.)

Both the measurement of function and the creation of an image are usually performed using a radioisotope of iodine. Stable iodine, which is found naturally in certain foods that we eat and may be added to others (such as table salt), is the substance that the thyroid extracts from the blood to convert to HORMONE. Your thyroid cannot discriminate the radioactive iodine from its stable cousin. Thus, substituting a radioactive isotope for the stable form results in the incorporation of the tracer into the gland.

There are several different ways in which the gland can be studied: RAI uptake and scan, Tc-99m scan, and hormone assay.

RAI Uptake and Scan R = radio; A = active; I = iodine; *uptake* = extraction rate ("extraction" is the term to identify the ability of a specific body part to remove a particular substance from the blood; rate is the amount removed in a given time); *scan* = picture.

For any given part of your body and any given substance, normal extraction rates are known. Measurement of uptake provides a reliable index of the health of the part. In this case the part to be measured is the thyroid, and the subtance extracted is iodine. A known amount of an isotope of iodine is given by mouth. After a period of time—usually 24 hours—the quantity removed by the thyroid can be easily calculated because the radioactivity of the isotope emits a signal that can be "heard" by an instrument called a PROBE. (A probe is like the Geiger counter used in all sci-fi flicks.) Another instrument, the gamma camera or scanner, can "see" the distribution of the isotope in the thyroid and take a picture of it—a scan.

The uptake and scan study require two days of your time.

Day One: After having had nothing by mouth after bedtime the night before, you will be seen by a doctor who will take a history of all your complaints as they refer to your thyroid. You will be asked about the medications you are taking now and may have used in the immediate past. You will also be asked whether you have had any recent X-rays in which "DYE" was used. These questions are to make sure that you have not taken or received anything that might interfere with the test, so bring a list of what you have taken or have had done in the last six months. Your neck will then be examined by gentle PALPATION. Then you will be given a tasteless liquid or one or two capsules to swallow, and instructed to refrain from eating or drinking for about two hours, after which you may resume your normal diet. Good-bye, until tomorrow.

Day Two: You will be taken into a room that has a probe and a gamma camera. You will be asked to sit or lie down so that the probe can be brought close to the front of your neck. The instrument will not touch you and will cause no discomfort. It is measuring the "uptake" of what your thyroid stored of the isotope you were given yesterday. This takes about five minutes. Then you will be asked to lie on a table on your back. The scanner will be positioned over your neck, but won't touch it; therefore, no discomfort. It is making a "picture" of your thyroid. Allow about 10 to 15 minutes.

Bottom Line: (+) Only the two visits are a chore.

Technetium (Tc-99m) Scan As discussed above under RAI uptake and scan, *scan* means "picture." In that case the picture was obtained 24 hours after your swallowing radioactive iodine and was part of a "two-fer" with the uptake. If your doctor wants you to have a scan only, this can be accomplished in one hour, thus saving you an extra day. A different isotope—technetium (Tc)—will be used. It is given by intravenous injection rather than by mouth. Scanning can commence in 20 minutes and you are out the door in less than one hour. The actual scanning experience is identical to that described for the RAI. There is no hazard. There is a (½ +) discomfort from the "stick" but you don't have to fast—and happy days, you don't have to come back tomorrow!

Bottom Line: (½ +) Fast and simple when it is the study for you.

Hormone Assay—T3, T4, TSH, TRH All of these abbreviations are for hormones that either are produced by the thyroid gland itself or regulate the thyroid's ability to function normally. For the record let's spell them out one time: T3 is triiodothyronine, T4 is tetraiodothyronine, TSH is thyroid stimulating hormone, and TRH is thyroid releasing hormone. The group is being lumped together because for our purpose of describing how a procedure affects you, the tests are all the same.

A sample of your blood will be drawn. That's it. So, it is a (½ +) discomfort for the "stick," a (−) for hazard, and about 10 minutes of your time. The only take-home is a Band-Aid.

Bottom Line: (+) "Ah say, 'Right on, Assay.' "

Parathyroids The parathyroids are organs located in the front of the neck, but behind the thyroid gland. Like the thyroid, they are glands. The particular hormone that the parathyroids produce regulates the body's calcium metabolism, which affects the SKELETAL SYSTEM. Abnormalities in parathyroid function cause widespread and diverse symptoms and problems. Hyperfunction often is first suspected because the sufferer experiences a sudden attack of acute pain found to be due to a kidney stone. The increase in circulating calcium has made that person a "stone former." The cause of this altered function may be benign tumors that are known as adenomas. Thus, when dysfunction of the parathyroids is suspected it is imperative to determine whether or not adenomas are the cause. If they are, surgical removal will correct the problem. Imaging techniques have recently been developed that are highly accurate not only in the detection of parathyroid tumors, but also in pinpointing their exact location.

No preparation is necessary. It all begins with the injection of an isotope (Tc-99m) into a vein, usually on the inside of your elbow. The needle will be taped onto your arm and left in the vein for later use. This will not bother you. Twenty minutes later you will be taken into the scanning room and asked to lie on your back. A pillow will be placed under your shoulders causing your head to fall back slightly. This stretches out the front of your neck. The gamma camera will be centered over your neck and as close to it as possible. You will be asked not to move. This is the most critical aspect of the entire study—keeping perfectly still. An image will be made. This requires only two to three minutes as a rule. While you remain in exactly the same position another injection, of a second isotope, thallium (Tl-201), will be made, using the needle that was left in so that a second "stick" won't be required. It is necessary to wait about five minutes—without moving—for this new material to localize. A second image is then made, also taking about three minutes. That's it. They will let you get up and you may leave. The exam takes about 30 to 45 minutes of your time, and has no hazard (−), but you'll experience some discomfort in your neck from holding still. No aftereffects.

Bottom Line: (+ +) The whole thing is a mild pain in the neck.

Chest

The chest extends from your neck to your abdomen—from that little notch under your Adam's apple to the bottom of your last rib. On the outside it is a kind of bony box called the chest cage. On the inside, protected by the box, are lots of good things like the heart, major blood vessels, blood, and the lungs. All of these can be studied.

Chest Cage The chest cage, or bony thorax, is formed by the ribs, breastbone (sternum), collarbones (clavicles), shoulder bones (scapulae), and a portion of the spine. These bones, like all of the other bones in the body, are subject to a variety of problems ranging from injury to infection and tumor. Usually these problems can be detected by conventional X-ray procedures.

But sometimes they cannot. When there is concern that SKELETAL PATHOLOGY is present and its cause is not revealed by X-ray, bone scanning is in order.

Note: Bone scanning is the same for all bones and therefore its description here is appropriatre not only for the chest cage but also for all other skeletal areas of the body.

As in all nuclear imaging procedures an appropriate ISOTOPE that will travel to the area or areas of interest must be introduced. In this case it is a bone-seeking nuclide that is injected into your vein. In some problem situations the part of concern is positioned under a gamma camera and the scanning is begun seconds after the injection. A series of rapid exposures is obtained in the next minute or two to show the appearance of blood to the examined area and how the part takes up the blood (phases 1 and 2). When the study is begun this way it is called a "three-phase" examination. Most examinations do not have this series. Most patients receive their injection without simultaneous imaging. Scanning is initiated two to four hours later. This later sequence (phase 3) is also performed on those who have had the early images as well. (On rare occasions, a 24-hour repeat of the four-hour adventure will be requested.) You can usually do anything you wish during the wait—leave and then return, grab a bite, whatever. Then it's into the scan room for pictures. Commonly, your entire body is imaged—both front and back. Occasionally, only the part of concern is imaged. The whole body requires about half an hour. After the initial injection there is no further discomfort. There is no hazard. Elapsed time from hello to good-bye is about four hours.

Bottom Line: (+) It's so boring you will be bone weary.

Heart Unlike some ORGANS that do not make the daily medical headlines and are therefore little known to the average reader—the spleen, the adrenal GLANDS, the seminal vesicles—the heart has no recognition problem. Besides its major function of symbolizing the greatest of our emotions, it also serves as the muscular pump that drives the body's CIRCULATION. "Pump failure," another term for heart disease, is the major cause of death in the U.S. Thus, examinations that pertain to the state of health of Big Red are of extreme value, particularly if they are accomplished easily, and especially if they identify disease *before* it has reached a stage at which no real correction is possible. Nuclear studies of the heart have these virtues. They can be performed with little discomfort or hazard and have a very high accuracy in both discovering early pathology and explaining advanced disease. These data are obtained both by imaging the heart wall and the heart's CAVITY, and by obtaining certain measurements of its function. Appropriate tests include infarct detection; an exercise stress test; wall motion; and ejection fraction.

Infarct Detection An INFARCT is an area of tissue destruction that is a consequence of a loss of the TISSUE's blood supply. In the heart wall, it occurs when a coronary artery (one of the blood vessels that supplies the heart wall) becomes OCCLUDED. It is the consequence of a heart attack. The severity of the attack is proportionate to the volume of affected wall. If it is massive then the victim will not survive. Immediate detection and appropriate management are often the difference in the ultimate outcome.

Fortunately, the vast majority of people who experience sudden and severe chest pain are not having a coronary occlusion. But which ones are? Which ones require immediate hospitalization and emergency treatment? There are techniques employing isotopic imaging that answer these questions quickly and with remarkable accuracy. The TRACER will depict the blood supply to the heart wall. If a vessel is occluded the picture will show the exact portion of the wall that is being deprived of blood. The level of correct detection is related to the time of the study after the onset of symptoms. If imaging can be performed within the first 12 to 24 hours after the onset of pain, a Yea: infarct—or a Nay: no infarct—can be offered with an accuracy in excess of 90 percent. The percentage falls the longer the delay, and after several days the test has questionable value.

How is the test done? An isotope—thallium-201—is injected into one of your veins. (In some situations another isotope might be used. This is the decision of the nuclear physician, but that is of little import here, since the procedure from your standpoint will be identical.) Five minutes later imaging is begun by positioning you under a gamma camera to image the left side of your chest. This takes about 10 minutes. Except for the injection ($\frac{1}{2}$ +) there is no other discomfort and no hazard (−). There may be a physician in attendance if you are acutely ill. If not, then you'll see only the technologist.

Bottom Line: (+) An important study achieved in a ho-hum style!

Exercise Stress Testing This is a procedure designed to detect in a NONINVASIVE manner the status of the coronary arteries in those individuals who are experiencing symptoms that might be due to artery diseease but have not as yet progressed to infarction, and in asymptomatic individuals who because of age, "lifestyle," or family history, or other conditions, are considered to be at risk for coronary artery disease. In both groups, a normal study will show that the blood supply to all portions of the heart wall is preserved and adequate and offers high confidence that there is no vessel pathology. When, however, the findings suggest disease, further investigation by ANGIOGRAPHY (see pages 194–200) is essential.

The rationale for, preparation for, and performance of this procedure are described in detail in Chapter 2 under Electrocardiogram—Exercise. There are two additions to that saga when the isotope (thallium-201) is included. First, at the time of the initial preparation, after you have been "wired," a small, thin, plastic tube will be inserted into a vein on the inside of your elbow or on the back of your hand, to which a syringe containing the thallium is attached. Second, when the cardiologist decides that you have exercised enough, the isotope will be injected. You will be moved to the scanning table, placed on your back under the gamma camera, and your heart will be imaged. It will take 20 to 30 minutes to complete the pictures. If a SPECT system (see page 234) is utilized you must remain motionless during the picture taking. With some cameras these images require that you get your arms up above your head so that the machine can get close to your chest. This doesn't seem like much the first few minutes, but by the tenth or fifteenth, or twentieth, it may really become a test of endurance. Forewarning is the best preparation. For some it may be minimal, but for others it can be a "bullet biter" (+) to (+ + +). That completes Part 1.

Part 2: You will be permitted to relax for the next three hours, after which your heart will again be imaged. This is identical to the picture taking of Part 1: You are on the table on your back with your arms up above your head. 20 to 30 minutes. The end.

Bottom Line: (+ +) to (+ + +) At some point you'll ask them to have a heart.

Wall Motion The heart is a remarkably efficient pump that drives the blood round a mighty loop—your body. This pumping action can be likened to the action of a bellows, but instead of filling and then expressing air, the heart fills with and expresses blood. Filling is accomplished by the relaxation of the heart walls as blood enters the heart's chambers (atria and ventricles). The expression is obtained by the muscular walls contracting and forcing the blood out. This relaxation and contraction is known as wall motion. The amount of blood actually expressed with each contraction (the heartbeat) is called its ejection fraction.

Evaluation of both the wall motion and the ejection fraction are of tremendous value in diagnosing particular cardiac pathologies. These data can be obtained in several ways: ventriculography (see pages 194–200), echocardiography (see pages 279–82), and nuclear imaging (see below). The decision of which to use resides in the able hands of your personal physician. Here's a description of the nuclear procedure. Let's go to the drawing board.

There is no required preparation. Two intravenous injections are made. The first is a nonradioactive PHARMACEUTICAL which acts to sensitize the surface of the red cells (erythrocytes), which are a major component of blood. ("Sensitize" is a simple term to explain a complex set of reactions that permit the surface of each red cell to accept a rider, the isotope.) Fifteen to 20 minutes later the nuclide is injected. It attaches itself to the erythrocytes in a process known as red cell or blood pool tagging; it is effective for about 12 hours. Once the "tagging" of the cells has occurred the rest is a snap. You are positioned under the gamma camera. The heart's blood pool is imaged in several views, each requiring about 10 minutes. No pain, no fuss. The obtained pictures are then computer-analyzed. They can be played back like a movie so that the actual movement of each portion of the heart wall can be examined. Alternatively, the computer can draw lines around the chamber when it is most distended (diastole) and when it is most contracted (systole). These lines should appear as two concentric circles (one centered within the other). If any portion of the wall fails to contract properly the outlines will reflect this variation. This test rates a discomfort index of (+) for the injections and a (−) for hazard, and takes one to two hours (Injection #1 plus Injection #2 plus pictures).

Bottom Line: (+ +) It beats catheters in your heart every time!

Ejection Fraction *Ejection* (the act of driving or throwing out) refers to the blood that leaves a chamber of the heart when that chamber contracts. *Fraction* refers to the percentage of the amount of blood that has been ejected as compared to the amount before the contraction. This is one of several measurements that are most helpful in determining "pump function."

The ejection fraction can be arrived at by using the data obtained in the wall motion study described above. The images that were obtained are now subjected to further computer wizardry. The volume of blood in a heart chamber (any or all chambers could be analyzed, but in practice it is always the left ventricle) is easily measured when it is most dilated with blood and again when it is most contracted. The difference between these volumes represents the percentage of ejection, or the ejection fraction. Since this measurement is really a "two-fer" with wall motion it adds no (+) or (−) to the above index.

Bottom Line: (−) Sometimes there is a "free lunch."

Blood Vessels Blood vessels come in two major flavors: arteries and veins. (A detailed discussion of these structures and their role in the circulatory system can be found on pages 194–200.) In most clinical problems of either, the examination is by X-ray, employing CONTRAST MEDIA ("DYE"). Those studies, particularly arterial imaging, are usually both painful and hazardous and may require hours to perform. In some diagnostic dilemmas visualization of either group of vessels by isotope techniques will be acceptable. When this is the case the studies are neither painful nor hazardous and often require no more than seconds to be accomplished. The decision of which way to go usually hinges on the necessity of anatomic detail. Nuclear images cannot compete with the quality obtained by X-rays. But some answers can be obtained driving a VW and leaving the Mercedes in the garage. When this is the case—hallelujah! Nuclear techniques lend themselves to the evaluation of circulatory integrity and the detection of thrombophlebitis.

Circulatory Integrity Testing for circulatory integrity is really only a fancy way of asking "Are the pipes open or is the plumbing in trouble?"

Here's how it's done: You are positioned under a gamma camera which is positioned over the suspected area of obstruction. The isotope is injected into the closest accessible vein—that is, the one closest to the part of concern. (In some special problems where the obstruction might be in the middle of the body the injection may be made from each side at the same time—thus two sticks rather than one.) Picture taking commences when the monitor shows the isotope reaching the target. (If you like that kind of thing, ask that the monitor—a small TV—be positioned so that you can watch too.) These images are rapid and sequential—they're taken about one to three seconds apart for perhaps 30 to 45 seconds.

That's it! It rates a (½ +) for discomfort for one injection, a (+) if you require two. Hazard is (−). Total time if a coffee break is thrown in may equal five minutes.

Bottom Line: (½ +) Talk about "nuthin'."

Venous Infection Infection in the veins is not an uncommon event. It is most frequently encountered where there has been previous vessel injury from any of a host of causes, and infection or inflammation is superimposed on the part (we are not talking about drug abusers here, among whom dirty needles are the most common cause). The inflammation affects the walls of the vein and often causes the blood moving against its inside surface to become attached and form a clot or THROMBUS. This combination of inflammation and clot formation is called *thrombophlebitis* and is a most serious problem. (See discussion of pulmonary embolus on pages 256–58.)

X-ray examination with the injection of contrast material ("dye") is the usual method of investigating this condition (and is described on pages 199–200). However, when this approach is inappropriate for any of several reasons —such as "dye" sensitivity or excessive swelling of the legs—similar images of the veins can be obtained by nuclear imaging.

Nonimaging (uptake measuring) techniques are also available that can identify areas within veins that are undergoing thrombus formation. The clot requires for its formation, among other things, a component known as fibrinogen, which is carried in the blood by small cells called platelets. It is possible to put a radioactive tag on fibrinogen. This tracer will seek out a forming clot and become part of it. This will result in a focally increased concentration of this material, which can be detected by an instrument called a probe.

Two methods of imaging exist. In one, the tracer is injected into a vein of one of your feet and pictures are taken as the material moves with your blood up your leg and into your pelvis. This is a (+) for the injection discomfort and a (−) for the hazard, and it takes about 15 minutes.

In the other, red cell "tagging" is performed. (See page 251.) You are asked to lie flat on the imaging couch while your legs are imaged with the gamma camera. The discomfort is (+) from the injections. There is no hazard, and it takes only an hour of your time.

Note: The pictures obtained in the second method are considered by many to be superior and of higher diagnostic quality than those of the first method, which is why this technique is becoming more popular. Its only "downside" is it requires two sticks and a longer wait. (But for every downside there may be a silver lining. The two-injection approach chooses the two easiest veins around. The one-sticker is in a foot vein, often difficult to get into, and often painful.)

Bottom Line: Both methods (+) Easy.

For the nonimaging technique, you will be asked to lie on an examining table after removing everything from your waist down and putting on a gown. The nuclear physician and technologist will trace with a marking pen the anticipated course that the major veins that drain your ankles, calves, knees, and thighs take to get to your groin. This will be a slightly curvy but basically straight line. They will paint this line on both the front and back of your leg. Then they will make a mark—frequently a number—at about every two inches along the line. This tattoo-job takes about five minutes to perform and should cause you no problem unless the marking part near your groin causes some embarrassment. A (+) at most. Then the isotope is injected into a vein in your arm. Expect (½ +) discomfort for the stick. Then you have a three-hour wait—bring a book or a pal to talk to. The delay is to permit the tracer to circulate and incorporate in any site of clot formation.

Then you head back into the examining room and get up on a table. The technologist will place the probe (it will look like a flashlight attached by a wire to a small hand-held box) against each of the marks that were previously painted on. Except for the first placement, which could be chilly, you will feel nothing but the mild pressure of the instrument on your skin. The probe measures the activity under each mark, which takes about one minute each. (The point of the whole thing is to see if there is a spot or perhaps even a group of spots that show a definitely higher count rate [the measurement] than the others next to them or than the same spots on the opposite leg. If so, then a clot is forming and treatment is begun.) Each leg, front and back, may take half an hour. The worst it can be is boring—the best is fun because it is a new experience. Once both sides are monitored and recorded the measurements are finished for that time. The kicker is that they will be repeated daily—exactly the same way each time—for several days. If the results become obviously positive even after the first day's measurement the study will end, but it is more common that it will continue for as long as five days. As a rule this procedure is done on a hospitalized patient so the daily visit is not as much of a drag as if you had to travel back and forth to the hospital. But, except for the length of the study, it's a laugher. The painted numbers wash off eventually, perhaps in one to two weeks.

Bottom Line: (+) The numbers, particularly at the beach, can become a real conversation piece.

Blood Volume Although blood is found throughout the body, the largest collection is in the heart. Therefore I have chosen this section to describe procedures that apply to blood in general. These are measurements of its total volume and of certain substances that are found in it.

Just about everyone knows that the blood is made up of cells—red and white, and some liquid stuff. Just about everyone at some time has had a blood count. And that's just about all everyone knows. Well, there are times that it is important to know just how much blood you have—your blood volume. For example, this may be important before contemplated surgery where significant blood loss might be expected. It helps to predict how the procedure will be tolerated and even if blood should be given before. Another situation in which this data may be of use is after that same surgery to help in correctly restoring the true loss. These measurements are accurately obtained by nuclear techniques.

The principles that underlie the procedure are simple and might be best understood by a simple analogy: Let's say you have a bottle of ink that is dark blue. The ink is poured into a tub of water. The water turns blue, but its hue is paler than the original ink. The ink has become diluted. The dilution is a function of how full the tub was, which in turn affects the final color. Less water—bluer, more water—paler.

The same principle is employed to determine blood volume but with minor variations: isotope is substituted for ink; you are substituted for the bathtub.

A known concentration of an isotope is placed in a known volume of water. A sample of this mixture (the "ink") is taken and counted. The two values are compared and a dilution ratio is calculated. A second sample of the mixture, identical in volume to the first, is then injected intravenously into you. After an appropriate time for circulation to occur—10 to 15 minutes—a sample of your blood of the same volume as what was injected is drawn and measured. The new measurement, which will be much lower than that of the injected sample, represents the dilution that has occurred in your blood pool ("the bathtub"). This value is compared by appropriate formulas to the earlier calculated dilution ratio and the answer is your blood volume.

Two sticks equal a (+) discomfort; there is no hazard. Total time for you is half an hour. (The counting and figuring is done long after you are gone.) One or two Band-Aids for your trouble.

Bottom Line (+) For those who enjoy the gruesome and macabre, the first recorded blood volume in medical lore was obtained by decapitating a convict who had just been executed, hanging him upside down, catching his blood in a bucket, and then measuring the volume of blood in the bucket. Given a choice he might have chosen the nuclear technique.

RIA *R* is for radio; *I* is for immuno; *A* is for assay. The term describes a method of directly measuring minute quantities of certain substances that circulate in the blood or might be found in the urine. The techniques employ antibodies that are tagged with an isotope. Although this procedure represented a monumental breakthrough in certain technologies and opened new ways of thinking about how to solve particular problems, it will appear no different than any other blood or urine test. It is beyond the scope of this primer to detail what goes on in the laboratory once the specimen arrives for analysis. Occasionally, however, you are told that an RIA is being done and for that reason this category of examination is mentioned.

Bottom Line: (+) From your standpoint—a blood test is a blood test is a blood test.

Lungs For those few who may not be up on things anatomic, the lungs are paired organs that live on either side of your chest. They are composed of trillions of tiny air sacs (alveoli). There are also tubes (bronchi) that bring air to these sacs when we inhale and return air to the outside world when we exhale, and blood vessels that "pick up" oxygen from the new air in each alveolus and deposit carbon dioxide back into the sac to be expelled with the next exhalation. So much for basics.

If there had ever been a mighty theoretical plan to build a body part that could best be examined by the common X-ray, the architect would have come up with a lung. And, indeed, X-rays are remarkably sensitive to abnormalities that are common to this organ. But there is always that exception that proves the rule, and in this case it is pulmonary embolus. ("Pulmonary" is a term that refers to the lungs; EMBOLUS is the blockage or occlusion of a vessel.) This problem is considered to be the most frequent ACUTE lung complication that befalls patients in hospitals, and ironically, it is almost never detected or identified in its early stages by routine X-ray examination. Since pulmonary embolus may be a life-threatening event, early detection and treatment is essential. It is most commonly caused by a blood clot, but may also be due to fat, or infected material, or even air that may be floating in the bloodstream. But let us just consider the blood clot and how it got into the stream of things. It originates, most commonly, in veins in the upper legs or pelvis, and in any of these locations, it is called a thrombus. It is usually the consequence of poor circulation or infection within the vessel. The clot forms and becomes attached to the inside wall of the vein. If for any reason the thrombus should break off, it begins to float and will travel with the blood until it reaches some other vessel whose diameter is too small to permit its continued transit. The vessel is thus occluded or embolized. All of the tissues supplied by this particular vessel beyond the point of occlusion will die if the circulation is not reinstituted. This eventuality is known as infarction. The reason the lung is the most common site for these events is because in the clot's travel from the leg vein, the vessels in the lung are the first it will encounter of a diameter too small for its continued passage. The early detection of the embolism and the initiation of treatment is often essential to life.

Enter again the mighty theoretical architect—the ultimate plan to detect these episodes came off the drawing board as the lung scan. It is a procedure best performed in two parts, called ventilation and perfusion. The study is remarkably accurate in its detection of embolization, and, joy of joys, it can be accomplished without discomfort or hazard.

Ventilation This portion of the study depicts the distribution of air that is taken in with a deep breath. When your air tubes (bronchi) are open (as they should be—both normally and in this condition, since emboli initially affect only the blood vessels), the air you inhale should be distributed throughout all portions of each of your lungs. If this is not the case then the problem may be something other than embolization, such as pneumonia or even a tumor.

No preparation is necessary for imaging. You will remove everything from the waist up and don a gown. Next, you will take a short study course from the technologist on how to breathe freely and comfortably with a mask over your nose and mouth, since it will be necessary, when you are ready, to wear this mask throughout the examination. This requirement stems from the need for you to inhale an isotope called xenon that is in gaseous form. The mask ensures that it will get into you and also that it will not get into the room air. The mask, which is plastic, is connected to a tube which in turn is connected to a machine that regulates the movement of the air that you breathe. The technologist will apply the mask to your face and you will practice breathing with it on. Take as long as you need to feel comfortable that you are getting all the air that you want. When you are comfortable with the mask in place, and are satisfied that you can breathe quite normally, you will be asked to sit in front of the gamma camera, and told, "Take in a deep breath, and hold it!" After about 15 seconds, you'll be told "Let it out, and breathe normally." At the moment of command 1, the technologist will introduce the xenon (sometimes another isotope is used but from your standpoint there will be no difference) into the tube that you are getting your air from, and the air with the isotope will be swept into your lungs. The camera will be activated and images will be obtained. Since the isotope has neither smell nor taste you will be completely unaware of its presence. There is discomfort (+) only from the mask. There is no hazard. The procedure requires about 10 to 15 minutes. Although not mandatory, most of these examinations are performed on hospitalized patients since the problem is usually one that is a complication of some preceding hospital event.

Bottom Line: (+) It's like a scuba dive on land.

Perfusion "Perfusion" is the term that describes the distribution of blood to a part. This portion of the study images the blood flow pattern in each of your lungs. If there has been an occlusion from an embolus there will be no blood delivered beyond the point of obstruction and the image will reveal this abnormality.

This portion of the examination usually follows the ventilation imaging described above. You are still sitting (occasionally lying) in front of the gan.ma camera. The mask will be taken away. The technologist will now give you an injection into a vein in your arm, which rates a (½ +) discomfort. Imaging will begin immediately and take about half an hour. You will be asked to change your position with each new picture—perhaps six to eight views will be obtained. Except for the discomfort of the injection there is no other grief. There is no hazard. Again, most people undergoing these studies are quite ill and therefore anything that is done to them is interpreted as an additional burden. But this burden must be borne since it provides the critical answer about a potentially life-threatening event.

Bottom Line: (+) Viva la lung scan!

Skeletal System

The SKELETAL SYSTEM means bones. It is composed of the skull, spine, pelvis, chest cage, upper extremities (arms), and lower extremities (legs).

The multitude of problems that may affect any of these structures— injury, infection, tumor, arthritis, and the one that is rapidly becoming Number 1 on the charts, osteoporosis—are all problems of bone. Typically, any complaint about these structures is studied first by some X-ray procedure. But often these examinations are found to be normal, and yet the symptoms persist. In these situations it is common to study further. Nuclear medicine provides two procedures to assist in the search: The bone scan and the bone density determinations. These studies are often more sensitive than the X-ray in confirming a true problem. As an example, a bone scan may identify tumor spread to bone months before this problem would be "X-ray-positive." Bone densitometry can confirm the existence of osteoporosis well before it is evident on X-rays. So, when there are unexplained complaints and all else has failed, a visit to your friendly nuclear medicine physician may be ordered.

Bone Scan All bone scans are performed in exactly the same way regardless of which bony part is of interest. The description of this procedure can be found earlier in this chapter under Chest (see pages 247–48.)

Bone Density Osteoporosis (*osteo* means "bone" and *porosis* refers to a loss of compactness; together they signify a decrease in the density of bone) has in the past few years become a household word. It has been recognized as a major cause of fractures in the elderly, particularly in women. It is a result of the changes that aging creates in how the body utilizes certain minerals—notably calcium—that are essential to skeletal strength. It is important to recognize the existence of this problem so that appropriate dietary and other corrective measures can be initiated before the process progresses to the stage of causing permanent debility. Nuclear techniques provide a splendid means for this detection.

The procedure to evaluate bone density goes by the tooth-rattling name of absorptiometry. All that that means is that if an energy source is passed through bone and then is captured and measured as it exits, the density of the part can be identified. If the bone is dense, less of the beam will get through to be captured. If the bone is porous, more. Thus a machine has been created that consists of a table with an L-shaped arm above it and a detector below it. The arm above contains a radioactive isotope that emits energy—like a beam of X-ray—that is neither seen nor felt. This arm is motor-driven so that it can move the length of your body. The detector, below the table, moves together with the arm, and is coupled to a computer. Thus you lie on the table and the isotope source passes back and forth above your lower spinal, pelvic, and hip regions. The entire study requires about half an hour. Except for keeping still on the table (½ +) it is without discomfort—it doesn't even have the usual ouch of the injection that initiates most nuclear studies—and there are no memories afterward.

Note: There are some nuclear physicians who may examine only your wrist. The procedure is otherwise identical with the above.

Bottom Line: (½ +) Talk about easy!

Abdomen and Pelvis

The abdomen and pelvis resemble the inner city with respect to high population density and congestion. There are seventeen specific ORGANS that reside in the space from the bottom of your breastbone to that hard little bone —the pubis—that lies just below your bladder. Many, as is common in such environments, join into gangs and call themselves by special names (such as "gastrointestinal tract" and "reproductive system"), while others are loners (such as the spleen and the adrenals). Therefore, it is best to study these various segments of the population individually.

Diagnostic procedures for the abdomen and pelvis concentrate on the gastrointestinal tract, the gall bladder, the liver and spleen, the genitourinary tract, and the lymphatic system.

Gastrointestinal Tract The DIGESTIVE SYSTEM is that group of organs that has to do with the intake of food, its absorption for use by your body, and the elimination of anything that is not processed. In essence, it is a continuous tube from the mouth to the anus composed of specialized sections where particular functions are performed. The gastrointestinal (GI) tract is that portion of the system that is within the abdomen. For the most part, conventional and special X-ray examinations are most effective in identifying any problems that may exist. However, certain specific difficulties may be better diagnosed by nuclear studies.

Gastroesophageal Reflux *Gastro* refers to the stomach. *Esophageal* refers to the esophagus, which is that portion of the digestive tract that lies in the chest—behind the heart—and connects the mouth and neck portions to the stomach. "REFLUX" is the term that describes the abnormal backward flow of liquid materials—vomiting is a form of reflux. Put all these things together and they spell "heartburn." Although the description of this misery varies from sufferer to sufferer, all agree that it is a most uncomfortable sensation that is located in the middle of the chest and that occurs after eating or at night, often awakening you from sleep. These symptoms are a result of liquid materials in the stomach being misdirected. Instead of being propelled forward, some amount moves backward into the esophagus. If the volume of liquid is large enough it may reach the mouth, but usually it only gets to the lower portion of the esophagus. Its presence sets up a reaction that we interpret as "burning." For proper diagnosis and treatment it is important to establish that reflux exists.

Imaging is used for this purpose. You must have nothing by mouth after bedtime the night before the exam. Before the examination begins a small balloon is placed over your stomach. It is held in place by a special inflatable belt, which is exactly like a blood pressure cuff but large enough to wrap around your abdomen. You are then asked to stand in front of a gamma camera and to drink a glass of orange juice to which a tasteless ISOTOPE has been added. Pictures are taken as the fluid moves from your mouth to your stomach. Then you are placed on your back on a table under the camera and the cuff is gradually inflated, applying pressure on the balloon which applies pressure on your stomach. While the cuff inflates, pictures are being taken to see if this pressure forces the juice in your stomach back into your esophagus.

If all is well, reflux should not occur. The entire procedure requires about half an hour. There may be discomfort (+) from the pressure, but there is no hazard.

Bottom Line: (+) Tough if you prefer tomato juice in the morning.

Gastric Emptying Time Certain GI complaints arise from some alteration in the normal time that is required for the stomach to perform its digestive function and then move its contents—both liquid and solid—along the tract. This transit is known as emptying time and it can be measured with relative ease.

Imaging is again used. Fasting for 8 to 12 hours before the examination is essential. You are given a sparse breakfast of juice, to which a tasteless isotope has been added, and some scrambled eggs, to which a different tasteless isotope has also been added. When the meal is over you are positioned on a table so that a gamma camera is over your upper abdomen. The camera can be adjusted so that it will "see" and take pictures of only the liquid isotope, and then readjusted to "see" only the solid isotope (the one that was added to the eggs) so that each can be measured individually. Pictures and measurements are taken at timed intervals. (Remember that an isotope emits a signal that is captured by the camera, which can translate it into either a picture or a number—or both. When your stomach is first filled the number of signals received is at its maximum. As your stomach empties the count rate lessens.) Thus a record is obtained: how long it takes your stomach to become completely free of counts, or empty, both of isotope A in the juice and isotope B in the eggs.

There is neither discomfort nor hazard. Study time averages almost three hours. No delayed complaints.

Bottom Line: (+) Ask for an after-breakfast mint on your way out.

Acute GI Bleeding ACUTE—meaning severe and going on right now—bleeding within the gastrointestinal tract is a common problem that arises from different causes—the most frequent being diverticuli (abnormal "outpocketings" or sacs that arise from hollow organs such as the colon), ulcers, and tumors. The bleeding may arise from any section of the tract. If it is severe it can be life-threatening and requires immediate attention—often surgical. However, the problem is characterized by a "start and stop" pattern. The sudden onset may be followed by a sudden cessation. Thus when bleeding is suspected two questions must be quickly and accurately addressed: First, is there bleeding now?; and second, where is the origin of the bleeding? Nuclear imaging is usually the first procedure invoked when these questions need answering.

There are two different approaches to investigate this problem. The whys and wherefores of which to use is a decision made by the nuclear physician after he or she reviews the given problem. From your standpoint the difference is either one injection or two. The one-stick method introduces the isotope into a vein and pictures are obtained over your abdomen at regular intervals—5 to 10 minutes apart—for approximately one hour, employing a gamma camera. The two-stick technique employs a blood cell labeling approach (see the description of this procedure on pages 250–51.) The only advantage of this method is that imaging through a longer interval—perhaps through 24 hours—is possible. The procedure is the same as in the one-stick —you are positioned on your back on a table under a gamma camera. Each picture requires about one minute to acquire, and they are taken at 5- to 10-minute intervals through one hour. If bleeding is seen, the study will be concluded. If the first series does not identify the problem, the whole thing may be repeated at various intervals throughout the remainder of the day, or even the next day. (If you are a candidate for this examination there is high probability that you will be a hospital patient, so the multiple series over time will not be too difficult since you will be returned to your room after each one.)

Discomfort rates a ($\frac{1}{2}$ +) for the one-stick approach, (+) for the other. No hazard, and no aftereffects.

Bottom Line: (+ +) Long and tiresome.

Schilling Test

Note: Try as one might to end the practice, there are still names used in medicine that honor a person—usually the creator or discoverer of something—rather than identify the examination by a more appropriate or descriptive title. The Schilling Test is such a dinosaur. It is named for Victor Schilling, the German hematologist (a specialist in diseases of the blood).

The Schilling test is a specific procedure capable of diagnosing pernicious anemia. *Pernicious* means "highly injurious or destructive." *Anemia* describes a deficiency in the number of red blood cells. Pernicious anemia is a blood disorder caused by an absence of a particular substance in the stomach known as intrinsic factor. This factor acts to facilitate the absorption of a B vitamin (vitamin B_{12}) essential to the normal development of the red blood cell. The presence or absence of this substance can be determined by the Schilling test.

For this technique, you are asked to swallow a capsule containing vitamin B_{12} to which an isotope has been added. One hour later an injection of B_{12} without isotope is given into one of your muscles, usually one in an upper arm. You are requested to collect *all* urine for the next 24 hours. The urine is then measured for the amount of the isotope that has been eliminated. If the quantity is within normal expectations the examination is over. If, however, the volume is abnormal, the study is taken to Part 2. The second procedure is exactly the same as the first except that in addition to the B_{12}-isotope capsule another capsule is also given. This capsule contains intrinsic factor. Urine is again collected for 24 hours and counted. If the original deficiency is corrected the explanation can be attributed to an absence of the factor, and a diagnosis of pernicious anemia (PA) is established. If, on the other hand, the addition of the factor in Part 2 did nothing to the urinary findings then the cause for the abnormality must be sought elsewhere. The total time for the examination (this does not include the urine collection) is about one hour. Except for the injection ($\frac{1}{2}$+) there is no discomfort, and there is no hazard. The only drag is toting those collection bottles.

Bottom Line: (+) Doesn't everyone carry gallon jugs of that yellow stuff around?

Gall Bladder The gall bladder is that component of the digestive system that concerns itself with fat digestion. It receives, stores, and concentrates a liquid made in the liver—bile. When you eat fatty foods it is the gall bladder's responsibility to send the bile into your intestine to aid in digestion.

Stones (calculi) are relatively common inhabitants of the gall bladder but they may live there for long periods without requiring more radical attention than careful dietary regulation. However, they may enter the neck of the gall bladder and completely block the exit of bile. This condition is followed by infection and is known as acute cholecystitis (again, *acute* means "active right now"; *cholecystitis* is an inflammation of the gall bladder and its ducts). This condition is often a surgical emergency. Although it can be diagnosed by conventional X-rays and ultrasound, the nuclear investigation is considered to be the most specific method of approach.

Fasting for at least four hours prior to the examination is desired. An intravenous injection of the appropriate isotope is the beginning of the imaging process. You are positioned on your back under the gamma camera. Pictures, each taking 1 minute to acquire, are made every 5 to 10 minutes for a half-hour and then every 15 minutes through the next one and a half hours. By the end of two hours a diagnosis of an acute problem is usually possible. If, for any reason, more images are deemed necesssary, they will be obtained in the same manner. The examination itself is most simple, but you are having it done because you are sick and hurting. Under these conditions anything that delays relief is viewed as *bad*. Come back another time and you will agree it is a snap. For now, rate it as a ($\frac{1}{2}$ +) discomfort for the injection and (−) hazard. You'll spend about two hours on the table.

Bottom Line: (+) If only we could be studied when we were well.

Liver and Spleen Nuclear studies examine the liver and spleen at the same time.

The liver is the largest solid organ in the body and perhaps the most complex. It performs multiple functions and is therefore a landlord of multiple systems. It is located in the upper right corner of your abdomen, tucked up under your lower ribs.

The spleen is another solid organ but not nearly as complex in its functions when compared to the liver. It concerns itself with matters of the blood —both the red and white cells. It lives tucked under your ribs in your upper left abdomen—to the left of and slightly behind your stomach.

The imaging process begins with one intravenous injection. Then, one 10-minute delay followed by three or four pictures acquired under the gamma camera over a 10-minute period. *That's it.* Total time one-half hour. Discomfort equals ($\frac{1}{2}$ +) for the injection. Hazard is (−). Take-home memory is a Band-Aid over the injection site.

Bottom Line: ($\frac{1}{2}$ +) Boring.

Genitourinary Tract Particular functions of the body are performed by groups of organs identified by the unique purpose they serve. The designation "genitourinary" combines two groups: those concerned with reproduction— genito—and those concerned with the elimination of bodily wastes through the urine—urinary. The genital system in women is composed of the ovaries, fallopian tubes, uterus (womb), and vagina. In men it is composed of the testicles, seminal ducts, prostate gland, and penis. The urinary system is the same for women and men: kidneys, ureters, bladder, and urethra. (The ureters are the tubes that carry urine, which is made in your kidneys, to your bladder. The urethra is the tube that carries urine from your bladder to the outside.) Not all of the component parts lend themselves to nuclear examinations. Only those that do and their studies are noted here.

Testicles The testicles are responsible for the production of sperm. There are two acute conditions that can affect them that may be clinically confusing—torsion and epididymitis. Torsion is another word for "twisting," and in medicine refers to problems such as a sudden rotation of the stalk of the testicles that reduces or even cuts off the blood supply. Epididymitis is an inflammation of a group of very specialized tubes that are located on the back of the testicles. The treatment for each condition is significantly different and thus an immediate diagnosis is urgent. These two entities can be readily separated from one another by nuclear imaging.

You will be asked to remove everything from the waist down (not including your socks and shoes) and to put on a gown that opens in the front. Then you will be positioned on an imaging table on your back, with your legs spread apart. The technologist or physician will apply wide strips of adhesive tape across the front of your thighs at the level of your scrotum (the sac that contains the testicles). This is called a "bridge." The scrotal sac is gently placed on this "little table" so that the testicles will lie side by side and thus each can be identified. The gamma camera is then brought down as close to the part as possible. When this has been accomplished—a matter of minutes —an injection of isotope is made in an arm vein. The TRACER will travel in the blood to those vessels that supply the testicles. Its arrival can be seen by a monitor—ask to watch if you think you'll find it interesting—and imaging is started. Pictures will be made through the next 10 to 15 minutes. All you need do is lie still. Discomfort rates a ($\frac{1}{2}$ +), hazard (−); the elapsed time is one-half hour. Depending on the findings you will either go home with medication or be admitted to the hospital for treatment.

Bottom Line: (+) Nothing to get into an uproar about.

Kidneys The kidneys are paired organs, each lying on either side of your spine, just behind and below your liver on the right, and just behind and below your stomach on the left. One of their major responsibilities is the awesome task of extracting certain waste materials that circulate in the blood, converting these wastes into a liquid called urine, and seeing to it that the stuff is eliminated from the body.

The conventional approach to the diagnosis of kidney problems is by X-ray, but as has been described in detail in Chapter 18, these examinations require the use of iodinated CONTRAST AGENTS. These materials ("DYE") impose mild to serious problems for some recipients and are absolutely contraindicated in others, such as those with advanced diabetes or those with certain kidney problems. Ultrasound, another excellent technique to examine the kidneys (see Chapter 20), does not require the use of "dye," but is limited in the scope of the information it can provide. Nuclear medicine studies provide images of structure and concepts of function not obtainable with ultrasound. These images lack the detail that can be obtained by X-rays, but—and a big but it is—*no* contrast material is required. Therefore, in many clinical settings, nuclear medicine becomes the method of choice. Although different problems require the use of different isotopes your experience will be the same regardless of what is used. Thus, one description fits all.

For imaging, you are positioned on a table lying on your back. The gamma camera is under the table at the level of your kidneys. One of your arms will be bared and a tourniquet—commonly a blood pressure cuff—will be applied above your elbow. The cuff will be inflated to a point of mild discomfort. A vein will be selected and the area cleansed with an antiseptic gauze. The technologist or physician will inject the isotope into your vein and the cuff will be snapped off. This maneuver permits the isotope solution to retain its concentration as it is propelled forward in the bloodstream. When the tracer reaches the major arteries that supply each kidney the camera is activated and a series of images is created. Each is one to two seconds in duration, and together they beautifully depict the blood supply to each kidney. (One of the many causes for high blood pressure is a difference in the amount of blood flow to each kidney. The technique just described can identify such an inequality if it exists.) The rapid-sequence pictures continue for about half a minute. You, of course, are completely unaware of these events unless you choose to watch on the monitor. If this is your kind of thing, ask that the monitor—it's like a small TV—be positioned so that you can watch too.

After the initial imaging, pictures are then taken at five-minute intervals for the next 20 to 30 minutes. These images are obtained exactly the same way as the first set. You remain on your back. The camera does the work.

Most of the time the visual data obtained from the picture sequence described above is enough. However, in some problems more detailed data of both individual and total kidney function is required. This is easily obtained from the information already available from the picture sequence. Each picture is computer-analyzed and the results provide an exact numerical value as to each kidney's capability. All of this computer stuff is done long after you have gone.

That is kidney imaging. The injection rates a ($\frac{1}{2}$ +) for discomfort. The process rates a (−) for hazard, and takes 30 to 45 minutes. You'll receive only a Band-Aid for your memory chest.

Bottom Line: (+) A big nothing.

Ureteric Reflux *Ureteric* refers to the ureters, which are the tubes connecting and carrying urine from your kidneys to your bladder. *Reflux* refers to a backward and inappropriate direction in the movement of a substance—in this case, urine moving back up the ureters from your bladder. The problem is found most commonly in infants and children, but may occur in adults.

The reflux occurs during the act of urination, and if severe may even reach your kidneys. It may occur in only one or even both ureters. The existence of reflux predisposes the sufferer to chronic infections of the urinary tract. Its detection is difficult by any other than isotopic techniques. Here is how the procedure is accomplished:

An isotope in solution must be instilled into your bladder. This is accompanied by inserting a flexible tube (CATHETER) into your bladder and instilling the tracer in the form of a liquid through it. The big deal in this study is the placement of the catheter. (See pages 163–64.) With the catheter in your bladder the solution will be run in. You will feel it as the sensation you well know of "having to go." When this fullness becomes really uncomfortable the technologist will turn off the flow. Your bladder is now full. That was the easy part! The tough job is to empty your bladder—to urinate—from a position that will permit pictures to be made simultaneously. This can be done while you're lying down—women into towels, men into a urinal—with the camera positioned above you. There is no argument that this is most awkward and embarrassing. But with understanding, patience, and appropriate draping by the technologist and effort by you, the mission is not impossible. The images will identify whether or not any urine moves backward and up the ureters while you are voiding. The ordeal varies in time. The variable is how soon after your bladder is filled you can "go." In some it is immediate and the experience, start to end, is about one-half hour. In others there may be coaxing, cajoling, faucet-running, whatever—of unpredictable duration—until the deed is done.

The combination of true physical discomfort from the catheterization and the mental trauma of urinating in public makes this a (+ +). The catheterization makes hazard a (+). There should be no aftereffects except for possible mild urethral irritation from the catheter for a day or so.

Bottom Line: (+ +) Not really a big deal, but for some—"Oh boy!"

Bladder Emptying It is assumed that in the normal state at the end of urination the bladder will be empty. There are certain conditions—an enlarged prostate (a GLAND found only in men that is part of their reproductive system and is located just behind and below the bladder) is one of the most common—that prevent complete emptying. It may be important to confirm this problem, if suspected. This information can be obtained by nuclear studies, both imaging and laboratory.

The initial steps in imaging are identical to those performed for ureteric reflux, described above; the isotope is instilled into your bladder by catheterization. Once your bladder is filled you are asked to lie on a table on your back under a gamma camera. A picture of the full bladder is taken. (One minute.) The catheter is removed and you are then asked to go to the bathroom and empty your bladder—to urinate. When you have performed what comes so naturally, you will return to the table where another picture is made. (One minute.) The two images identify your bladder when full, and when you have emptied it. If more than a "trace" is seen on the "after" image, it suggests that emptying is incomplete. If this should be the case, each picture is subjected to computer analysis, and the exact percentage of retention and even its volume can be easily calculated.

This process rates a (+ +) discomfort and (+) hazard. It takes about 30 minutes. You may experience some mild irritation when urinating for the next day, and maybe even a faint trace of pink. If it should persist, or the pink turns to red, get thee back to thy medic.

Bottom Line: (+ +) No fun.

Lymph Glands Everything you ever wanted to know about lymph glands and the LYMPHATIC SYSTEM has been described in Chapter 18. It is the place to start since the most common approach to imaging this system—lymphangiography—is an X-ray procedure.

However, the areas that can be evaluated by that methodology are limited to certain portions of the pelvis, abdomen, and chest. There are some nuclear physicians who champion the cause of visualizing and thus evaluating the lymphatics in other areas, notably the drainage sites from the breasts, rectum, and prostate. Nuclear imaging can accomplish this end. The images obtained from these studies do not rival in beauty or detail those that result from the direct "dye" injection methods or even those seen on CT, but there are no acceptable ways to inject the lymphatics that drain these parts. So it's isotope or "nuthin'." Nuclear is the only show in town for those parts, and it can be accomplished in a far simpler manner than the more conventional methods.

The isotope will be picked up by the lymphatic vessels adjacent to the site into which it is injected. Therefore the injection is made as close to the area of interest as is possible. For studies of your breasts, the injection is made into the muscles of the front of your abdomen just below the lowest rib on each side. The prostate gland is studied after injections are made through the rectum into the region of the prostate. The rectum is evaluated by injecting the TISSUES that surround it.

So, if your advisers say do it, this is how it is done.

The injection sites are bared and "prepped" by cleansing them with an antiseptic solution. The nuclear physician will make the injection, and the discomfort index is: breasts (+); rectum (+ +); prostate (+ + +). All pain is gone in less than a minute. There is no hazard. You can now redress and prepare to wait one to three hours—until the nuclide has localized satisfactorily. After this time, you will be asked to disrobe and regown. Picture taking is then begun. You lie on a table and the gamma camera and technologist do the work. The imaging series takes about 30 to 45 minutes. Elapsed time for the whole thing is about a half-day. There should be no aftereffects. Take a pal along—you will be tired when it is over.

Bottom Line: (+ +) It really is easy—so why does it seem hard?

Miscellaneous

Miscellaneous is defined as "consisting of diverse things."

Below, two diverse things remain—two diagnostic procedures that are helpful in detecting problems that may occur anywhere in the body and thus cannot easily be fitted into any one of the individual-area categories. One of the procedures is for suspected but "hidden" infection; the other, for early tumor recognition.

Infections There are infections and there are infections. There are the kind where you scratch your finger and in a day or two it becomes red and swollen and painful. That's an infection. Then there are the kind where you just don't feel well. Nothing that you can put your finger on—maybe you're just tired, maybe you're achy, perhaps you've got a headache—something's just not right. A blood count shows certain changes. A thermometer identifies that you have an increased temperature. This is often called F.U.O. —fever of unknown origin. Somewhere in your body is a seat of infection. How to find it?

There are two different *isotopes* that are used to find areas of inflammation. (Infection and inflammation are not exactly the same thing, but I think we can use the two terms interchangeably here.) These isotopes differ somewhat in how they function. One of them—gallium—is particularly helpful in confirming the presence of a particular type of pneumonia that some patients suffering with AIDS are subject to well before it becomes evident on X-rays. The other, indium, is particularly useful in finding pockets of infection that may be a complication of recent surgery. But which isotope is used when is the decision of the physicians who are studying your problem. From your standpoint they differ only slightly from one another.

Gallium When this TRACER is chosen, the test is a one-stick, intravenous event, with a (½ +) discomfort rating. Picture taking does not usually begin until at least the next day; more often, not until 48 hours later. It takes that long for the isotope to localize in any abnormal area. You will lie on your back on a scanning table and the gamma camera will be above you for the frontal views and under you for views of the back. Commonly, most of your body is imaged since the doctors don't know where the problem is located. You will feel nothing. It may take as long as an hour to do the whole thing. They may even repeat the picture taking the next day in the same way. Some imagers demand that you take a laxative the night before picture time. Others don't. There is no hazard, and there are no symptoms afterward.

Bottom Line: (+) There is only Tedium (with a capital T).

Indium For this tracer to do its duty it must first be attached to the white cells in your blood. This is accomplished by taking a small sample of your blood—Stick 1—and "cooking" it up with the indium in the laboratory. When the brew is ready—a matter of about an hour—it is injected back into you—stick 2. Imaging will begin in several hours and can be repeated several times through the next 24 hours. Picture taking is with you on your back on a table with the gamma camera doing the job. There is no discomfort. There is no hazard. It is slightly less tedious than gallium because it is over sooner.

Bottom Line: (+) There's tedium (with a little t).

Tumor Detection—Monoclonal Antibodies As of this writing this procedure is limited in both its scope and its availability. It holds remarkable promise for the future, however, and thus deserves a nod of recognition.

Monoclonal (single clone) ANTIBODIES can now be engineered to detect the presence of certain tumors. These antibodies can also be given a radioactive isotope marker. This combination of tumor specific plus marker provides a new method for tumor detection. Here is how it works: You are suspected of having a tumor in your breast. Breast-tumor-specific radioactive monoclonal antibodies exist. You will be given an appropriate amount of these antibodies by injection, and after the appropriate amount of time, perhaps days, you will be placed under a scanning camera and images will be obtained. If you have a breast tumor the antibodies will have attached themselves to the breast tumor cells and the image will show this collection. If, on the other hand, you do not have a tumor the image will be free of localized areas of activity. If the antibodies find no cells of their sensitivity they will be eliminated from the body, thus constituting no radiation hazard to you.

The same radioactive antibodies can perform an additional diagnostic service. If the tumor has spread from its original site—say, the breast tumor has spread to bone, liver, or elsewhere in the body, a condition known as metastasis—the same antibody mission of seek and locate will occur, and images will detect the different locations involved.

And finally, the same mechanism can be used for treatment purposes. The isotope that is tagged to the antibody can be further modified to irradiate the tumor after their contact has been made. The mission becomes seek and destroy.

If you are a candidate for this procedure, all that is required is injection of the material, a ($\frac{1}{2}$ +) discomfort. The time of imaging after receipt of the antibodies is highly variable and may only be hours but could be days. Actual imaging time is also variable but usually averages about an hour for each session. Yes, you may have to return one or more times. There is no hazard and no aftereffects.

Bottom Line: (+) Let's hope this one gets off the drawing board soon.

20

Go Get
an Ultrasound

Ultrasound (abbreviated US) is what the hi-fi fanatic spends a lifetime seeking. It is also the name of a remarkable technology that permits images to be made without ionizing radiation, which is another way of saying "without hazard." If you are going to have one you might like to know more about how it works.

Perhaps the easiest way to understand this technology is to use a source of reference that is familiar to each of us—the echo. Who has not had the fun of hollering into the wind only to have the words come back at him sounding a bit hollow or strange? Who has not had that "spooky" experience of walking in some confined place and hearing her own footsteps? These are echoes.

When we speak we are really making very specialized cords in our throats vibrate. This vibration also causes movement of the air that is adjacent to these cords. This movement of air assumes a special character that we call sound waves. When someone speaks, the waves leave his or her mouth and move away. Eventually, they will strike something. If the something is someone's eardrum the waves will be absorbed, further processed, and eventually "heard." If the same waves strike another surface and are incompletely absorbed they will be reflected or "bounced off," only to strike another surface— and so forth until their energy is spent. If the sound wave should strike a non-absorbing surface such as a neighboring canyon wall it will be reflected back to the ear of the one who initiated the wave, and this ricochet is the echo.

This principle is the basis for radar and sonar. It is also the basis for the medical technology known as ultrasonography. The waves used are similar to the sound waves that we can hear in that both are mechanical vibrations. These vibrations possess measurable physical characteristics such as wavelength, wave period, velocity, intensity, and frequency. Frequency refers to the number of vibrations per unit of time and is measured in hertz units. When the sound wave is audible to the human ear its frequency is between 20 and 20,000 hertz. Any wave that has a frequency greater than this is inaudible and is designated as ultrasonic.

Waves in the ultrasonic range are used in imaging. They can be generated by a unique physical phenomenon known as piezoelectricity. When an electrical voltage is applied to certain substances—of those found in nature the best known is quartz—those substances will expand in such a way as to create these waves. Equally important, when waves return—echo—and strike these elements they will be compressed and, in turn, generate an electrical impulse that can be transposed into a picture. Certain synthetic ceramics, such as lead zirconate tetanate, have also been found to generate and receive ultrasound waves, and in medicine they have, for the most part, replaced the naturally occurring substances. Regardless of which is used, the material can be fashioned into a piece of equipment that looks something like a flashlight and is called a TRANSDUCER.

Images are obtained by placing the transducer over the part to be examined and energizing it to produce the sound waves. These then enter the body. They will pass through the first layer of TISSUE, which will be the skin. As they encounter the next layer, some of the waves will be reflected back and be captured by the transducer while the rest will continue forward. At the next tissue layer the same events will occur—some waves will be reflected backward and the remainder will continue forward. And so on, and so on . . . until all of the original energy is expended.

Each tissue type and substance affects the wave differently. This is known as the reflective coefficient. Air, for example, does not permit any wave to pass through it. The impinging wave striking air will be totally reflected back, making air's coefficient 100 percent. Water is at the other end of the scale, permitting the entire wave to pass, and thereby having a coefficient of zero percent. Thus the final image will be a mirror of the various tissues and any other substances through which the beam has passed.

The image can be presented as a static picture of a body part, or, utilizing a technology known as realtime, in which there is rapid sequencing of images, the image can be presented as a movie. The part can be visualized in motion, and thus internal body movements such as the heartbeat can be seen and studied. And, wonder of wonders, all of this good stuff without imposing a radiation load!

Most, but not all, examinations employing the ultrasound modality are similar. Let's start with what's common to all:

The Room The ultrasound suite is quite simple. It consists only of a couch on which you lie or sit, and the machine that creates the images. The unit is a cabinet-like piece of furniture whose front incorporates a keyboard like a typewriter, or even more like the keyboard of a personal computer. There is also a small monitor, or TV screen, above the keyboard. There are attachments like foot pedals and other stuff that the technologist uses but that are barely noticeable. Add a cabinet or two, and perhaps a small desk, and that's the usual room.

Transducers A *transducer* is a device that receives its power to operate from one system and supplies power, usually in another form, to a second system. This is the instrument that transmits the ultrasound wave into your body and captures the returning echo to create a picture. These devices come in different sizes and shapes. Some look like pocket flashlights. Some are more like regular flashlights. Others resemble a TV remote controller. Which will be used is a decision based on the nature of the problem to be solved and need not concern you. From your standpoint they are all the same in how they are employed, and more importantly, how they feel. Each is hand-held by either the technologist or physician, and will be gently moved back and forth, up and down, round and round—I think you get the idea—on your skin over the part of your body that is being studied. The sensation is actually pleasant.

Lubrication Everyone gets a lube job. It consists of the technologist applying a warm oil or gel to your skin over the area of interest. The purpose of this application is to ensure that there is a tight seal between the transducer and you. Any air space will essentially prevent sound transmission and thus prevent a diagnostic study. So—the oil. Additionally, LUBRICATION permits the transducer to be moved more smoothly. Most people find the oil and the mild pressure of the transducer to be like a minimassage. It really feels "real good."

Picture Taker The image that is the end product of an ultrasonic examination is created, for the most part, by a specially trained individual known as a US technologist who is carefully and thoroughly trained in the methodology inherent in achieving the goal for each examination—an image. Such a person is not a physician. However, when the picture has been obtained it is then given to another trained specialist who will interpret it so that it has medical meaning.

Picture Reader   The trained specialist who interprets the images is a physician. After graduating from both college and medical school, this person has spent an additional four or five years becoming versed in some specialty —usually internal medicine or radiology. When the physician has satisfactorily mastered this study as attested by successful passage of examinations known as boards, he or she is awarded a degree proclaiming certification. The physician then begins a second period of study, requiring approximately one year, exploring and mastering the mysteries of ultrasonography.

Most examinations are done by the technologist alone. All images are reviewed by the physician. If something is seen on this review that is unclear or that might be improved upon by additional views, the physician will appear and get into the act. But even if you don't physically see the "person in the white coat," rest assured that there is a highly trained medical specialist who will make the final decision on your ultrasound.

For the particulars of each examination, start with the accompanying tables. It divides the body into five general sections. Within each major area are listed the parts that are found there that are commonly studied by this technique. (Some body areas do not lend themselves to this modality, which explains their absence from the table.) For example, if your doctor said: "Go have an ultrasound of your gall bladder," you would refer to the table and find abdomen, the general body section in which the gall bladder is found. You would find gall bladder and read across its entire line. A quick synopsis of the pertinent data inherent in this study, i.e., discomfort, hazard, informed consent, extras, etc., is listed. (These data are elaborated upon in the Appendix.) The last item on the line is the page number where the study is described in detail.

And finally, after you have read about the particular examination that you are preparing for, reread pages xiv through xvi, General Events Common to All Adult Diagnostic Procedures.

Head

In the adult, ultrasound examinations of the head are limited almost entirely to investigations of the eye.

Ultrasound

Body Part/ Procedure	Discomfort* (−) to (++++)	Hazard* (−) to (+++)	Hospital (Incl. Short Procedure)	Special Prep.	Physician	Extras*	Informed Consent*	Exam Time* (Hrs.)	Bottom Line* (−) to (++++)	Exam Description (Page)
Head										
Eye	(+)	(−)	N	Y	N	Y	N	½	(+)	278
Neck										
Thyroid										
Lumps & bumps	(½+)	(−)	N	N	N	N	N	½	(½+)	278
Biopsy control	(++)	(++)	N	N	Y	Y	Y	1	(++)	279
Carotid arteries	(+)	(−)	N	N	Y	N	N	1	(+)	279
Chest										
Heart	(+)	(−)	N	N	Y	N	N	1	(+)	280
Blood vessels	(++)	(−)	N	N	Y	N	N	½	(+)	282
Breasts	(+)	(−)	N	N	N	N	N	½	(+)	282
Abdomen										
Gall bladder	(½+)	(−)	N	Y	N	N	N	½	(½+)	283
Liver	(½+)	(−)	N	Y	N	N	N	½	(½+)	283
Spleen	(½+)	(−)	N	Y	N	N	N	½	(½+)	283
Pancreas	(½+)	(−)	N	Y	N	N	N	½	(½+)	283
Kidneys	(½+)	(−)	N	Y	N	N	N	½	(½+)	283

Body Part/ Procedure	Discomfort* (−) to (++++)	Hazard* (−) to (+++)	Hospital (Incl. Short Procedure)	Special Prep.	Physician	Extras*	Informed Consent*	Exam Time* (Hrs.)	Bottom Line* (−) to (++++)	Exam Description (Page)
Pelvis										
Uterus & ovaries										
Nonpregnant	(++)	(−)	N	Y	Y/N	Y	N	½	(++)	285
Pregnant Routine	(++)	(−)	N	Y	Y/N	Y	N	½	(++)	286
Amniocentesis	(++)	(+++)	N	Y	Y	Y	Y	½	(++) to (+++)	286
Chorionic villus	(++) to (+++)	(++) to (+++)	N	Y	Y	Y	Y	½	(++) to (+++)	288
Prostate										
Transabdominal	(+)	(−)	N	Y	Y/N	Y	N	½	(+)	289
Transrectal	(++)	(−)	N	N	Y	Y	N	½	(++)	289
Testicles	(½+)	(−)	N	N	Y/N	Y	N	½	(+)	290

* See Appendix, Table Details.

Eye The ultrasonic examination of the eye is, almost without exception, a study that is performed by an ophthalmologist (a specialist in diseases of the eye) as a consequence of something you are complaining about or something that has been found in an examination of your eyes. See Diseases of the Retina in Chapter 11.

Neck

Diagnostic procedures for the neck concentrate on the thyroid gland and the carotid artery.

Thyroid Gland The thyroid is one of the major GLANDS of the body. It is located in the front of your neck, just below the "Adam's Apple." Its role is to regulate your body's METABOLISM.

Most examinations to evaluate thyroid function and status are a combination of blood studies and nuclear medicine imaging. These are described in detail in Chapter 19. However, this gland is prone to a relatively common problem that requires a big assist from ultrasound. This problem is the development of "lumps and bumps." A lump or a bump is just what it says it is— "something" that appears suddenly (or over time) that wasn't there before. If it contains fluid it is probably a CYST and, except for possibly causing discomfort, is of no serious concern. If it is a solid collection of abnormal cells—a NODULE—there is cause for some real concern that it could be MALIGNANT. Ultrasound images are uniquely suited to differentiate between these two possibilities. If the lump is fluid-filled it will be treated according to the degree of discomfort it evokes. If the bump is solid a BIOPSY may be necessary. When this is the decision ultrasound also can assist in directing the tissue collection.

Note: The description that follows, although specific to the thyroid gland, is essentially that which would be performed anywhere in your body where a lump or bump needed further investigation.

Ultrasound imaging is often a two-part examination. Part 1 is the identification of the character of the lump. Part 2 is when the lump is found to be suspicious and a biopsy is indicated and you have said Yes to the procedure.

Part 1: There is no preparation necessary. You will be asked to remove any clothing or jewelry that prevents the front of your neck from being completely exposed. Then the technologist will ask you to lie on your back with a pillow under your shoulders. This will result in "stretching out" your neck and bringing it forward. This position is mildly uncomfortable but usually well tolerated. Then warm oil will be spread over your neck and the TRANSDUCER gently moved over your skin. You may be asked to turn your head from side to side, to swallow occasionally, and to hold your breath on command. That's *it!* The lump or bump is identified. The whole procedure takes about 15 minutes. Give discomfort a (½ +). Hazard gets nothing.

Part 2: (The lump has been found to be solid and with your approval a biopsy will be done.) You are placed in the same position as above. The skin over your neck is prepared by antiseptic cleansing and draping with sterile towels. The lump is again imaged as above and a local anesthetic is injected under the skin that overlies it, which results in a slight prick and a slight burn. Additional anesthesia is injected at deeper levels until the entire area is numb. A longer needle is then inserted with the intention of placing its tip in the TISSUE requiring biopsy. Your neck is again imaged with the needle in place to check the needle's position. This is repeated, with adjustments in positioning, until the placement is precise. Suction is then applied to the other end of the needle by a glass syringe sufficient to draw up some cells from the area of abnormality. These acts of needle placement and suction are felt, in most cases, only as sensations of pressure and tugging (+). The needle is then withdrawn and a dressing applied. Your neck is reexamined for the last time to see whether the procedure has caused any undesirable new problems. If everything is cool—that's it. It usually requires half an hour. Both discomfort and hazard score (+). Except for mild soreness or even some black and blue marks for a few days there is usually no other unhappiness.

Bottom Line: For Part 1 (½ +) A piece of cake! For Part 2 (+ +) the cake is a tad lumpy.

Carotid Arteries   The carotid artery is the largest artery (one of those blood vessels that carry blood from the heart to the rest of the body) of the neck and transports blood to the head. It is particularly prone to ARTERIOSCLEROSIS. The condition results in the building up of PLAQUES that gradually narrow the inside diameter of the vessel even to the point of total OCCLUSION (it's like rust forming on the inside of pipes). Additionally, pieces of the plaques may break off and float in the blood until they reach a smaller vessel, usually in the brain, where they become lodged, thus completely occluding that smaller vessel.

When a carotid artery becomes narrowed, the blood supply to the brain is affected. This may produce a condition known as TIA (transient ischemic attack), which is a momentary loss of some brain function. It is estimated that one-third of all individuals who experience TIAs will, some time within the following five years, progress to complete occlusion. (When vascular occlusion occurs in the brain the condition is called stroke or apoplexy, and the sufferer experiences a sudden diminution or loss of consciousness, sensation, and voluntary motion.)

Frightening statistics time: There are approximately 2 million stroke victims in the United States each year. Of these about 200,000 will die—some 50 percent immediately. Of the remainder, approximately 30 percent suffer sufficient permanent damage that they lose their independence and must be cared for. Consequently, discovering the existence of changes in a carotid artery is most important. This evaluation is possible by X-ray (see pages 194–200). It may also be accomplished, in many situations, by ultrasound.

No preparation is required. You will be asked to remove anything that makes getting to your neck difficult. (Leave your necklaces and chains at home.) You will either sit or lie back on the examining table. Your neck will be given the warm oil treatment and the examination will begin. Two different techniques will probably be used: one in which images are made (called duplex) and another in which measurements of movement—the rate and quality of blood flow—are made (called Doppler). From your standpoint they will be almost identical—the transducer will be gently moved about each side of your neck. The only difference will be that the Doppler phase of the "neck stroking" is associated with *noise*. It can be loud; it can be high-pitched; it can be thumping, whooping, or hammering. Just don't let it frighten you. The sound is produced by the movement of your blood through the vessel and varies in pitch and intensity with both the velocity and character of its movement. Often a physician will perform the Doppler portion of the study. The whole number takes about 30 minutes. No to discomfort and hazard. No to aftereffects.

Bottom Line: (+) *Yes!* to the whole thing, particularly if it can be done instead of ARTERIOGRAPHY.

Chest

Diagnostic procedures for the chest look at the heart, blood vessels, and breasts.

Heart Although the heart is perhaps the most familiar of all of the body ORGANS—we all know it as the Big Red Machine that drives the blood through our body and controls our CIRCULATION, and we also know that it is subject to "attacks"—we might need to review (or learn) some of its functions.

The "old pump" is really a very special kind of muscle whose ability to contract and drive the blood forward, and relax and let blood enter, is the one-two punch of successful circulation. Thus in the overall evaluation of your heart's function it is essential to know just how well it contracts and moves blood—this performance is called ejection fraction—and just how orderly and at what speed these contractions and relaxations occur (heart rate and rhythm).

We should also know that the heart is composed of four compartments called chambers. The chambers are separated from each other by swinging doors called valves. Blood enters the first chamber and remains there until the valve opens to permit it to enter the second, and so on until it leaves the heart. The correct opening and closing of these doors is crucial to appropriate function. So, valve action is also a critical determinant of the cardiac condition and must be evaluated.

And we should know that the heart is surrounded by a special covering called the pericardial membrane, which sometimes produces abnormal amounts of fluid. When this occurs, this problem—known as pericardial effusion—increases the load on the heart.

Ultrasound imaging of the heart, commonly referred to as echocardiography, is a spectacularly simple, accurate, and NONINVASIVE way to go for the examination of excessive pericardial fluid, the calculation of the ejection fraction, and particularly for the evaluation of valvular function.

The procedure for echocardiography is almost exactly like that described for the examination of the carotid artery, above, except that it is your chest rather than your neck that will be imaged. You will be asked to remove everything from the waist up and to don the proffered gown so that it opens in the front. You will be asked to lie on an examining table or couch and the technologist will anoint your chest with warm oil. Then he or she will gently move a hand-held TRANSDUCER over your heart, taking pictures from time to time. Often, each snap is accompanied by a bleeping sound. You will be asked to change your position—from lying on your back to lying on your side or even to sitting. After the portraits are obtained, a different transducer will be substituted and the same gliding movements performed. This portion of the study is accompanied by much louder sound effects—whooshing and rushing noises. But except for the stroking and the background music, that is all that you will experience. There is neither discomfort nor hazard. The whole event requires 30 to 60 minutes. The only aftereffect is a nicely LUBRI-

CATED chest. Oh, yes, if such things interest you, the technologist can probably position the monitor—a small TV screen—so that you can see your own "ticker."

Bottom Line: (+) The sound of the heart you just heard was your own.

Blood Vessels The blood vessels (the arteries and veins), together with the heart, comprise the circulatory system. This system addresses the need that every living tissue in the body has to receive oxygen to survive. This service is provided by the arteries (those vessels that carry blood from the heart to all parts of the body), with a helpful push from the heart. However, once that oxygen has been used at the tissue level there is a new product formed—carbon dioxide—that must be gotten rid of. This service is provided by the veins (those vessels that carry blood from all parts of the body to the heart). They haul off the carbon dioxide and deliver it to its dump site, the lungs, where it gets "blown away."

Imaging of a particular vessel, be it artery or vein, is requested, as a rule, when there is reason to be concerned about the condition of the circulation of a given area. US lends itself to this investigation, in many instances, by providing information not only about the vessel's appearance but also, in many locations, by revealing the characteristics of the way the blood is flowing. It is important to verify the appearance of a vessel—usually an artery— if there is any concern that it may be enlarging abnormally (aneurysm) and therefore might eventually burst. It is important to evaluate the possibility that there might be "something" within a vessel—usually a vein—that might possibly break off (THROMBUS) and float in the blood to eventually lodge and obstruct the circulation to all parts beyond it (EMBOLUS).

Each area of concern becomes the target for examination and the study is requested by the name of the particular vessel in question. Such an example has been discussed in detail in the section entitled Neck—the carotid arteries. The technique of examination of that vessel has been described above. Since all vessels—arteries and veins—are all examined in the same manner, that discussion will suffice for all. Just substitute the name of the part your doctor sends you to have done—your femoral artery, or the varicose veins in your calf, or the aorta . . . whatever—for carotid arteries, and substitute the part of your body in which the vessel is located (your thigh for the femoral artery, for example) whenever neck is mentioned, and that's it.

Breasts At this moment in diagnostic history the premier investigative study for problems of the breast (after the good old physical examination done by both you and your physician) is mammography—pictures of the breast made by X-ray. (See discussion of mammography on pages 190–92.) But even after both of those have been done, there may still be questions to be answered. What are the questions, and what are the answers?

The following is a common scenario: You discover a lump in your breast. Your doctor confirms your fears. You have a mammogram, and it, too, shows a lump. But there are lumps and there are lumps. Many exhibit characteristics that require immediate attention—usually some form of surgery. Many exhibit changes that are not nearly as ominous, but are suspicious and bear watching. These are managed by reexamination, by both physicals and X-rays, after some time interval (commonly six months) to see what, if anything, has changed. And there are still other lumps that are thought to be CYSTS because of their history of being tender, painful, and/or enlarging around the time of your period. These lumps are, with rare exception, BENIGN so they can be either left alone or if troublesome, drained by simple ASPIRA-TION. Differentiation of a cystic from a solid lump can be made by ultrasound. So—what are we waiting for?

No preparation is necessary. It will be necessary to bare your breast. You will probably be in a sitting position. The technologist will apply warm oil, and gently move the transducer over your breast. There should be no unhappiness on your part unless the lump being studied happens to be particularly tender to pressure, or unless you are embarrassed by the procedure. There is no hazard. Examination time is less than a half-hour. There are no after-symptoms.

Bottom Line: (+) You literally have made a clean breast of it.

Note: The above description represents what is usual and average. There are some US centers that have very specialized equipment for this study. This equipment may look like a large bathtub filled with water. You might be asked to lie on your stomach on a platform with your breast in the water. Another variation of the "water bath" approach is a smaller device, also water-filled, that may be placed onto your breast. Neither of these variations will bother you any more than the more commonly performed method described above, except that the positioning is more awkward and may take a bit longer to do.

Abdomen

In the X-ray and nuclear medicine chapters the abdomen and pelvis are considered together because some systems, such as the urinary tract, contain ORGANS that are located in both the abdomen and pelvis. But the nature of the ultrasonic imaging techniques makes it more appropriate to consider each area separately. However, of the many organs that are found in the abdomen, only the gall bladder, liver, spleen, pancreas, and kidneys lend themselves to this methodology (note the exclusion of the stomach and several other DIGESTIVE SYSTEM structures). A brief description of the nature and function of the gall bladder can be found in Chapter 5; of the liver, spleen, and pancreas in Chapter 18; and the kidneys in Chapter 7. Each of the parts can be found in Chapter 18. See the tables in each chapter for the page number reference for the organ.

The motto for imaging of these parts is "One size fits all." For all parts, you should fast for at least eight hours before the study. You will be given a glass of a whitish liquid to drink. This material will identify the stomach and small intestines, diminishing the confusion that these structures often create because of the air that they contain. (The drink doesn't even taste too bad.) Next, you will be asked to lie down on the couch after having gotten into an appropriate gown which will permit your abdomen to be exposed. Then the lube job—warm oil will be applied to the skin. The technologist (sometimes the physician, too) will move the TRANSDUCER over your belly. You will probably be asked to turn from side to side, hold your breath on command, and try not to be bored. (Ask to watch the monitor that the technologist is looking at, if that is of interest to you.) Very infrequently, patients experience minor pain (+) if something hurts and the technologist presses the transducer firmly into that area. That is the extent of the discomfort. There is no hazard. The time of examination varies and is dependent on your complaints and what is found. It averages about half an hour. No aftershocks.

Bottom Line: (½ +) Another ho-hummer.

Pelvis

The ORGANS found in the pelvis (the genital or reproductive systems of both women and men) and ultrasound, were—like bacon and eggs, Elvis and rock, or Steinbrenner and the Yankees—*made for each other!*

Read on to find out why this is so, and how the examinations are performed.

Genital System—Female The genital system in the female is composed of the ovaries, fallopian tubes, uterus, and vagina. Until the advent of ultrasound it was a system in search of an imaging technique! Of all of the organs of the body, those concerned with reproduction are far and away the most sensitive to the harmful effects of radiation—the stuff that X-rays and nuclear medicine require to make their pictures. Until the development of US, they were the only picture show in town. But no more! US provides a technology that permits imaging without risk! Wow! The female pelvis can now be evaluated for such problems as excessive bleeding, discharge, pain, "irregularity," infertility, and infection—to mention only the tip of the iceberg— without fear of harmful effects.

Pregnancy can also be studied now. Investigations that were impossible by other techniques can now be performed without hazard. It is now possible to answer the question: Is there really a uterine pregnancy? And if Yes: Is the age of the pregnancy in agreement with the woman's records? If there is disagreement is it due to the mother's error or an error in fetal growth? What is the condition of the fetus? Is there more than one fetus? Where is the placenta (the organ that unites the fetus to its mother in her uterus) located in the womb, and what is its condition? Are there any GENETIC defects? And if No: Is there evidence of an ECTOPIC pregnancy? Is there evidence of a spontaneous abortion (miscarriage—the expulsion of the fetus from the uterus)?

Unlike other areas examined by US, where the same technique is appropriate regardless of the clinical problem being investigated, the study of the female pelvis differs depending on whether or not pregnancy exists. Therefore, the techniques are discussed under these two categories: nonpregnant and pregnant.

Nonpregnant Prepreparation is essential. Your bladder must be full. This condition is non-negotiable. The distended bladder serves to push the portion of your bowel that lives in the pelvis "up, up, and away" so that it does not interfere with the picture taking of the genital structures. (Remember that "gas" and US don't go well together.) It requires about 32 to 40 ounces of fluid (four to five glasses of your choice) to fill the bladder, and it takes about one hour for it to happen. So, start drinking! You will know that the deed is done when you "really, really, gotta go!"

Once the above has been accomplished and you are quite miserable, you will be invited to remove everything from the waist down, hop up on the table, have warm oil applied to your abdomen, and then lean back and relax. The technologist (sometimes the physician as well) will then gently move a TRANSDUCER about your lower belly. Although you have to urinate—and the feeling is getting worse with each passing moment—and there may be pressure applied by the image-taker over your bladder, there is no other discomfort, but score it a **(+)** or even a **(+ +)**. There is no hazard. Remember that you can watch what is going on, if that is your pleasure, just by asking. The study averages about one-half hour and there are no memories afterward.

Bottom Line: **(+ +)** Joy is when they let you go to the bathroom.

Pregnant

Routine Whether or not any "prep" is necessary will depend on just how long you've been pregnant. If it is still early in your pregnancy and your uterus is still small, the same prepreparation as described for the nonpregnant group applies to you, too. And for the same reason—getting the bowel out of the way. All of the other events described above are also identical. However, if you're late enough in your pregnancy for your uterus to have grown large enough to do its own bowel pushing, the full-bladder misery is avoided. *Don't forget:* ask the technologist to adjust the monitor (TV screen) so that you can see your baby! It is an experience that you'll remember forever! You can actually see your child, in you, and watch its heart beat, its hands and feet move. Perhaps you'll see your baby make a face, and on occasion you can even see if it is a he or a she. So—discomfort equals **(+ +)**, hazard **(−)**, and it takes half an hour.

Bottom Line: **(+ +)** This one is *joy!*

Note: At this writing there is another method just beginning to become popular called transvaginal sonography. The initial reviews are raves. It differs from the method described above in that the transducer is introduced into your vagina and the pictures are obtained from there rather than from the front of your belly. The pluses are far superior images, because the sound waves have a shorter distance to travel and their echo is freer of interference from other parts, and there is no need for the grossly distended bladder so that discomfort is thus eliminated. The negatives are only singular —just one. Some women find the thought of the instrument *in them* to be repugnant. But if that can be overcome, the rest is all positive. You put the transducer in yourself. You do this with the aid of the technologist and your privacy is otherwise respected. Then when you are as comfortable as this condition permits, you will be draped (covered appropriately with sheets or towels) and the physician will be called. That person—whether a radiologist, a gynecologist, or an obstetrician—is well skilled and will move the transducer, whose handle extends to the outside, gently and carefully. Pictures will be made by the technologist. Remember: watch on the monitor. The discomfort caused by this technique is less than that of the routine method. Give it a **(½ +)** for the insertion. Hazard is zero. Allot about one hour. No aftereffects.

Bottom Line: **(+ +)** The vast majority of the women I have spoken to who have been examined each way prefer this method.

Special—Amniocentesis Explanatory note: The fetus in utero is surrounded by several layers of MEMBRANE. The innermost layer, called the amnion, forms a sac containing fluid, also called amnion (or amniotic fluid), around the baby and in which the baby floats. (It's like a huge transparent bag.) The fluid contains cells and other materials shed by the developing child. These materials, when analyzed by trained physicians, can provide a remarkably accurate picture of possible genetic abnormalities such as Down's syndrome and such possible defects of development as spina bifida (a failure of closure of the spine, so that the cord is exposed) and anencephaly (failure of the brain to develop). These problems are incurable. For those women who believe in "free choice" the knowledge of whether or not their babies are at high risk is most important. High risk exists when there is a history of certain problems in families, or when the woman is having her first child and is 35 years old (or older), or the obstetrician is concerned by certain findings. If the findings indicate that a problem is present a therapeutic abortion can then be considered. If no problem exists then the remainder of the pregnancy can be spent without those fears.

Amniocentesis is usually done early in pregnancy, around the fourteenth to eighteenth week. It starts out just like the preceding description although the amount of water necessary is usually not too great and will depend on how well your uterus can be seen. Your abdomen is bared by the technologist. The lower portion is cleansed or "prepped" with an antiseptic solution (always cold) and then the part is draped with sterile towels. Warm oil is applied to your skin. But now, the person with the transducer is a physician (radiologist, gynecologist, or obstetrician). The examination will be made by moving the transducer over your lower belly, looking for a "clear space" between the wall of your uterus and the baby, and avoiding the placenta. This clear space is the amniotic fluid. When this is located, the doctor will prick the skin over the spot with a very short, fine needle and inject a small amount of local anesthetic. There is an instantaneous burning (+) and then numbness. Then the doctor will take a longer needle, perhaps four to five inches long, and gently but firmly push it through your skin and into your uterus. You will certainly feel the event. Most women rate the pain with that of having blood taken from a vein (+). Some equate it with a severe menstrual cramp (+ +). Then there will be a mild sensation of pulling as the fluid is drawn up into the syringe. This takes but a minute or two and the needle is then withdrawn. If that is it—and it almost always goes that way—the whole thing requires only 15 to 20 minutes. It rates a (+ +) for discomfort and a (+ +) for hazard. Yes, there is a hazard for this one. There is always the risk that there could be bleeding or that the procedure might induce labor. The risk is small, but real. Occasionally, the first "stick" does not strike the fluid. Then, the maneuver must be repeated. It happens, but fortunately not too often. Except for some lingering soreness from the poking around you should have no other problem. If, however, you experience other things—like increasing pain, or cramping, or leakage, or anything, get thee to thy doctor, *pronto!*

Bottom Line: (+ +) or (+ + +) This reads worse than it usually is.

Extra Special—Chorionic Villi Biopsy Explanatory note 2: See note on page 286 about membranes. There is an outer layer that surrounds the amniotic sac, called the chorion. This membrane is composed of many small spike-like projections called villi. These villi contain cells that can provide the same information as is obtainable from amniotic fluid. Thus, a sample of a chorionic villus serves the same purpose as an amniocentesis. It has several important advantages to commend it over amniocentesis. These are that it can be performed earlier in the pregnancy—between the eighth and ninth weeks—and that its results can be available in a day or two. This compares with waiting until the fourteenth to eighteenth week, and an additional three to six weeks' wait for a "readout" of the "amnio" method. Thus, if remedial action is required it can be accomplished much sooner. But (always a but) the technique of examination is more demanding and the risks are reported as somewhat greater. *Discuss it with your doctor!*

Chorionic villi sampling is done two different ways.

The first is identical to amniocentesis, except you must add a (+) to the discomfort (it just seems to hurt a bit more), and add a (+) to the hazard. However, some claim that the two studies are indistinguishable from each other.

The second method is different from amniocentesis. Some obstetricians obtain the sample by passing a fine CATHETER through the vagina, through the cervix (the opening of the uterus), and into the uterus. The villi are then pulled into the catheter by suction. When this is the method of procedure no addition to the discomfort index is necessary—the rigor of the catheter placement is about equal to the needle ASPIRATION described for amniocentesis— but add another (½ +) to the hazard score. The risk of infection and/or spontaneous abortion is increased slightly.

Either way, it's a long hard day. Although the whole thing won't take an hour, try to spend the rest of the day "at leisure." And, invoke the rule of BAP—Bring a Pal!

Bottom Line: (+ +) or (+ + +) Let's hope the results set your mind at ease.

Genital System—Male In the male, the genital system is composed of the prostate gland, the seminal ducts, the testicles, and the penis. Of these, only the prostate gland and testicles lend themselves to examination by US.

Prostate Gland The prostate gland is a structure that resides just below your bladder. It manufactures a milky-colored fluid that is combined with the sperm from your testicles and the fluid from your seminal vesicles to make semen.

There are two ultrasound methods now available to examine the gland. The more common is through the front of the abdomen, and is known as transabdominal. The second is a relatively new technique in which the transducer, instead of being positioned on the front of your lower abdomen, is inserted into your rectum, and the prostate is imaged from this location. This method is called transrectal, and requires a special instrument not yet found in all centers. Those that are doing the examination in this latter manner assert that the images obtained are far superior to ones from the abdominal approach. Additionally, they state that if there is anything in the study that is suspicious, a piece of TISSUE (a BIOPSY) can be obtained through the same instrument at the same time, thus saving one an additional and far more difficult procedure. Those that don't do this procedure claim that the advantages do not warrant the additional patient discomfort or cost. Discuss this one with your doctor!

Transabdominal You must get your bladder really filled by drinking a great deal of fluid about an hour before the study. Four to five glasses of your choice are the minimum. Once you're ready, you'll get up on the table with your lower abdomen bare. The technologist will have you lie down on your back and apply some nice warm oil on your skin. A transducer will then be moved around the area in a firm but gentle fashion as images are being made. Except for the discomfort of your DISTENDED bladder and the additional pressure from the transducer, that is the extent of it. A big (+) for discomfort. The hazard rating is (−). Give it a half-hour max. No lingering memories.

Bottom Line: (+) Only those of you who have had this part examined by the usual methods in the past will know *how grand this is!*

Transrectal The technologist will have you strip from the waist down and give you a gown that opens in the rear. You will be placed on the scanning couch on your side with your upper leg rolled forward. The transducer will be LUBRICATED and either you or the technician will gently insert it into your rectum. Give this a (+) for discomfort. The ultrasonographer will then enter the action. The transducer will be gently moved about and positioned for pictures to be made. Add another (½ +). There is no hazard. Give it about

15 minutes. If a biopsy is to be done add the following: (+) to discomfort; (+) to hazard; one-half hour to time. Except for the lingering discomfort for a couple of hours that's the whole thing.

Bottom Line: (+ +) Not the worst, but getting close.

Testicles Your testicles lie outside of the pelvis within the sac known as the scrotum. One or both may be subject to enlargement from multiple different causes. US can help to identify the nature of the enlargement— whether it is CYSTIC or solid. The technique may also be helpful in determining the cause, in those cases in which there is a sudden onset of severe pain.

You are asked to lie flat on your back on the imaging table and to spread your legs. The technologist or physician will apply wide strips of adhesive tape across the front of your thighs at the level of your scrotum. This is called a "bridge." The scrotal sac is gently placed on this "little table" so that your testicles will lie side by side and thus each can be identified. Warm oil will then be applied and a transducer gently moved over the part. There is mild discomfort (½+) but no hazard. It may take as long as half an hour. No aftereffects.

Bottom Line: (+) Good for a locker-room laugh or two.

CHAPTER

21

Go Get a Magnetic Resonance Image (MRI)

MRI is the abbreviation for magnetic resonance imaging, and your doctor has told you to have one. But unless you are the exception that proves the rule, you don't know what those words mean or what you have been directed to "go get." However, if you are going to have one, you just might like to know more about how it works.

First the hype: MRI is without doubt or contention the hottest ticket in town. It is to the world of imaging what Babe Ruth was to baseball, and Larry Bird was to basketball—a *superstar!* It has added a new dimension to medical diagnosis of inestimable importance and value, and it is still a virtual toddler, having been out there only a few years and available to only a relative few.

Magnetic resonance is a specific form of radiowave that is emitted by protons when they are within a magnetic field and are excited by the absorption of energy from an applied radiofrequency pulse.

To understand this sentence and grasp the basis of MRI, you must know a smattering of basic physics. So here goes . . .

All things found in nature are composed of combinations of fundamental building blocks called elements. For example, oxygen is an element, as is hydrogen. Together, in the appropriate combination, these two elements make water. Each has a unique configuration that makes it oxygen or hydrogen and not iron or copper, or a Big Mac. That configuration is its atomic structure. The atom is the smallest particle of an element that can exist alone. An atom is composed of a nucleus (the nucleus is the central portion of the atom and comprises almost all of its weight) and electrons (an electron is an elementary particle that is negatively charged) which orbit around the nucleus. Thus, an atom can be thought of as similar to our solar system in which the sun is the nucleus and the planets such as Earth and Mars are the orbiting electrons.

The nucleus of the atom is our main interest. It is composed of two fundamental particles: protons (a proton is an elementary particle of matter that possesses a positive charge and a mass greater than that of an electron) and neutrons (a neutron is an elementary particle of matter that possesses no charge but has a mass almost equal to that of a proton). For our discussion of MRI, only the protons need to be considered. Not only do they have a charge, they also have motion—they spin. (Remember charge. Remember spin.) In their everyday environment the protons' alignment in the atom and their spinning characteristics are essentially random. However, if they are placed within a strong magnetic field, since they have a charge, protons will line up in a very specific fashion. (Think of the protons as a group of pins lying in a scattered array on a sheet of cardboard, pointing in all directions. If you carefully place a magnet beneath the surface of the sheet the pins will line up in a very specific direction with relationship to the North and South poles of the magnet. Protons will behave in the same manner. They will behave like individual bar magnets or the needle of a compass. They differ from the pins in that even as they align they continue to spin.) It is this physical principle that is utilized as Step 1 in creation of an image: The body part that is to be examined is placed within a very powerful magnetic field and the protons in that field align themselves pointing either North or South.

Now, another ingredient is added. A radiofrequency pulse is applied to the part of the magnetic field in which the protons are now aligned within their atoms. This pulse imparts additional energy to the protons so that they are rearranged—both their alignment and their spin characteristics change. The pattern of this new position can be controlled by the strength and the timing of the radiofrequency pulse applied. This is Step 2: Initiation of a radiofrequency pulse.

In Step 3, the pulse is removed and the protons return to their earlier alignment within the magnetic field. This movement results in the discharge of the energy that they had acquired from the radiofrequency pulse. This energy release is in the form of a radiowave. This wave, with appropriate instrumental and computer genius, can be converted into an image that will reflect the configuration of the parts from which it was derived.

Not only has this picture been created without the patient being exposed to radiation, but it has many other marvelous virtues to commend it. Suffice it to say, as of this writing, that although this technology is hardly out of its swaddling-clothes stage of development, it has already established itself as a giant step for mankind in diagnostic imaging.

Now that you are completely conversant with the basics let's get on to the particulars. Most examinations employing MRI are similar. Let's start with what's common to all:

Picture Taker The image that is the end product of an MRI examination is created, for the most part, by a specially trained individual known as an MRI technologist. This person is specifically, carefully, and thoroughly trained in the methodology inherent in achieving the goal of each examination—an image. This person is not a physician. However, when the picture has been obtained it is then given to another trained specialist who will interpret it so that it has medical meaning.

Picture Reader The trained specialist who interprets the images is a physician. That person has graduated from both college and medical school, and has spent an additional four or five years becoming versed in the specialty of radiology. When the physician has satisfactorily mastered that study as attested by successful passage of examinations known as boards, a degree proclaiming that he or she is a certified radiologist is awarded. The physician then begins a second period of study, requiring approximately one year, to explore and master the mysteries of magnetic resonance.

Most examinations are done by the technologist alone. All images are reviewed by the physician. If there is something seen on this review that is unclear, or if something might be improved upon by additional views, the physician will appear and get into the act. But even if you don't physically see the "person in the white coat," rest asssured that there is a highly trained medical specialist who will make the final decision on your MRI.

The Room The MR suite is virtually indistinguishable from the CT suite described in Chapter 18. It differs only in that the machine is a huge magnet and not multiple X-ray tubes.

The MRI Experience Whereas imaging procedures done by the conventional X-ray, nuclear medicine, or ultrasound techniques often vary significantly, those done by MR vary only on whether you enter the doughnut (the porthole in the wall) head or feet first. (In the very near future, but not yet permitted as routine, an injection may be part of certain studies. The injection story will be told shortly.) It would therefore be redundant to repeat the same words to describe each MR procedure. So, a one-time walk through the MR experience will suffice for all.

All imaging procedures are essentially the same. You will be helped onto the imaging table and asked to lie on your back. When you have been made comfortable, a surface coil (the device that applies the radiofrequency pulse) will usually be applied to the area of your body that is to be examined. These coils take different forms depending on the part that is to be examined. If the head or neck is the target, you will don a helmet that resembles that worn by an astronaut or deep sea diver. If the part to be examined is an extremity, such as your knee, that part will be placed in a special holder that is lined by a foam material so that there is no discomfort. For imaging of the spine the coils are built into a pad that you lie on. Other areas may require the placement of a small thin doughnut-shaped device to just touch the part of concern. *None hurt!*

You are now almost ready. A device to monitor either your heartbeat or your rate of respiration is added to your gear. For certain studies it takes the form of a Velcro band that is applied to one of your fingers. For other studies it looks like a coiled rubber belt that is placed around your middle. Neither cause stress or fuss. Now you are ready!

The table will begin to move (sometimes noisily) into the magnet. You will feel like you are entering and then are in a tunnel. The couch will move you to a depth that corresponds to the part of your body that is to be imaged. Each exposure requires several seconds. After each, the table will move slightly (about one-quarter to one-half inch) and the next exposure will be made. (MRI images, like those of CT, are a composite of very thin individual "slices" through an area of interest.) You will not experience any sensation from the exposures, but you will definitely experience noise and you may experience anxiety!

Noise Be prepared. Once you are in the magnet it will begin. If you are a hi-fi type you will be able to distinguish four distinctly different qualities that have been variously described as "galloping horses," "clanking," "a knocking radiator," and a "jackhammer." All have a pulsing character. All are intrusive and, if you're not forewarned of their coming, can be frightening. Foam earplugs can be had for the asking. Ask! If your head is not encased in the helmet you can even have earphones that will deliver music to diminish—but not entirely exclude—the racket.

Anxiety The anxiety that may be experienced in this situation is an overwhelming sense of apprehension and fear. It may be triggered by a CLAUSTROPHOBIC reaction. Some patients react in this fashion when they are moved into the tunnel of the magnet. There is no question that the space is both closed and narrow. In its favor is a mirror arrangement over your head that permits you to see out. Additionally, there is a built-in intercom that allows you to speak to the technologist. But if you still feel anxious, or can anticipate anxiety based on some earlier similar event, holler! Medication can be given that will diminish or even control your fear.

That's it! That is what an MR study is about. But, before we call it a closed chapter, let's review the other vital statistics (since all examinations are similar, no tables—as found in previous chapters—are necessary):

Discomfort (+) Lying on the table for 40 to 60 minutes can get uncomfortable because you must lie very, very still. The noise can be a drag. But, hey, you have to have something to talk about.

Hazard (−) Hardly any. As of now, except for the exceptions that will follow, there are no recognized dangers of this form of examination, making it far safer than conventional X-rays. The exceptions are

Pregnancy—It is unknown whether being in a magnetic field is harmful to the fetus. So, until sufficient research clarifies this question, discretion dictates no!

Cardiac pacemakers—the magnetic field will affect pacemakers and cause them to malfunction. The same no-no applies to any implanted stimulatory devices.

Hospitalization required No.

Special Preparation None.

Physician Attendance No.

Extras No (as of now) but almost certainly yes in the near future. There is an injectable material, gadolinium by name, which is still in the research stage but will shortly be released for use, and which holds great promise for improving image contrast and thus quality. It will be analogous to the iodine used in X-rays, and by all present reports, less hazardous than that CONTRAST AGENT. If and when gadolinium is approved, you will be told when it is appropriate for your particular examination and probably will be asked to sign an informed consent. It will be given intravenously by the radiologist (you'll finally get to see the person in the white coat).

Informed Consent Maybe. Some centers require your signature, others do not.

Examination Time Anywhere from 30 to 90 minutes. Techniques vary and with them, time. The average study is about 45 minutes, but figure that you won't be average, and allot at least one hour. (The time is only for the actual examination. Add the usual delays that have been described earlier in the section General Events Common to All Adult Diagnostic Procedures; see pages xiv–xvi. Follow the rule that will help keep you tranquil: Double or triple the examination minutes for a realistic "Hello"-to-"Good-bye" total.)

Aftereffects None.

Bring a Pal Always a good idea. Although you should have no problems there is always the outside shot that you might need medication to allay anxiety, which might then make you unable to drive or get home easily. Also, since there is no radiation hazard your pal may even be able to stay in the room with you while the examination is going on.

Precautions Unique to the MRI Experience

• Metal of any sort—The magnetic field will affect only certain metals, but it is wiser to consider all as evil and have the technologist decide what is or is not O.K. This metal prohibition applies to what's in you as well as what's on your person. The latter is easy. Just leave everything in your dressing booth. This includes your watch, jewelry, hairpins, eyeglasses with metal frames, and even removable dentures. What's in you is tougher. Fillings in your teeth may cause some minor distortion if they get into the area of examination, but will not cause you harm. Certain surgical implants such as hip and knee prostheses are also all right, but metallic clips such as those used in certain brain surgery are an absolute No! So—what to do to be safe? *Ask!* If you have any question, the rule is "check with the tech."

• Credit cards—leave your wallet with your pal or in the dressing room. Most "plastic" has a magnetic strip on it which goes bye-bye inside the big magnet.

Bottom Line: (+) High-tech at its highest!

Table Details

Discomfort When a particular study produces discomfort, it is scored in the following way: (½ +) very mild, (+) mild, (+ +) moderate, (+ + +) severe, or (+ + + +) very severe. These designations represent both my personal observations and ratings obtained from many thousands of patients. A (−) suggests no anticipated problem.

Having said the above, let me now qualify it, since the grading of discomfort is the most subjective category in the entire list. What one person endures stoically is another's "the worst." Thus, it is difficult, if not impossible, to fully and correctly extrapolate from my average rating to your actual experience. And, there is another catch. The gradings represent the anticipation of the "normal" individual—normal being here defined as "having no complaint in the area to be examined." This criterion may evoke an immediate howl of "how foolish," since except for those having a SCREENING procedure or a routine check, who sees a physician for no complaint? However, there is a good reason why these ratings are formulated this way.

If you are asked to bend your elbow, this act can be performed without discomfort. If you've sustained an injury to your elbow, bending it will elicit pain. Without the trauma, the act of bending would be rated (−) for discomfort. This is the rationale for my ratings: Does the study, by its own nature, induce discomfort? If the answer is no, I rate the examination (−), knowing full well that the sore-elbowed sufferer will find the experience a (+ + +). This yardstick acknowledges that there isn't a living human who can undergo an X-ray of the bowel, a spinal tap, an internal examination, a catheterization, and many other examinations without big-time misery. Here it isn't the patient—it's the nature of the study. So I rate the study itself, not what the person brings to it.

Just so we have some frame of reference for the grading, compare your experiences to mine as they relate to the dentist.

(−) is not going for a six-month check.

(½ +) is going, and although everything is "looking pretty good," the sticks and pricks elicit a gagging "ouch."

(+) is what happens when the "sticker" finds a hole and the digging begins. This is a real *"ouch."*

(+ +) is when the dentist says, "Found a little cavity here which I'll just go ahead and fill. It will only take me a couple of minutes, so let's skip the local."

(+ + +) is the visit after two days of increasing pain and throbbing, hoping it would go away, but it only kept getting worse. The dentist says, "This looks like you've got yourself a little abscess here. Please bear with me. I have to poke about a little to see just how extensive it is. This may hurt a mite." The "mite," as we who have been there well know, is severe! Severe, although most uncomfortable, is tolerable. Tolerable is here defined as not representing cruel or unusual punishment, and if the duration is not too long, can usually be endured without "big-time" medication or anesthesia. (Let's say the "big time" is something that might make you lose consciousness.)

(+ + + +) is when the dentist pokes that abscess a tad deeper than he or she intended, or how it would feel if it were attacked without anesthesia. It's the type of thing for which long ago they supplied bullets to bite down on. This one demands some up-front help of the "big-time" class.

Hazard   Hazard, as used here, refers only to the probability of complication, or risk, inherent in a procedure, *not* the degree of seriousness of a complication if one should occur. A (−) suggests no anticipated or known risk of a problem is associated with the study. A (+) indicates a mild risk, perhaps in the order of falling out of bed—it has been known to happen. A (+ +) points to a true possibility of a problem, but one that is no more likely than that which is accepted whenever one rides in or drives a car. A (+ + +) identifies a more than theoretical possibility that a complication will occur. The probability, however, is less than 10 percent, which is a value less than the complication rate faced by the long-term smoker.

To repeat: Hazard equals probability, not degree. It is conceivable that a serious complication might develop in a procedure listed as (+) and conversely that the event in a (+ + +) study could be minor. The range of seriousness should be discussed with and explained to you by the physician prior to any examination with a (+ +) or (+ + +) rating.

Physician Attendance   In procedures covered in Part I, you will always see a physician, although certain procedures may be done by a highly trained nonphysician—a technologist.

In Part II, you will always be attended by a highly trained nonphysician, the technologist, and certain procedures will demand the presence and participation of a physician. This physician, a specialist in either imaging or clinical laboratory tests, will always interpret the meaning and significance of any examination you undergo, even if you don't see the doctor. His or her absence must not be a source of concern that you "didn't even see a doctor." These specialists are like movie directors—they create the picture without ever being seen.

An N says probably no physician; a Y says he or she will be there.

Extras It is often necessary to put something into you. The something could be an instrument that will permit or enhance a particular examination—this might be a SPECULUM for an internal examination or an arthroscope to examine the knee—or it might be one of many available contrast materials, such as barium in X-rays, that will improve the visualization of certain body parts. Let's discuss these extras.

Catheters and Tubes CATHETERS and tubes are essentially the same, differing only in diameteer. When the tube is thin it is called a "catheter." When fat, a "tube." The terms are interchangeable for all of our purposes. These devices are commonly used to deliver or remove things from different body parts. Perhaps the best known to many is the catheter that is inserted into the bladder to remove urine. The same tube, just by having the direction of flow reversed, could bring something such as a contrast agent to the bladder. Similarly, these tubes (lovingly referred to as "spaghetti" by their users) can be inserted almost anywhere for the same purpose.

Other Instruments "Other instruments" refers to all of the various things that may be necessary to accomplish the same goal of providing a means to better examine a part, but that don't use catheters or tubes. These might be speculums (permitting better visualization of the nasal chamber or vagina), or special wires inserted into the breast to localize a lump found on an earlier X-ray. There are other such helpers, and each will be noted when the particular examination requires their use.

Contrast Agents Certain body parts may not be seen when X-ray alone is used. When this is the case, such as in examinations of the kidneys, stomach, colon, or blood vessels, certain extra things must be done to make these organs visible. These extras are usually in the form of substances best referred to as contrast agents. Each substance may be added by way of a direct injection (usually by vein), by your swallowing it, or by instillation (having it put into you). CONTRAST AGENTS possess two general characteristics: they have a significantly different density than the part they are put into or will be adjacent to, and they are relatively PHYSIOLOGICALLY INERT. There are three common agents used —iodine ("DYE"), barium, and air.

Iodine ("dye") Iodine is an element found in nature. It has all (well, almost all) of the properties demanded of a contrast material. It is readily available. It can be made in different combinations. It provides excellent increased density in the part of the body in which it is placed or into which it will move. It is injectable, and to this end, provides an excellent way to "see" blood.

Iodine, in its various combinations, is used extensively. For reasons based more on simplicity of communication than on absolute accuracy, it has become common practice to refer to these compounds as "dyes." Since this is common usage and since the word *dye* is far easier to write than "iodinated compounds," I have used this term throughout the book, but will doff my hat to the purists and acknowledge the technical inaccuracy by setting it off as "dye."

Unfortunately, iodine is not completely inert. There are some who are sensitive (perhaps a better word than "ALLERGIC," since it is not always clear what is happening) to it. There is a wide range of possible reactions in people who exhibit sensitivity. In the vast majority the reaction is minor (minor means no serious consequence is anticipated; it does not refer to a degree of discomfort), such as nausea, vomiting, sneezing, itching or hives. For a few, it can be severe. Severe reactions include such events as marked wheezing with difficulty in breathing, marked drop in blood pressure, unconsciousness, and yes, even death. The incidence of a fatal outcome has been reported as 1 in every 40,000 to 60,000 injections. (A contrast agent is used only after considered deliberation by professionals fully knowledgeable of its dangers, and who have deemed the action to be essential to your health.) The minor reactions are treated with an antiallergic type of medication, an antihistamine. This usually solves the problem, although it makes some patients sleepy for several hours. Driving should be postponed until the antihistamine's effects are gone. The more serious complications require hospitalization.

If this is your first time, all of the above are possible. If you have had "dye" before without any difficulty, you are probably home free. If you have had a previous reaction, then the radiologist will decide whether or not you should have "dye" again. If the indications for this examination are compelling, premedication for several days prior to the study can be instituted and this will prevent any reaction. But, in most cases, alternative studies are available that make the risk unnecessary. And finally, there are people who are better served with alternative studies. These include the very elderly, those with known serious kidney disease, people who have sickle cell anemia, and those with multiple myeloma.

Before this agent is given, the radiologist will attempt to determine whether or not you have a predictable sensitivity—rarely possible unless you have been given this material before. The risk should be explained and you may be asked to sign a form known as informed consent (see below).

Medical professionals wish that there was something better than iodine available, and someday there will be. But, despite all of the things mentioned above that seem so scary, iodine is a substance that has proven itself to be of such tremendous value in diagnosis that at present its downside has to be accepted.

Barium Barium is a mineral found in nature. In the sulfate form it is soluble in water and forms a white, chalky liquid that can be swallowed (nicer when flavored than plain) or INSTILLED by enema. It is completely inert and thus absolutely safe. It is used almost exclusively in studies of the digestive tract—from the mouth to the anus. It is dense and will cast a white shadow.

Air Air, like barium, is inert, and being less dense than most tissue will cast a black shadow. There is no hazard in its use.

These "extras" are noted as follows: a Y if anything is added to the examination; otherwise (if it's you alone), an N.

Informed Consent Simply stated, informed consent is the name of a document that is to be signed by you after the details of a given procedure have been explained. It is your signed permission. But, *know what you are signing!* This permission is formally requested only when the nature of the examination is such that there is a risk element in its performance. After these risks have been identified and you are satisfied that you understand them—ask, ask, ask until you do—then the decision is yours: "No" is equivalent to "Good-bye"; "Yes, where do I sign?" gets the show on the road.

Your yes says that you understand that there are inherent hazards that you are willing to accept because you and your medical advisers believe that the benefits of the procedure warrant the risk. Additionally, your yes serves to protect the performer if there should be a complication as a result of the study.

One last word about informed consent. Physicians agree that in most situations there is either no need for such a consent or that it is mandatory. However, there is a small group of studies that fall into a "gray zone." Some doctors say "I need it"; others say "I won't bother." Once the discussions begin, only the most intrepid or foolish patient is not shaken by the disclosures. Therefore, when the risks seem minor or of low probability, some examiners elect to take their chances rather than open the Pandora's box of "what might be." Thus the listing of informed consent is N, Y, or ?

Examination Time   The average length of a study is listed in hours. This time refers to the actual procedure and does not include other elements: clerical processing, delays, redo's, or other unanticipated miseries. These "others" cannot be given a time factor, but commonly average out to be at least equal to the examination time. A good rule of thumb to predict how long the whole thing will take is to at least double or, more safely, triple the examination time.

Bottom Line: This relatively new addition to our vernacular by way of Wall Street connotes a "quick and dirty" final opinion on impact. Here, the bottom line attempts to add and subtract all the components of the diagnostic experience: the preparation, the time of involvement, the discomfort, the hazard, the possible embarrassment, the probable irritations, the failures of communication, the requirement of additional outside assistance, the delayed and lingering effects, and more.

It goes without saying that each individual's bottom line is uniquely personal and idiosyncratic, but a general averaging does exist and is offered in the hope that it will give you a ballpark range of what the procedure will be like. The rating system is as follows:

(−): an experience that is actually fun and that you would enjoy repeating. These are few and far between but do occasionally appear on one's shopping list. As an example, most people enjoy hypnosis.

(½ +): an experience that has no built-in aversive aspects except the mere inconvenience of having it done. An example is a urine analysis or chest X-ray.

(+): an experience that, besides the inconvenience of having it done, also has some additional, though minor, element that evokes moodiness: it may hurt a little, it may cause mild embarrassment, it might require more than a single visit, etc. Some examples of these are: having blood drawn or receiving an injection for a procedure; having an upper GI X-ray, because of having to drink that "stuff"; having your pupils dilated.

(+ +): an experience that is more involved, with additions that are more stressful, but still not of a severe nature: for instance, an exercise stress test of your heart, because it is physically demanding and fatiguing; an X-ray exmination of your kidneys where "dye" is injected; the passage of an instrument to "see" your vocal cords.

(+ + +): an experience that is totally aversive—one that has nothing about it that you will like. It contains elements of serious discomfort, probably hazard, and may have lingering effects. It is one that invokes the rule of BAP—Bring a Pal—to help you get home. Some of these "baddies" are: a spinal tap for the collection of fluid; the instillation of "dye" for certain X-rays; the obtaining of certain tissues (BIOPSIES); the analysis of certain nerve and muscle functions.

(+ + + +): an experience that is just out-and-out tough. The only consolation is that it is extremely important to your diagnosis. Often medications are offered or given. Often anesthesia is possible. Absolutely bring a pal! Some tests that live in infamy are an X-ray study of your bowel, the insertion of an instrument through the back wall of your vagina to detect the presence of blood, the passage of certain tubes, and the injection of certain "dyes" to examine blood vessels.

Acute: of a disease, reaching a crisis point rapidly

Acute process: a problem of sudden onset that requires immediate—often surgical—attention

Allergy: abnormal sensitivity to certain substances

Anesthesia: loss of sensation with or without the loss of consciousness

Anesthesiologist: physician trained in administering anesthetic agents ·

Angiography: X-ray visualization of blood vessels

Antibody: specialized substance produced by the lymphatic system that defends the body against foreign materials

Arterial line: a thin tube or needle inserted into an artery that allows substances to be introduced into the bloodstream or blood to be removed

Arteriography: X-ray visualization of arteries

Arteriosclerosis: disease characterized by thickening and hardening of the inside walls of arteries

Arthritides: diseases of the joints

Aspiration: type of BIOPSY in which a needle is used to suck back samples of suspicious fluids or cells, which are then analyzed

Auscultation: diagnostic monitoring of the sounds made by an internal bodily part; most commonly done with a stethoscope

Bacteria: microscopic, single-celled organisms that may exist in the body as useful PARASITES or may cause infection

Benign: not cancerous

Biopsy: removal of suspicious tissues or fluids for analysis; may be excisional, in which the material is cut from the body, or done with a needle (*see* ASPIRATION)

Brain stem: portion of the brain composed of the midbrain, pons, and medulla oblongata

Cardiovascular: related to the heart and blood vessels

Cartilage: a type of connective tissue that is hard and bone-like

CAT or CT: abbreviations for computerized axial tomography, a type of X-ray whose images of a body part are composites of multiple thin, cross-sectional slices

Catheter: thin, flexible tube that is inserted into a body cavity or vessel to permit injection or withdrawal of fluids

Cavity: hollow space

Cell: smallest unit of living matter that is capable of functioning independently

Centesis: technique of draining large abnormal quantities of fluid from a body cavity, usually with a special needle; a form of ASPIRATION

Cholesterol: steroid necessary in digestion but which when present in excess can cause disease in blood vessels

Chromosome: body in the cell nucleus that carries GENETIC material

Chronic: of a disease, long-standing and recurrent

Circulation: in anatomy, movement of blood through the vessels of the body

Circulatory system: network of blood vessels that is responsible for supplying oxygen and nutrients to and removing waste products from all parts of the body

Claustrophobia: dread of being in a closed or narrow space

Congenital: existing at birth but not hereditary; usually refers to a defect

arising from a fault in fetal development

Contraindication: reason not to proceed

Contrast media: substances that can act as a "dye" of organs, allowing them to be visualized more accurately

CT: *see* CAT

Culture: growing of certain cells or fluids on special laboratory preparations for analytic purposes

Curettage: excision with the use of a surgical instrument, a curette, which is shaped like a small spoon and has sharp edges

Cyst: closed, fluid-filled sac

Diabetes: disease in which there is a loss of sugar regulation

Digestive system: group of organs responsible for breaking food into its component nutrients and removing waste products from the body

Dilate: enlarge; become wide

Distend: inflate, make bigger

Drape: surround a body part with sterile sheets or towels

"Dye": any solution that, when injected, creates a shadow on X-ray film, improving visualization of parts of the body

Ectopic: occurring in an abnormal location, particularly a pregnancy

Electrocardiogram: tracing made by an ELECTROCARDIOGRAPH

Electrocardiograph: instrument capable of producing traces of the electrical patterns of the heart

Electrode: small metal disk that is capable of detecting electrical impulses originating in portions of the body

Embolism: condition in which an EMBOLUS reaches a blood vessel too small for it to pass through and the vessel is blocked

Embolus: any abnormal substance, such as a blood clot or air bubble, that is carried by the blood

Emergent: requiring immediate attention

Endocrine system: network of ductless GLANDS that manufacture, store, and secrete HORMONES to regulate many organs and functions

Endoscopy: examination with any instrument that allows for direct visualization of internal organs

Enzyme: complex protein substance that acts as an essential catalyst for certain bodily functions

Excision: removal by cutting

Excisional biopsy: *see* BIOPSY

Fluoroscopy: form of X-ray visualization that permits the body part to be seen in motion on a screen rather than as a static image on film

Genetic: inherited from the parent; hereditary

Genitourinary system: group of organs that are responsible for reproduction in both men and women and the elimination of certain body wastes through the urine

Gland: specialized cells capable of synthesizing, storing, and releasing HORMONES

Hematoma: localized swelling filled with blood

Hernia: abnormal protrusion of a body part through the wall of a CAVITY that contains the part

Hollow organ: body organ that has a CAVITY, such as the stomach or heart

Hormone: chemical substance, manufactured and secreted by a gland, that produces specific and often regulatory effects on tissues and organs distant from its site of origin

Hypertension: high blood pressure

Hypertrophy: increase of the size of an organ, especially the heart, often due to overexertion of the muscle

Immune system: those structures consisting of both organs, such as the thymus gland, and cells, such as the lymphocytes, that function together to protect the body against infection (*see* LYMPHATIC SYSTEM)

Incision: surgical cut

Infarction: death of TISSUE as a result of the loss of its blood supply

Inspection: examination by direct visualization

Instill: put a liquid into something, usually slowly, sometimes drop by drop

Intravenous: within a vein

Intravenous injection: introduction of a fluid into a vein through a needle that has first been inserted into the vein

Intubation: passing a tube into an ORGAN or body CAVITY

Ischemia: inadequate circulation of blood to a particular body area or part

Isotope: any of two or more forms of the same element having related atomic structures but different physical properties; when RADIOACTIVE, an isotope may be used as a tracer in certain testing procedures

IV line: needle and thin tube inserted into a vein to allow for continuous provision of fluid or medication

Laminography: type of X-ray examination that permits a selected body area to be in sharper focus than the parts both in front of and behind it

Lance: pierce or cut with a sharp, pointed instrument, a lancet

Lesion: patch of diseased tissue

Lubricant: thick, slippery material, such as petroleum jelly; in medicine, used on the skin during certain examinations and on instruments or gloved fingers when inserted into a body CAVITY

Lumen: inside diameter of a tubular organ, such as a blood vessel

Lymphatic system: specialized cells that manufacture and distribute ANTIBODIES throughout the body

Lymphoma: any of a group of different abnormalities, usually MALIGNANT in type, that affect lymphoid tissues

Malignant: cancer or cancer-like; life-threatening

Membrane: thin sheet of specialized TISSUE that acts as a covering of a part

Metabolism: sum of the processes that build up and break down cells in the body

Musculoskeletal system: system of the body composed of bones, joints, and muscles

Needle biopsy: *see* ASPIRATION

Neoplasm: abnormal growth of TISSUE that is either MALIGNANT or BENIGN

Nervous system: specialized structures, such as the brain, spinal cord, and nerves, that both receive and interpret stimuli and also transmit impulses to other organs

Nodule: small, rounded lump of abnormal cells

Noninvasive: of a medical procedure: carrying no significantly painful or hazardous aspects

Occlude: block or obstruct

Opacified: of a body part: having "DYE" added to appear denser when X-rayed

Organ: any part of the body that performs a specific function or functions

Organic: of or relating to a body organ, often used to imply a physical deficiency

Palpation: examination by touch

Parasite: organism living within another organism and dependent on its host for survival

Pathologist: physician who specializes in the microscopic analysis of cells and tissue

Pathology: deviation from normal; disease

Percussion: in physical examination of the body, tapping the skin over an internal body part of concern and using the sound thus created to judge its condition

Percutaneous: through the skin

Perforation: poking a hole, such as through the wall of an organ

Pharmaceutical: drug useful in medicine

Physiologically inert: not inducing a response or a reaction in the body

Plaque: abnormal layer of material that may OCCLUDE the vessel or ORGAN in which it accumulates

Polyp: abnormal growth with a hemispheroidal shape, arising from a mucous MEMBRANE

Probe: thin, flexible instrument used for examining body CAVITIES; instrument used to detect electrical or RADIOACTIVE impulses arising within the body

Radioactive: emitting certain forms of energy, such as gamma rays

Radiologist: physician who specializes in X-ray imaging

Radiopharmaceutical: PHARMACEUTICAL to which a RADIOACTIVE ISOTOPE has been chemically attached so that the action of the drug can be traced by special instruments as it moves through the body

Reflex: response that occurs involuntarily to a particular stimulus

Reflux: backward flow; an example in medicine is the flow of stomach juices into the esophagus, causing heartburn

Respiratory system: system of the body that is responsible for breathing

Retrograde: against the normal flow

Scraping: in medical diagnosis, method of cell collection in which an applicator is scraped across the surface of a body part to obtain cells for analysis

Screen: study routinely, even in the absence of symptoms

Section: a thin, cross-sectional image segment or "slice" of the body as obtained in imaging by CAT, laminography, or MRI

Sedative: drug used to induce a relaxed state that often leads to sleep

Sensor: detector of activity; in medical diagnosis, a metal disk ranging in size from that of an aspirin tablet to that of a nickel (*see* ELECTRODE)

Skeletal system: support system of the body, composed of bones and cartilage

SMA-12: instrument capable of twelve different analyses from a single blood sample (S = sequential, M = multiphasic, A = analyzer)

Solid organ: body ORGAN that has no CAVITY, such as the liver or pancreas

Spatula: small applicator with an end that can be used for SCRAPING

Speculum: metal instrument consisting of two blades that can be spread apart

to improve visualization of a canal or CAVITY

Stenosis: narrowing, especially of blood vessels

Stirrups: metal poles attached to the end of an examination table and constructed to support the heels or the back of the knees during medical examinations that require elevation of the legs and separation of the thighs

Superficial: on or near the skin

Suppress: inhibit normal function

Sutures: stitches

Syndrome: group of signs and symptoms that occur together and that characterize a particular abnormality

Tenaculum: instrument that resembles a long forceps with small prongs or teeth at the end, used to grasp and steady an organ for examination

Thrombus: clot of coagulated blood that OCCLUDES a vessel or fills the heart CAVITY

Tinnitus: ringing noise heard in the ears that originates inside one's head, not from an outside source

Tissue: in anatomy, aggregate of cells, usually of the same type, performing a similar function and constituting a basic structural material of the body

Tonometry: measurement of the tension of a body part

Tracer: radioisotope used to analyze or visualize a body part (*see* RADIO-PHARMACEUTICAL)

Transducer: device actuated by power from one system that supplies power in another form to a second system

Vascular: related to the blood vessels

Vertigo: dizziness

cystoscopy, 147–48
cytology, 167
  vaginal, 65
cytoscope, flexible, 148

deglutition (swallowing function), 40, 189
dementia, 242
dermatitis, contact, 7
dermatologists, 5, 23–24
diabetes, 32, 33, 104, 150
Digital Subtraction Angiography (DSA), 199
dilation and curettage, 60, 61–62
direct ophthalmoscopy, 102
diverticuli, 261
Doppler blood flow, 151, 152, 280
DSA (Digital Subtraction Angiography), 199
ductography, 191–92
dye injection, 194, 196
dyspnea, 134

ear problems, diagnostic procedures for, 119–24
ecchymoses, 79
echocardiography, 250–51, 281
ectopic pregnancy, 62, 285
edrophonium (tensilon) test, 42
EEG (electroencephalography), 76–78, 80, 151
ejection fraction, 251
electrocardiograms (EKGs), 14, 68
  ambulatory (Holter monitoring), 18, 19, 21
  for congenital heart disease, 22
  for ischemic (coronary artery) heart disease, 15–17
  for kidney problems, 68
  for myocardial heart disease, 19
  resting, 15–16, 18, 19, 22, 68
  for valvular heart disease, 21
electroencephalography (EEG), 76–78, 80, 151
electromyograms (EMGs), 78–80
  for joints and muscles, 142
electronystagmograms, for ear problems, 123–24
electroretinograms:
  for neuro-ophthalmic diseases, 111
  for retinal diseases, 106–7
EMGs, see electromyograms
endocrinologists, 26–35
endometrial biopsy, 60, 61–62
Endoscopic Retrograde Cholangiopancreatography (ERCP), 212
endoscopy:
  for lower gastrointestinal tract, 45–48
  for upper gastrointestinal tract, 40–42
EP (evoked potentials), 80–82
epididymitis, 264–65
ERCP (Endoscopic Retrograde Cholangiopancreatography), 212
esophageal function studies:
  procedure for, 43–44
  types of, 42
esophageal reflux, 40
esophagus:
  examination of, 40
  X-rays of, 201–2
evoked potentials (EP), 80–82
excisional biopsy, 93, 114, 126, 140, 168

exercise stress tests, 16–17, 249–50
exophthalmometry, 110
eye diseases, 95–102, 109–11
  ultrasound for, 278

fallopian tubes, X-rays of, 215–17
FAST (fluorogenic allergosorbent) tests, 6
feces, 164–65
female genital system, diagnostic procedures for, 284–88
fertility tests, 65, 151
fetal monitoring, 88–89
fever of unknown origin (F.U.O.), 269
finger stick, 162
flexible cystoscope, 148
fluids, laboratory tests for, 168–71
fluorescein angiography, for retinal diseases, 106
fluorogenic allergosorbent (FAST) tests, 6
fluoroscopic equipment rooms, 176
fluoroscopy, 50, 176, 189
F.U.O. (fever of unknown origin), 269

gadolinium, 295
gall bladder, 49
  nuclear studies of, 263–64
  X-rays of, 210–12
gall bladder stones, 49, 263
gallium, 269, 270
gamma cameras, 234–35
gantry, 176, 179, 234–35
gastric emptying, 40, 261
gastroenterologists, 36–51
gastroesophageal reflux, 260–61
gastrointestinal (GI) tract:
  nuclear studies of, 260–64
  X-rays for, 207–10
gastroscopes, 41
genitals:
  female, 284–88
  male, 288–90
  see also specific organs
genitourinary tract, 143, 145
  nuclear studies of, 264–68
X-rays of, 215–22
GI bleeding, acute, 261–62
GI tract, see gastrointestinal tract
glaucoma, 94, 101, 108–9
  symptoms of, 107–8
glucagon, 209–10
goiter, 30, 244
gynecologists, 52–65

head:
  nuclear studies of, 237–44
  ultrasound of, 275–78
heart, 13
  CT scan of, 194
  nuclear studies of, 248–51
  ultrasound of, 280–81
  X-rays of, 193–200
heart attacks, 16
heart disease:
  congenital, 10, 21–22
  myocardial, 10, 18–20
  valvular, 10, 20–21
hematoma, 198
hernias, 146